Pancreaticobiliary Maljunction and Congenital Biliary Dilatation

Terumi Kamisawa • Hisami Ando
Editors

Pancreaticobiliary Maljunction and Congenital Biliary Dilatation

Springer

Editors
Terumi Kamisawa
Department of Internal Medicine
Tokyo Metropolitan Komagome Hospital
Bunkyo-ku
Tokyo
Japan

Hisami Ando
Aichi Prefectural Colony
Kasugai
Aichi
Japan

ISBN 978-981-10-8653-3 ISBN 978-981-10-8654-0 (eBook)
https://doi.org/10.1007/978-981-10-8654-0

Library of Congress Control Number: 2018941815

Printed on acid-free paper

This Springer imprint is published by the registered company Springer Nature Singapore Pte Ltd.
part of Springer Nature
The registered company address is: 152 Beach Road, #21-01/04 Gateway East, Singapore 189721, Singapore

Preface

Pancreaticobiliary maljunction (PBM) is a congenital malformation in which the pancreatic and bile ducts join outside the duodenal wall, usually forming a markedly long common channel. The sphincter of Oddi is normally located at the distal end of the pancreatic and bile ducts and regulates the outflow of bile and pancreatic juice. As the action of the sphincter of Oddi does not functionally affect the pancreaticobiliary junction in PBM, reciprocal reflux between pancreatic juice and bile (pancreaticobiliary reflux and biliopancreatic reflux) occurs, resulting in various pathologic conditions such as biliary cancer and pancreatitis. The fluid pressure in the pancreatic duct usually exceeds that in the bile duct, and reflux of pancreatic juice into the biliary tract frequently occurs. PBM is diagnosed when an abnormally long common channel is evident on imaging studies.

PBM is divided into congenital biliary dilatation (CBD) and PBM without biliary dilatation. CBD, the so-called choledochal cyst, was first well documented in a clinical case, which was treated by Douglas in 1852. Anomalous arrangement of the pancreaticobiliary ductal system, which is currently called PBM, was first described in an autopsy case of CBD by Arnolds in 1906. Although Babbitt suspected that reflux of pancreatic juice into the common bile duct leads to its dilatation in CBD, this theory is not accepted currently. CBD had been recognized as a congenital malformation of the bile duct associated with different degrees of dilatation at various sites in the bile duct and had been classified into three types in the classic Alonso-Lej's classification, and five types in the Todani's classification. However, CBD is recently recognized as a malformation involving local dilatation of the extrahepatic bile duct including the common bile duct and PBM.

Once PBM is diagnosed, prophylactic surgery is recommended before malignant changes can take place in the biliary tract. Extrahepatic bile duct resection is a standard operation for CBD, but complete excision of the intrapancreatic bile duct and removal of stenoses of the hepatic ducts are necessary to prevent serious complications after surgery. On the other hand, the optimal treatment of adult patients with PBM without biliary dilatation is under debate.

The goal of this book is to provide readers with the opportunity to obtain a complete understanding of PBM and principles for the diagnosis and management of

PBM and CBD with imaging features. We are deeply grateful to all the authors for their painstaking writing and contributions in preparing this concise and informative book. The publisher has also made a significant contribution to this book and has turned out an impressive volume with illustrations of the highest quality.

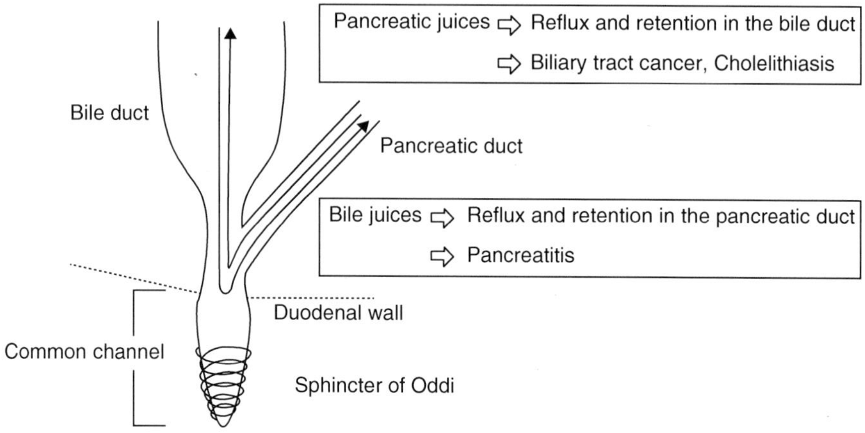

Pathophysiology of pancreaticobiliary maljunction (cited from J Gastroenterol 2012;47:731-759)

Tokyo, Japan — Terumi Kamisawa
Aichi, Japan — Hisami Ando

Contents

Chapter 1
Outline of Congenital Biliary Dilatation and Pancreaticobiliary Maljunction

Hisami Ando

Abstract Congenital biliary dilatation (CBD) is a congenital malformation involving both local dilatation of the extrahepatic bile duct, including the common bile duct, and pancreaticobiliary maljunction (PBM) that is thought to develop as a misarrangement of the embryonic connections in the pancreaticobiliary ductal system. Patients can be diagnosed with CBD at any age, but more than two-thirds of cases are diagnosed in children younger than 10 years of age. The major clinical symptoms are recurrent abdominal pain, nausea and vomiting, and mild jaundice. The occurrence of signs and symptoms is explained by the bile and pancreatic flow being disturbed by protein plugs. In PBM, the sphincters of the pancreatic duct and the bile duct cannot work, and this long common channel permits reflux of pancreatic juice freely into the biliary tract. This free reflux may be a key factor in the pathogenesis of malignant changes in the bile duct. According to a nationwide survey performed in Japan, cancer of the biliary tract was found in 21.6% of 997 patients with CBD/PBM diagnosed in adulthood and was developed biliary tract cancer 15–20 years earlier than individuals without PBM. Immediate extrahepatic bile duct resection is recommended once a definitive diagnosis is established because juvenile patients with CBD can develop cholangitis and/or cancer even if asymptomatic. However, reports of intrahepatic stones and/or bile duct carcinoma after surgery are gradually increasing. Therefore, careful long-term follow-up is very important.

Keywords Congenital biliary dilatation · Pancreaticobiliary maljunction Long common channel · Protein plug · Extrahepatic bile duct resection

H. Ando
Welfare Center for Persons with Developmental Disabilities, Aichi Prefectural Colony, Kasugai, Aichi, Japan
e-mail: hando@med.nagoya-u.ac.jp

T. Kamisawa, H. Ando (eds.), *Pancreaticobiliary Maljunction and Congenital Biliary Dilatation*, https://doi.org/10.1007/978-981-10-8654-0_1

1.1 History and Epidemiology

Congenital biliary dilatation (CBD) is a congenital malformation involving both local dilatation of the extrahepatic bile duct, including the common bile duct, and pancreaticobiliary maljunction (PBM) [1]. CBD is known by various other names, including congenital bile duct dilatation, congenital choledochal cyst, congenital bile duct cyst, and choledochal cyst. PBM is a congenital anomaly defined as a union of the pancreatic and biliary duct that is located outside the duodenal wall, away from the ampulla of Vater. PBM is also known by various other names, such as anomalous arrangement of the pancreaticobiliary ducts, anomalous arrangement of the pancreaticobiliary ductal system, anomalous pancreaticobiliary ductal union, anomalous union of the biliopancreatic ducts, and abnormal junction of the pancreaticobiliary ductal system. Japanese clinical practice guidelines recommended using the terms "congenital biliary dilatation" and "pancreaticobiliary maljunction" for these conditions [2].

The first description of a fusiform dilatation of the common bile duct was by Vater in 1723 [3]. According to McConnel, the first successful report of treatment was that by Swain et al., who performed a cholecystojejunostomy in 1894 [4]. PBM was first noted by Arnold in 1804 [5], and Kozumi and Kodama [6] reported in detail an abnormal union of the pancreatic and bile ducts in an autopsy case in 1916 (Fig. 1.1). Irwin and Morison reported the first case of malignancy associated with a CBD in 1944 [7]. Alonso-Lej [8] classified cystic dilatation of the extrahepatic bile duct into three types, and Todani et al. [9] refined the classification of the bile duct cystic disorders into five types including the concept of PBM. In Todani's classification, types Ia and Ic and type IV-A, which is associated with intrahepatic duct dilatation, are CBD accompanied with PBM, but types Ib, II, III, IV-B, and V are not accompanied by PBM in almost all cases. Davenport and Basu [10] categorized CBD into only two types—cystic malformation and fusiform malformation—because Todani's classification of five types and sub-types was complex and confusing.

Cases of CBD are relatively uncommon in Western Europe and North America but are appreciably more common in Asia. Approximately 1 in every 1000 persons in Japan is affected [11], whereas only 1 in every 50,000–150,000 persons is affected in Western countries [12]. The preponderance in female patients is shown, with the female-to-male ratio being 3 or 4 to 1. Patients can be diagnosed with CBD at any age, but more than two-thirds of cases are diagnosed in children younger than 10 years of age [2].

1.2 Embryology

There are many theories to explain the occurrence of bile duct dilatation: it arises due to a bile flow disturbance caused by congenital stenosis of the terminal common bile duct; it arises due to a weakness of the common bile duct itself; it arises

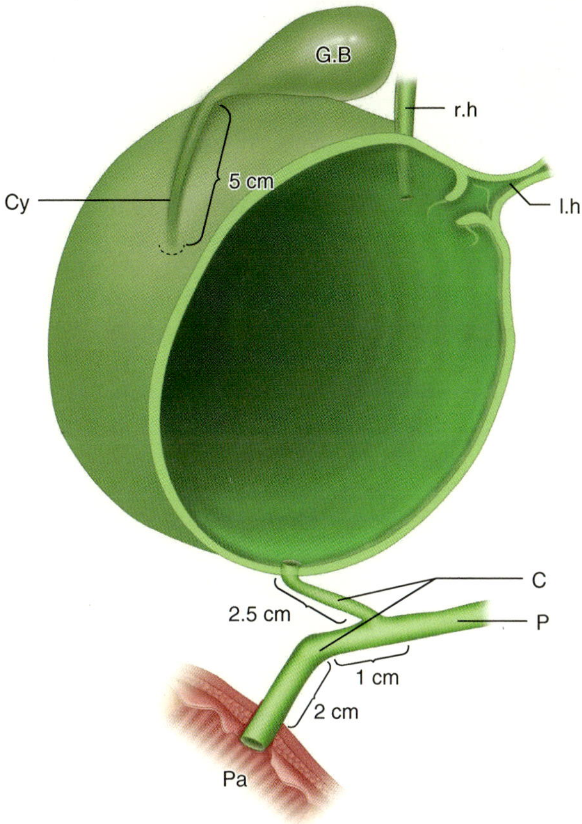

Fig. 1.1 Figure of PBM by Kozumi and Kodama (quote from [6]). An abnormal union of the pancreatic and bile ducts is shown clearly. *GB* Gallbladder, *Cy* cystic duct, *r.h* and *l.h* right hepatic duct and left hepatic duct, *C* choledochal duct, *P* pancreatic duct, *Pa* papilla (ampulla) of Vater

due to an inequality between the proliferation of epithelial cells in the upper portion and the lower portion of the common bile duct [13]. PBM is thought to develop as a misarrangement of the embryonic connections in the pancreaticobiliary ductal system. Suda et al. [14] suggested that with PBM the lower portion of the bile duct originates as a branch of the ventral pancreatic duct because there is a second branch in the lower portion of the bile duct. The lower part of the bile duct may become narrow or atretic with a disturbance of the biliary recanalization if abnormal fusion between the branch of the ventral pancreatic duct and the lower part of the bile duct occurs during the recanalization process of the embryonic stage. In other words, when normal recanalization of the bile duct does not take place in the lower part, the result is CBD; when the recanalization disorder is minor, the result is PBM with minor dilatation of the bile duct; and if there is no recanalization disorder in the part of an abnormal fusion, the result is PBM without bile duct dilatation [15]. As noted above, there are many theories for CBD and PBM; however, the true origins of bile duct dilatation and PBM remain obscure.

1.3 Pathophysiology

Usually, the bile duct and the pancreatic duct open into the duodenum through the ampulla of Vater. The sphincter of the bile duct, the sphincter of the pancreatic duct, and the sphincter of the ampulla regulate the flow of bile and pancreatic juice through the ampulla. When these sphincters work properly, the ampulla opens to allow bile and pancreatic juice to flow through and then closes again. However, with PBM, the sphincters of the pancreatic duct and the bile duct cannot work because there is a long common channel after the pancreaticobiliary junction of bile duct and the pancreatic duct. This long common channel permits reflux of pancreatic juice into the biliary tract and reflux of bile into the pancreatic duct. Pancreatic juice frequently refluxes into the biliary tract because the pressure in the pancreatic duct is usually higher than in the bile duct. Free reflux of pancreatic juice into the bile duct may be a key factor in the pathogenesis of malignant changes in the bile duct. Bile mixed with regurgitated pancreatic juice produces substances that are hazardous to the biliary epithelium, including activated pancreatic enzymes, lysolecithin, bile acids, and mutagens. Activated pancreatic enzymes include phospholipase A2, which is itself cytotoxic and converts phosphatidylcholine in bile to lysophosphatidylcholine, a strong cytotoxic substance [16]. Biliary carcinogenesis in patients with PBM is thought to involve the hyperplasia–dysplasia–carcinoma sequence caused by chronic inflammation resulting from pancreaticobiliary reflux, which differs from the adenoma–carcinoma sequence or de novo carcinogenesis associated with biliary tract cancer in patients without PBM [12]. In addition, the pancreas secretes trypsinogen and a protein called lithostathine, which is regurgitated into the biliary tract in patients with PBM. Refluxed trypsinogen is activated to trypsin and cleaves soluble lithostathine into insoluble forms, protein plugs that interfere with bile and pancreatic flow [17].

1.4 Signs and Symptoms and Complications

Abdominal pain, jaundice, and an abdominal mass are the classical triad; this meant that in the past, diagnosis and treatment were performed at a later stage, resulting in poor outcomes. These days, most patients with CBD are identified in childhood. However, few patients with PBM without bile duct dilatation have symptoms in childhood, and they are not usually diagnosed until adulthood and might be diagnosed simultaneously with advanced-stage gallbladder cancer. In children with CBD, the major clinical symptoms are recurrent abdominal pain (82%) that may occur repeatedly for several days, nausea and vomiting (66%), mild jaundice (44%), an abdominal mass (29%), and fever (29%) [17]. In adults, too, recurrent abdominal pains are major clinical symptom. The occurrence of signs and symptoms is explained by the bile and pancreatic flow being disturbed by protein plugs (Fig. 1.2) [17]. Most plugs are fragile and disappear

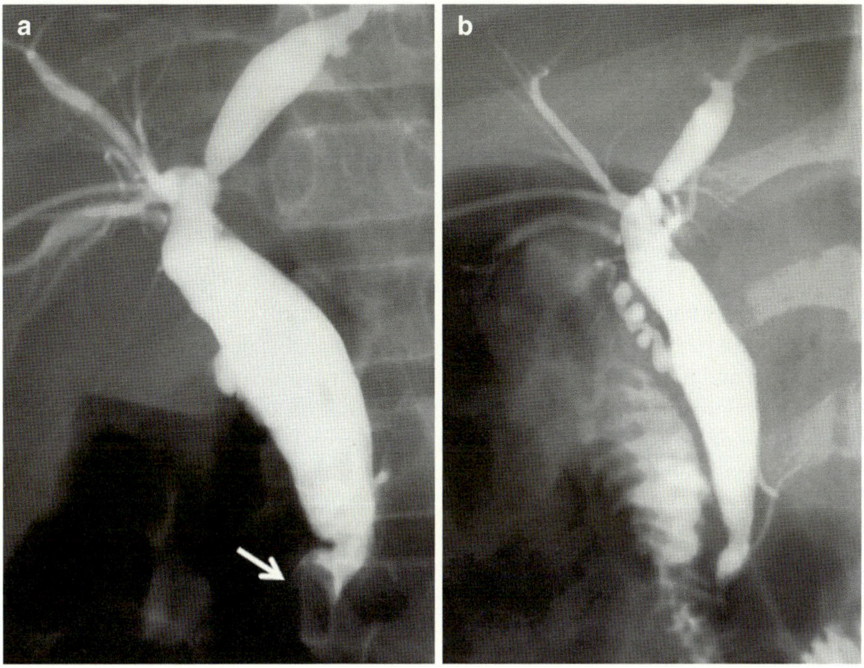

Fig. 1.2 Regression of protein plugs. Protein plugs (*arrows*) become incarcerated in the common channel and disturb the flow of bile and pancreatic juice (**a**). Protein plugs disappeared from the common channel (**b**)

spontaneously, but they are produced repeatedly, so although symptoms are usually mild and self-limiting, they are also recurring. In most cases, abnormal results appear in blood tests (amylase, elastase 1, trypsin, phospholipase A2, total bilirubin, direct bilirubin, alkaline phosphatase, and γ-glutamyl transpeptidase) during symptomatic periods, but these abnormalities are transient, and they are only evident during the symptomatic phase. Patients with CBD are more predisposed to forming biliary tract stones than individuals without CBD, and biliary tract stones are observed in 24.1% of adults and 9.0% of pediatric patients [18]. However, there is no difference in these symptoms and signs among the types of CBD.

Patients with CBD/PBM have a high rate of biliary tract cancers. According to a nationwide survey performed in Japan, cancer of the biliary tract was found in 21.6% of 997 adult patients with CBD and was in the extrahepatic bile duct in 32.1% and in the gallbladder in 62.3%. These rates are significantly higher than the 0.01–0.05% incidence of bile duct cancer in the general population [19]. The ages at which patients with CBD become predisposed to develop biliary tract cancer are 60.1 ± 10.4 years for gallbladder cancer and 52.0 ± 15.0 years for bile duct cancer [19]. Patients with CBD/PBM may develop biliary tract cancer 15–20 years earlier than individuals without PBM.

1.5 Morphological Feature and Diagnosis

Most cases of CBD show the characteristic form: localized bile duct dilatation involving the common bile duct, abrupt caliber change between the common bile duct and the hepatic duct, abrupt narrowing at the lower portion of the dilated bile duct (narrow segment), dilatation of the cystic duct, stenosis at the porta hepatis in cases of intrahepatic duct dilatation, abnormal junction of the pancreatic and bile duct away from the ampulla, dilated common channel, and normal dorsal pancreatic duct (Fig. 1.3) [12]. In healthy individuals, imaging of the common channel usually depicts the papillary sphincter in the relaxation phase, not in the contraction phase. In contrast, in patients with PBM, the common channel is depicted during both the contraction and relaxation phases of papillary sphincter activity.

For a diagnosis of CBD, both abnormal dilatation of the bile duct and PBM (long common channel [>9 mm] and/or an abnormal union between the pancreatic and bile ducts) must be evident either by imaging (e.g., endoscopic retrograde cholangiopancreatography [ERCP], magnetic resonance cholangiopancreatography [MRCP], multi-detector row computed tomography, endoscopic ultrasonography) or by anatomical examination. The presence of the following items casts doubt on the diagnosis of CBD: a cystic lesion adjoining the tubular structure heading toward the lower surface of the liver in prenatal fetal ultrasound checkups, intermittent jaundice with predominance of direct bilirubin in the neonatal period, recurrent abdominal pain since childhood, pediatric patients with abdominal pain and hyperamylasemia, and biliary peritonitis by perforation of the bile duct in children [1].

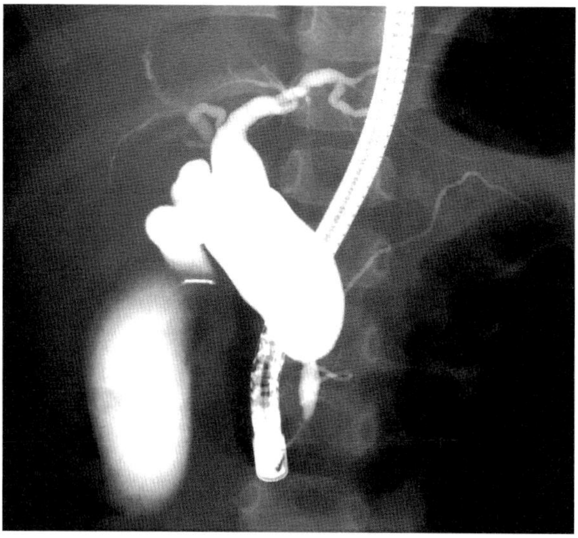

Fig. 1.3 Morphological findings of CBD by ERCP. Localized bile duct dilatation involving the common bile duct, abrupt caliber change between the common bile duct and the hepatic duct, abrupt narrowing at the lower portion of the dilated bile duct, dilatation of the cystic duct, abnormal junction of the pancreatic and bile ducts away from the ampulla, dilated common channel, and normal dorsal pancreatic duct are recognized in this ERCP image

1.6 Treatment

There is no clear evidence-based recommendation as to when a patient with CBD should undergo surgery. However, immediate surgery is recommended once a definitive diagnosis is established because juvenile patients with CBD can develop cholangitis and/or cancer even if asymptomatic. In patients whose cholangitis or jaundice fails to resolve with conservative therapy, percutaneous or endoscopic biliary drainage should be performed, and the cholangitis or jaundice should be controlled prior to the definitive operation. In patients with spontaneous perforation of the bile duct, emergency treatment of the biliary peritonitis is conducted, usually by means of T-tube drainage, followed by radical operation once the inflammation has subsided and after the anomalous anatomy has been clarified. However, the standard treatment for spontaneous perforation of the bile duct is currently undefined.

Extrahepatic bile duct resection and Roux-en-Y hepaticojejunostomy is recommended as a standard operation for patients with CBD. The results of this operation are almost always good after a short-term follow-up. However, reports of cholangitis, intrahepatic stones, and/or bile duct carcinoma after long-term follow-up are gradually increasing [20]. To prevent these serious complications after surgery, it is crucial that the pancreatic portion of the common bile duct be dissected at the level immediately above the pancreaticobiliary junction and that the stenosis of the porta hepatis be resected during the initial operation [20]. Meanwhile, the optimum treatment for patients with PBM without bile duct dilatation is debatable. In adult patients with PBM without bile duct dilatation, excision of the common bile duct may be regarded as unnecessary because bile duct cancer only rarely develops. By contrast, a simple cholecystectomy as performed for adult patients is not justified in children given their long life span because pancreatic secretions continue to come into contact with the bile duct due to PBM. In any case, careful long-term follow-up is very important, because the outcome needs long time.

References

1. Hamada Y, Ando H, Kamisawa T, et al. Diagnostic criteria for congenital biliary dilatation 2015. J Hepatobiliary Pancreat Sci. 2016;23:342–6.
2. Kamisawa T, Ando H, Suyama M, et al. Japanese clinical practice guidelines for pancreraticobiliary maljunction. J Gastroenterl. 2012;47:731–59.
3. Vater A. Dissertation in auguralis media, poes diss. Qua Scirris viscerum dissert, c.s. ezlerus, vol. 70. Edinburgh: University Library; 1723. p. 19.
4. McConnell AA. Cyst of the common bile duct. Br J Surg. 1919;7:520–4.
5. Arnolds. Eine manneskopfgroβen Retentionszyste des Choledochus. Dtsch Med Wochenschr. 1906;32:1804.
6. Kozumi I, Kodama T. A case report and the etiology of choledochal cystic dilatation (in Japanese). J Tokyo Med Assoc. 1916;30:1413–23.
7. Irwin ST, Morison JE. Congenital cyst of common bile duct containing stones and undergoing cancerous change. Br J Surg. 1944;32:319–21.

8. Alonso-Lej F, Rever EB Jr, Pessagno DJ. Congenital choledochal cyst, with a report of 2, and an analysis of 94, cases. Int Abstr Surg. 1959;108:1–30.
9. Todani T. Congenital choledochal dilatation: classification, clinical features, and long-term results. J Hepatobiliary Pancreat Surg. 1997;4:276–82.
10. Davenport M, Basu R. Under pressure: choledochal malformation manometry. J Pediatr Surg. 2005;40:331–5.
11. Yamaguchi M. Congenital choledochal cyst. Analysis of 1,433 patients in the Japanese literature. Am J Surg. 1980;140:653–7.
12. Ishibashi H, Shimada M, Kamisawa T, et al. Japanese clinical practice guidelines for congenital biliary dilatation. J Hepatobiliary Pancreat Sci. 2017;24:1–16.
13. Yotuyanagi S. Contributions to the aetiology and pathogeny of idiopathic cystic dilatation of the common bile-duct with report of 3 cases: new aetiological theory based on supposed unequal epithelial proliferation at stage of physiological epithelial occlusion of primitive choledochus. Gann. 1936;30:601–50.
14. Suda K, Matsumoto Y, Miyano T. Narrow duct segment distal to choledochal cyst. Am J Gastroenterol. 1991;86:1259–63.
15. Ando H, Kaneko K, Ito F, Seo T, et al. Embryogenesis of pancreaticobiliary maljunction inferred from development of duodenal atresia. J Hepatobiliary Pancreat Surg. 1999;6:50–4.
16. Kamisawa T, Kuruma S, Tabata T, et al. Pancreaticobiliary maljunction and biliary cancer. J Gastroenterol. 2015;50:273–9.
17. Kaneko K, Ando H, Ito T, et al. Protein plugs cause symptoms in patients with choledochal cysts. Am J Gastroenterol. 1997;92:1018–21.
18. Tashiro S, Imaizumi T, Ohkawa H, Committee for Registration of the Japanese Study Group on Pancreaticobiliary Maljunction, et al. Pancreaticobiliary maljunction: retrospective and nationwide survey in Japan. J Hepatobiliary Pancreat Surg. 2003;10:345–51.
19. Morine Y, Shimada M, Takamatsu H, et al. Clinical features of pancreaticobiliary maljunction: update analysis of 2nd Japan-nationwide survey. J Hepatobiliary Pancreat Sci. 2013;20:472–80.
20. Kamisawa T, Kaneko K, Itoi T, Ando H. Pancreaticobiliary maljunction and congenital biliary dilatation. Lancet Gastroenterol Hepatol. 2017;2:610–8.

Part I
Embryology

Chapter 2
Embryology of Pancreaticobiliary Maljunction

Naohiro Hosomura and Hideki Fujii

Abstract In normal pancreaticobiliary junction, the common bile duct and the main pancreatic duct penetrate the muscle layer of the duodenum obliquely and parallel to each other and make a junction in the submucosal layer just before opening into the duodenum. While in the case of pancreaticobiliary maljunction, the junction of the ducts is external of the muscle layer of the duodenum, thus forming an extension to the muscularis propria of the duodenum and thus forming an extended common channel. It is clarified that both the long common channel and narrowed duct segment in pancreaticobiliary maljunction originate from the pancreatic duct in ventral pancreas. In conclusion, pancreaticobiliary maljunction is an embryological disorder that the terminal bile duct join to the pancreatic duct in the ventral pancreas. This misconnection of both ducts occurs during the fifth week of gestation as the proximal portion of the hepatic diverticulum elongates and the ventral primordium has been carried away from the duodenum by elongation of the proximal part of the diverticulum.

Keywords Pancreaticobiliary maljunction · Embryology · Long common channel Narrowed duct segment

In the normal pancreaticobiliary junction, the main pancreatic duct (Wirsung's duct) joins with the common bile duct inside the muscle layer of the duodenum to form the ampulla of Vater. On the other hand, in pancreaticobiliary maljunction which is a congenital anomaly, the junction of the pancreatic duct and biliary duct is located outside the duodenal wall. Pancreaticobiliary maljunction is almost always seen in patients with congenital biliary dilatation (congenital choledochal cyst). However,

---

N. Hosomura (✉)
First Department of Surgery, Yamanashi University, Chuo, Yamanashi, Japan
e-mail: naohiroh@yamanashi.ac.jp

H. Fujii
First Department of Surgery, Yamanashi University, Chuo, Yamanashi, Japan

Department of Surgery, Kofu Municipal Hospital, Kofu, Yamanashi, Japan
e-mail: hfujii@yamanashi.ac.jp

T. Kamisawa, H. Ando (eds.), *Pancreaticobiliary Maljunction and Congenital Biliary Dilatation*, https://doi.org/10.1007/978-981-10-8654-0_2

pancreaticobiliary maljunction may occur independently of any other developmental anomaly in the common bile duct.

The reason why pancreaticobiliary maljunction is not normal may possibly be explained more clearly by the reconstruction study by Suda et al. [1]. In normal pancreaticobiliary junction, the common bile duct and the main pancreatic duct penetrate the muscle layer of the duodenum obliquely and parallel to each other and make a junction in the submucosal layer just before opening into the duodenum. The angle of the ductal junction is therefore very sharp. The sphincter of Oddi, which surrounds both ducts and the common channel, normally consists of three sections: the sphincter choledochus, the sphincter pancreaticus, and the sphincter ampullae [2]. Of these, the sphincter muscle at the distal end of the choledochus (sphincter choledochus) is the best developed. It regulates the outflow of bile and prevents free communication between the bile duct and pancreatic duct.

In the case of pancreaticobiliary maljunction, however, the junction of the ducts is external of the muscle layer of the duodenum, thus forming an extension to the muscularis propria of the duodenum and thus forming an extended common channel [3]. The angle of the ductal junction is less sharp in these patients than in control cases. The well-developed sphincter muscle in the submucosal layer is seen in patients with pancreaticobiliary maljunction. It mainly surrounds the common channel (sphincter ampullae), but the sphincter choledochus is extremely hypoplastic. The anatomical findings suggest the possibility of the communication between the ducts in cases of pancreaticobiliary maljunction.

It is very important to understand the normal human development (normal embryology) of the hepatobiliary system and pancreas to better understand pancreaticobiliary maljunction. Akin [4] described the process of normal development of the hepatobiliary system and pancreas (Fig. 2.1). The extrahepatic bile duct system and the ventral anlage (primordium) of the pancreas arise from the hepatic diverticulum, which is first visible on the ventral surface of the anterior intestinal portal of the embryo early in the fourth week of gestation. By the end of the fourth week, ventral anlage of the pancreas arises from the base of the hepatic diverticulum itself, and the dorsal anlage of the pancreas arises directly from the dorsal side of the duodenum almost opposite the liver primordium. By the beginning of the fifth week, the pancreatic duct, gallbladder, cystic duct, and common bile duct are demarcated, and during the fifth week, the proximal portion of the hepatic diverticulum elongates but does not increase greatly in diameter, in contrast to the tremendous growth of the distal end. During this stage, the future common bile duct system is in an incomplete or solid cord state. By the sixth week, the ventral primordium has been carried away from the duodenum by elongation of the proximal part of the diverticulum. During the seventh week, duodenal torsion brings the two pancreatic primordia side by side, and the smaller, ventral primordium fuses with the proximal part of the dorsal pancreas. No solid stage seems to occur in the pancreatic ducts. Reestablishment of the lumen of the hepatic diverticulum commences with the common bile duct in the sixth week of gestation and progresses slowly to the distal portion. The lumen extends into the cystic duct by the seventh week. During the eighth week, the proximal portion of the diverticulum is usually absorbed into the intestinal wall, so that the common bile duct and the pancreatic duct enter the duodenum side by side. The duodenal wall thickens, and the confluence point of the

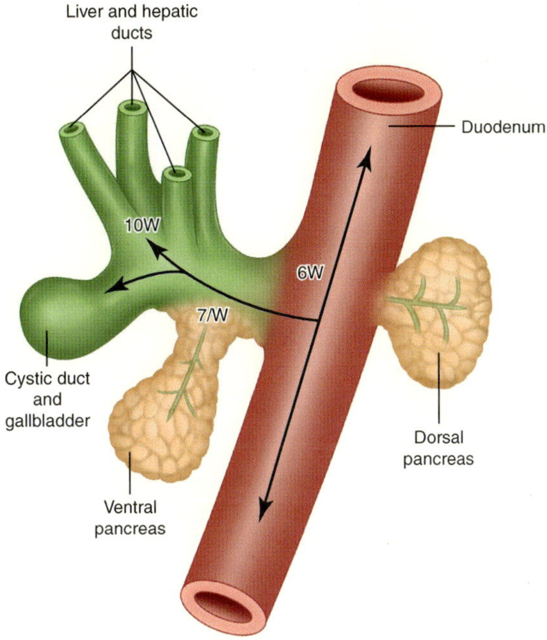

Fig. 2.1 The process of normal development of the hepatobiliary system and pancreas

pancreatic duct and common bile duct moves to the duodenal lumen. Then the papilla of Vater is formed. The muscle fibers of the sphincter of Oddi are derived directly from the mesenchyme around the common bile duct during the 11th week of gestation. In short, during the normal course of development of the hepatobiliary system and the pancreas, the main pancreatic duct joins to the common bile duct to form a "common channel" (the ampulla of Vater), and the common channel moves inside the muscle layer of the duodenum after the 12th week of gestation.

Alonso-Lej et al. [5] and Yotuyanagi [6] described the narrowed duct segment distal to the dilated bile duct as a "narrow part of the terminal bile duct." Babbitt [7] described it as a "long common channel" that was thought to arrest the normal inward migration of the junction of the main pancreatic duct and the common bile duct [8], similar to the occurrence of congenital biliary atresia. We clarified that the "long common channel" actually represents pancreatic duct system [9], based on a radiological and anatomical analysis of patients with pancreaticobiliary maljunction. We have some cases that show small radicles that are thought to be branches of the pancreatic duct arising from so-called long common channel. Figure 2.2 shows a surgical (pancreaticoduodenectomy) specimen associated with congenital biliary dilatation and with gallbladder carcinoma that invades the duodenum. In this specimen, the junction of the main pancreatic duct and the common bile duct is external of the muscle layer of the duodenum and forms a "long common channel." This condition refers to pancreaticobiliary maljunction. Also in this surgical specimen, the minute orifice is found in the narrowed duct segment. It is identified as a small pancreatic duct from the pancreatic parenchyma by microscope. These small pancreatic ducts are derived from the ventral pancreas, based on the distribution of islet

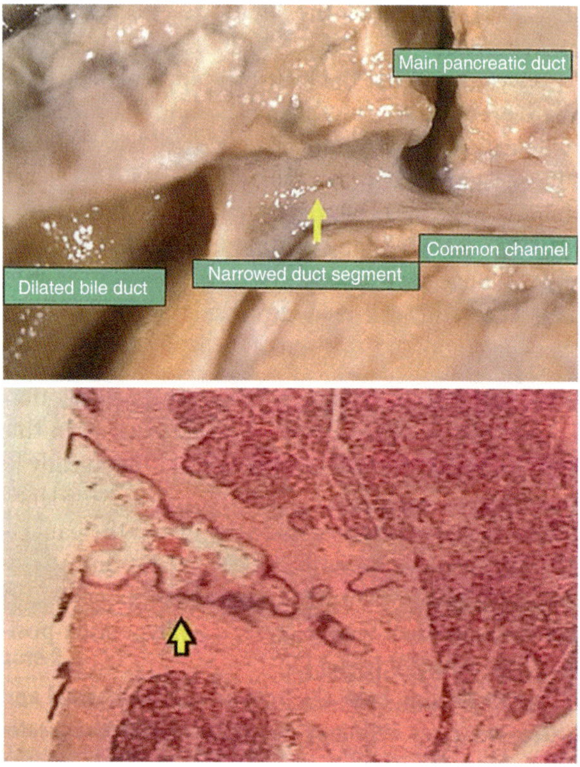

Fig. 2.2 The junction of the main pancreatic duct and the common bile duct is external to the muscle layer of the duodenum. A minute orifice can be found in the narrowed duct segment macroscopically. Furthermore, It is identified microscopically as a small duct in the pancreatic parenchyma that can be recognized as a pancreatic duct

with pancreatic polypeptide cells [10]. In conclusion, both the "long common channel" and "narrowed duct segment" originate from the pancreatic duct in the ventral pancreas. By anatomical and radiological analysis, a variation of pancreaticobiliary maljunction derives from the location of the union of the terminal bile duct to the ventral pancreatic ducts.

Sometimes, we experience the pancreaticobiliary maljunction with the pancreas divisum. In this case, the shape of the union of the pancreatic duct and common bile duct looks very complex. In the pancreas divisum, the parenchyma of the ventral pancreas and the dorsal pancreas are separated as a double pancreas. Recently, however, the term pancreas divisum has been used widely to describe two ductal systems, the ventral pancreatic duct and the dorsal pancreatic duct, which do not unite or communicate and separately drain to the two duodenal papillae [10]. In this condition, pancreatic juice from the dominant dorsal moiety flows out only through the minor papilla, in which the outlet is notably small in most cases. This raises the question of whether this variation plays a role in the development of pancreatic pain or pancreatitis. The clinical relevance of pancreas divisum has been argued repeatedly [11]. Figure 2.3 shows an example of isolated dorsal pancreatitis associated with pancreas divisum. This condition strongly suggests inadequate drainage from the minor papilla. In this case, fusion via two so-called inferior branches

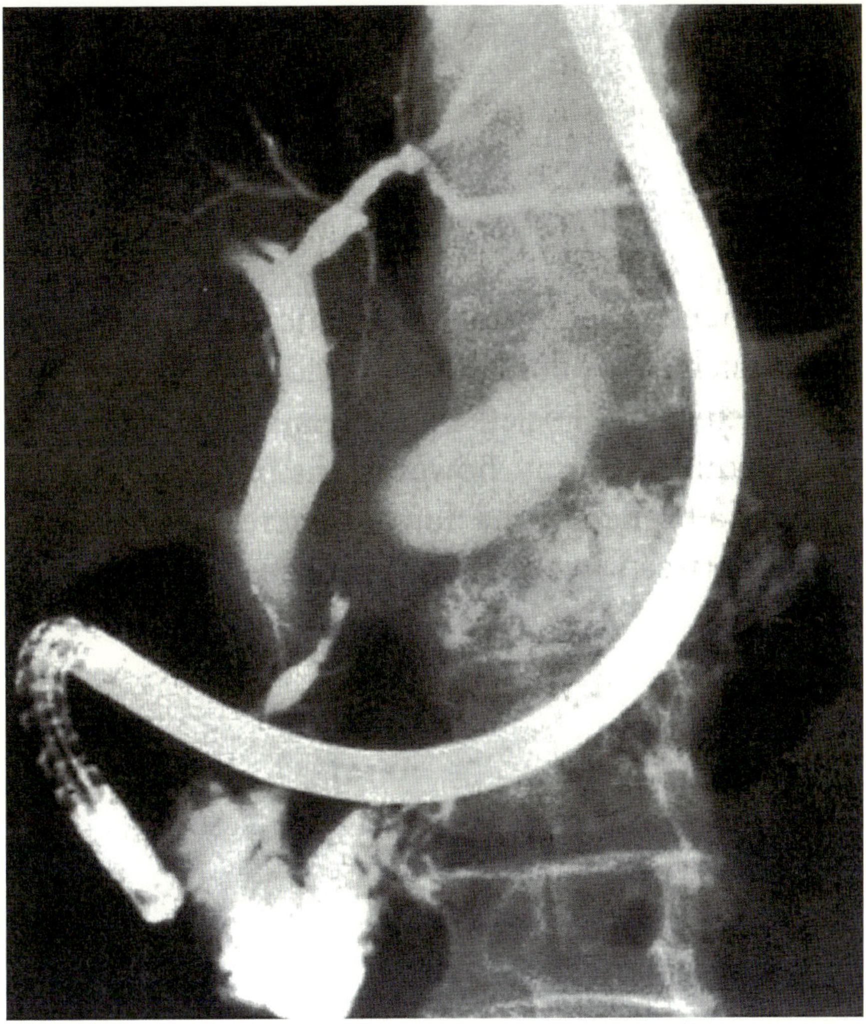

Fig. 2.3 A case of isolated dorsal pancreatitis associated with pancreas divisum. The branch fusion seems to be composed of an inferior branch of the ventral pancreatic duct and an inferior branch of the dorsal pancreatic duct

between the ventral pancreatic duct and dorsal pancreatic duct was studied based on organogenesis of the pancreas [12]. Radiologically, the branch fusion seems to be composed of an inferior branch of the ventral pancreatic duct and an inferior branch of the dorsal pancreatic duct. By mapping the locations of pancreatic polypeptide islets in material obtained by pancreaticoduodenectomy, however, the branch was identified as a branch of the dorsal pancreatic duct. Thus fusion between two inferior branches was not established but was found to consist of an inferior branch of the dorsal pancreatic duct connected with the ventral pancreatic duct.

References

1. Suda K, Miyano T, Hashimoto K. The choledocho-pancreatico-ductal junction in infantile obstructive jaundice disease. Acta Pathol Jpn. 1980;30:187–94.
2. Boyden EA. The anatomy of the choledochoduodenal junction in man. Surg Gynecol Obst. 1996;104:641–52.
3. Frierson HF Jr. The gross anatomy and histology of the gallbladder, extrahepatic bile ducts, Vaterian system, and minor papilla. Am J Surg Pathol. 1989;13:146–62.
4. Akin JT. The liver. Anomalies of extrahepatic biliary ducts and the gallbladder. In: Gray SW, Skandalakis JE, editors. Embryology for surgeons. Philadelphia: Saunders; 1972. p. 217–62.
5. Alonso-Lej F, Rever WB, Pessagno DJ. Congenital choledochal cyst with a report of two and analysis of 94 cases. Intern Abstr Surg. 1959;108:1–23.
6. Yotuyanagi S. Contribution to aetiology and pathology of idiopathic cystic dilatation of common bile duct with report of three cases: new aetiologic theory. Gann. 1936;30:601–50.
7. Babbitt DP. Congenital choledochal cyst: new etiological concept based on anomalous relationships of common bile duct and pancreatic bulb. Ann Radiol. 1969;12:231–41.
8. Arey LB. Developmental anatomy: a textbook and laboratory manual of embryology. 7th ed. Philadelphia: Saunders; 1974. p. 255–62.
9. Matsumoto Y, Fujii H, Itakura J, et al. Pancreaticobiliary maljunction: etiologic concepts based on radiologic aspects. Gastrointest Endosc. 2001;53:614–9.
10. Suda K, Matsumoto Y, Miyano T. Narrowed duct segment distal to choledochal cyst. Am J Gastroenterol. 1991;86:1259–63.
11. Cotton PB. Congenital anomaly of pancreas divisum as cause of obstructive pain and pancreatitis. Gut. 1980;21:105–14.
12. Suda K, Mogaki M, Matsumoto Y, et al. Gross dissection and immunohistochemical studies on branch fusion type of ventral and dorsal pancreatic ducts: a case report. Surg Radiol Anat. 1991;13:333–7.

Part II
Epidemiology

Chapter 3
Most Recent Analysis of a Japanese Nationwide Survey of Pancreaticobiliary Maljunction over a Quarter of a Century

Yuji Morine, Mitsuo Shimada, and Hiroki Ishibashi

Abstract We herein present the most recent data on pancreaticobiliary maljunction (PBM) from a nationwide survey, which 3,303 individuals with PBM were registered at over 100 medical institutions in Japan for over 25 years. In this analysis, clinical features of eligible patients ($n = 3,184$) were compared according to age and presence of biliary dilatation (BD), and key points of this analysis were the coexistence of associated cancers and the surgical procedure including postoperative complication. Of the adults with CBD, 7.0 and 13.5% had gallbladder or bile duct cancers, whereas 4.0 and 37.2% of those with PBM without BD had these cancers. Three children with congenital biliary dilatation (CBD) had bile duct cancers (0.24%). As to individuals without asociated cancers, cholecystectomy combined with extrahepatic bile duct resection had been performed on 94.3% of children with CBD and on 90.7% of those with PBM with BD. In contrast, this procedure had been performed on 29.8% of adults with PBM without BD but on 87.1% of those with CBD. Postoperative complication rates of this procedure ranged from 10 to 20%. Thus, this largest and most recent series could be widely used to assist in making decisions about treatment strategies and understanding the pathophysiology of PBM.

Keywords Nationwide survey · Biliary dilatation · Biliary tract cancer
Extrahepatic bile duct resection

Y. Morine (✉) · M. Shimada · H. Ishibashi
Department of Surgery, Institute of Health Biosciences, University of Tokushima Graduate School, Tokushima, Japan

Japanese Study Group on Pancreaticobiliary Maljunction, Tokushima, Japan
e-mail: ymorine@tokushima-u.ac.jp

T. Kamisawa, H. Ando (eds.), *Pancreaticobiliary Maljunction and Congenital Biliary Dilatation*, https://doi.org/10.1007/978-981-10-8654-0_3

Abbreviations

BD	Biliary dilatation
CBD	Congenital biliary dilatation
JSPBM	Japanese Study Group on Pancreaticobiliary Maljunction
PBM	Pancreaticobiliary maljunction

3.1 Introduction

Pancreaticobiliary maljunction (PBM), in which the junction of the pancreatic and biliary ducts is located outside the duodenal wall [1–3], has been defined as a congenital anomaly by the Japanese Study Group on Pancreaticobiliary Maljunction (JSPBM). This condition was first described by Komi et al. in Japan in 1976 [4] and is now widely recognized as an anomalous arrangement or abnormal junction of the pancreaticobiliary ductal system. The JSPBM was developed at a small conference and founded in 1983 to discuss the diagnosis and treatment of this anomaly. The JSPBM has classified this anomaly into two categories according to the presence of biliary dilatation (BD). Until now, PBM with BD has been recognized as the congenital biliary dilatation (CBD) worldwide. Almost all individuals with CBD of Todani Type I (except for Type Ib) and Type IV-A have associated PBM [5]. The principal project of the JSPBM has been to collect clinical data on patients with PBM from 1990, and they have twice reported the clinical characteristics of this anomaly [6, 7]. as well as publishing Japanese clinical practice guidelines for this condition [5].

The most important clinical feature of this condition is the high frequency of associated biliary tract cancers, which was revealed by the JSPBM nationwide survey. Furthermore, biliary carcinogenesis in individuals with PBM arises as a result of reflux and stasis of bile mixed with pancreatic fluid in the bile duct and gallbladder and is associated with various epithelial gene mutations, such as *K-ras* and *p53* [5, 8–12]. Another important issue investigated by the JSPBM is the optimal surgical strategy for PBM without BD, which may not strongly associated with bile duct cancers, because the treatment strategy differs between CBD and PBM without BD in adults [7]. A worldwide consensus has been reached that CBD without associated cancers is best treated by cholecystectomy combined with extrahepatic bile duct resection. However, for PBM without BD and no associated biliary tract cancer, the prophylactic combined resection of the extrahepatic bile ducts is generally not recommended because of the comparatively low risk of bile duct cancer.

The JSPBM has continued to collect data on PBM in its nationwide survey, 3,303 individuals with PBM in this Japan having been registered during the 25 years from 1 January 1990 to 31 December 2014. This chapter presents the most recent analysis of this large cohort of individuals with PBM.

3.2 Methods

3.2.1 Patients and Methods

As reported previously, the JSPBM via its Registration Committee enrolled 3,303 individuals who had been diagnosed with PBM and treated for it from 1 January 1990 to 31 December 2014 at over 100 institutions throughout Japan. The registration system did not have a definition of dilatation of the extrahepatic bile duct throughout the period of data collection, the diagnostic criteria for CBD having been established only in 2015 [13]. Therefore, the attending doctors at each institute had determined whether the bile duct was dilated according to their own criteria referring the Registration Committee recommended criteria for BD in 2006.

It is unknown whether 26 of the 3,303 individuals with PBM had BD; additionally, the ages on initial diagnosis of a further 93 cases are unknown because of loss of detailed registration records. In this registry, adults are defined as aged 15 years or more. Consequently, after exclusion of those with unknown BD status or age, 3,184 individuals were analyzed after allocating them to one of four groups (Fig. 3.1a).

To facilitate registration, the JSPBM Registration Committee has designated three types of PBM according to the type of confluence between the terminal common bile duct and pancreatic duct (Fig. 3.1b) [6] as follows: in Type A (known as C-P, choledochal, or right-angle type), the common bile duct seems to join the pancreatic duct; in Type B (known as P-C, pancreatic, or acute-angle type), the pancreatic duct seems to join the common bile duct; and in Type C (known as complex type) junction of the pancreaticobiliary ductal system is complex.

Using the above criteria, the clinical features of PBM, including biliopancreatic disease and associated biliary tract cancers, were evaluated in individuals with and without BD. Additionally, the pancreatic enzymes in the bile were examined when available and the surgical procedures and postoperative complications investigated in individuals without associated cancers.

3.2.2 Statistics

All statistical analysis was performed using statistical software (JMP 8.0.1, SAS Campus Drive, Cary, 27513 NC, USA). The significance of differences between groups in clinical features was analyzed with the χ^2 test. Amylase, lipase, and phospholipase A2 concentrations in bile juice are expressed as median and range and analyzed using one-way ANOVA and the Bonferroni correction. $P \leq 0.05$ was considered to denote significance.

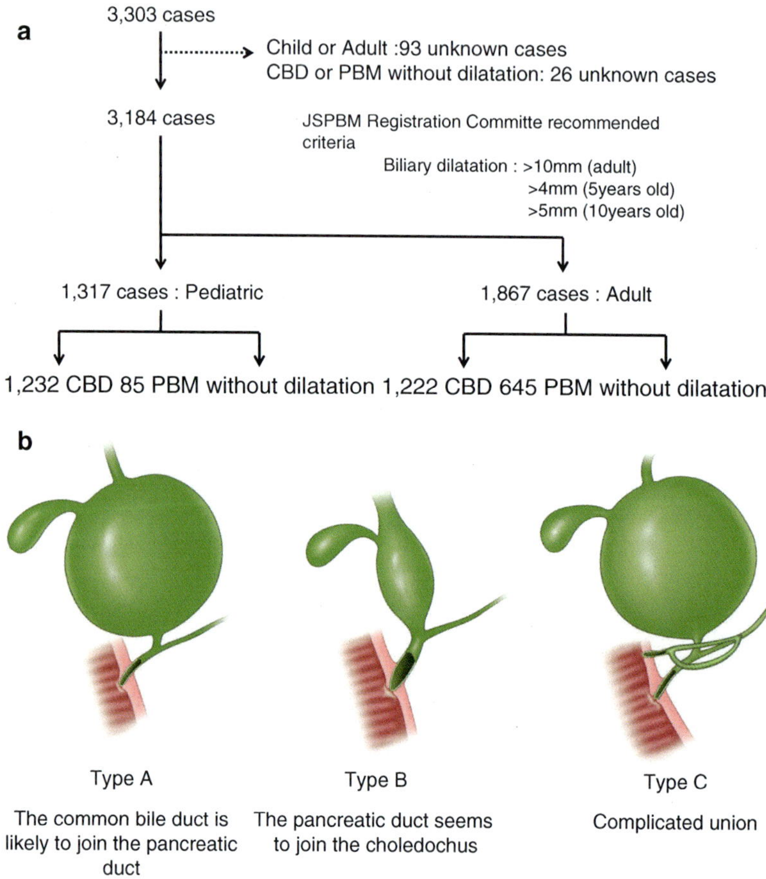

Fig. 3.1 (**a**) Flow chart showing patient enrollment and grouping according to age and presence of biliary dilatation. (**b**) Classification of pancreaticobiliary maljunction

3.3 Results

3.3.1 Patients' Distribution and Clinical Features

Using the specified cutoff age of 15 years, there were 1,317 pediatric and 1,867 adult patients. Of the pediatric patients, 1,232 had CBD (PBM with BD) and 85 PBM without BD. Of the adult patients, 1,222 had CBD and 645 PBM without BD; thus, BD was more frequently absent in adult than in pediatric patients. Figure 3.2 shows the age distribution of the registered PBM patients and that the adults frequently had PBM without BD.

Clinical features according to age and presence of BD are summarized in Table 3.1. Regarding confluence type, Type A (C-P type) occurred more frequently in individuals with CBD and Type B in those with PBM without BD, regardless of age. Pediatric patients more frequently had clinical symptoms than adults regardless

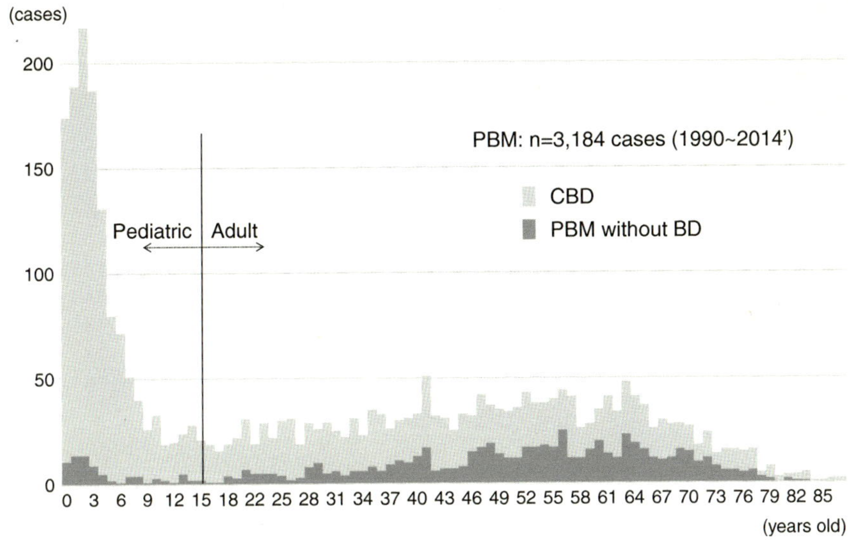

Fig. 3.2 Age distribution of registered individuals with PBM

Table 3.1 Clinical features of PBM according to age and presence of BD

	Pediatric (n = 1,018)		Adult (n = 1,511)	
Factors	CBD (n = 1,232)	PBM without BD (n = 85)	CBD (n = 1,222)	PBM without BD (n = 645)
Gender male:female (unknown)	298:924 (10)	23:62	310:894 (18)	173:463 (9)
PBM type A:B:C (unknown)	708:390:53 (81)	26:44:10 (5)	677:431:76 (38)	201:387:31 (26)
Common channel dilatation	354 (28.73%)	19 (22.35%)	317 (25.94%)	112 (17.36%)
Clinical symptom	1144 (92.86%)	77 (90.59%)	869 (71.12%)	441 (68.37%)
Abdominal pain	1140 (92.53%)	61 (71.76%)	726 (59.41%)	348 (53.95%)
Back pain	40 (3.25%)	3 (3.53%)	139 (11.37%)	82 (12.71%)
Jaundice	339 (27.52%)	19 (22.35%)	132 (10.80%)	90 (13.95%)
Tumor palpation	148 (12.01%)	6 (7.06%)	28 (2.29%)	14 (2.17%)
Fever	295 (23.94%)	17 (20.00%)	158 (12.93%)	73 (11.32%)
Vomiting	629 (51.06%)	47 (55.29%)	114 (9.33%)	42 (6.51%)
Nausea	435 (35.31%)	28 (32.94%)	143 (11.70%)	57 (8.84%)
Whitish stool	190 (15.42%)	11 (12.94%)	28 (2.29%)	12 (1.86%)
Preoperative complication				
Acute pancreatitis	327 (26.54%)	22 (25.88%)	100 (8.18%)	52 (8.06%)
Chronic pancreatitis	21 (1.70%)	3 (3.53%)	32 (2.62%)	6 (0.93%)
Biliary perforation	44 (3.57%)	3 (3.53%)	3 (0.25%)	1 (0.16%)

(continued)

Table 3.1 (continued)

Factors	Pediatric (n = 1,018)		Adult (n = 1,511)	
	CBD (n = 1,232)	PBM without BD (n = 85)	CBD (n = 1,222)	PBM without BD (n = 645)
Cholangitis	174 (14.12%)	8 (9.41%)	140 (11.47%)	48 (7.44%)
Liver dysfunction	410 (33.28%)	16 (18.82%)	162 (13.26%)	62 (9.61%)
Biliary stone	136 (11.04%)	7 (8.24%)	268 (21.93%)	152 (23.57%)
Gall bladder	26 (2.11%)	1 (1.18%)	112 (9.17%)	114 (17.67%)
Extrahepatic	96 (7.79%)	4 (4.71%)	161 (13.18%)	26 (4.03%)
Intrahepatic	10 (0.81%)	0 (0%)	24 (1.96%)	13 (2.02%)
Pancreatic stone	164 (13.31%)	12 (14.12%)	65 (5.32%)	10 (1.55%)
Calcium calculus	3 (0.24%)	0 (0%)	23 (1.88%)	3 (0.47%)
Protein plug	152 (12.34%)	10 (11.76%)	39 (3.19%)	4 (0.62%)

of the presence of BD (pediatric CBD, 92.8%; pediatric PBM without BD, 90.6%; adult CBD, 71.1%; adult PBM without BD, 68.4%). Also, there was no difference in the incidence of clinical symptoms according to the presence of BD regardless of age. The most common clinical symptom in all patients was abdominal pain, whereas nausea and vomiting occurred more frequently in pediatric than adult patients, regardless of the presence of BD.

The main preoperative complications were liver dysfunction, acute pancreatitis, and biliary perforation. In particular, acute pancreatitis and liver dysfunction were more frequent complications in pediatric than in adult patients, regardless of the presence of BD. Over 20% of adults had coexisting biliopancreatic stones, regardless of the presence of BD, whereas only about 10% of pediatric patients had such stones, regardless of whether they had CBD or PBM without BD. Conversely, coexistence of pancreatic stone was more frequent in pediatric than in adult patients, the stones most often comprising a protein plug in the former.

Regarding pancreatic enzymes in bile, amylase, lipase, and phospholipase A2 concentrations were investigated (Table 3.2). Amylase and lipase concentrations were significantly higher in both the gallbladder and bile duct in adults with CBD than in children with CBD; no other significant relationships were identified.

3.3.2 *Prevalence of Associated Cancers*

The prevalence of associated cancers according to patient group is shown in Table 3.3. Only three pediatric patients with CBD developed associated biliary tract cancers, and there were no other types of associated cancer. However, in adults, the prevalence of associated biliary tract cancers was extremely high, being 21.9% in those with CBD and 43.7% in those with PBM without BD; this difference was significant ($p < 0.0001$). Meanwhile, the prevalence of liver cancer was 0.65% in adults with CBD and 1.9% in those without BD ($p < 0.05$), whereas the prevalence of pancreatic cancer was 0.82% in adults with CBD and 1.4% in those with PBM without BD.

Table 3.2 Pancreatic enzymes in bile in individuals with PBM

	Pediatric		Adult	
Factors	CBD	PBM without BD	CBD	PBM without BD
Amylase: IU/L				
Gallbladder (range)	32,903 (0–6,633,000) $n = 772$	24,235 (0–1,266,399) $n = 42$	87,850 (0–6,920,000)* $n = 542$	55,977 (0–5,845,900) $n = 237$
Bile duct (range)	15,800 (0–958,000) $n = 631$	16,069 (0–592,000) $n = 30$	76,000 (0–6,730,000)** $n = 609$	53,400 (0–6,600,500) $n = 183$
Lipase: IU/L				
Gallbladder (range)	8,350 (0–1,059,156) $n = 453$	16,000 (2–841,400) $n = 21$	39,424 (0–1,332,500)** $n = 213$	55,006 (1–650,025) $n = 98$
Bile duct (range)	6,000 (0–2,149,688) $n = 335$	35,470 (138–606,810) $n = 16$	41,050 (0–1,873,000)* $n = 222$	60,550 (0–3,087,315) $n = 56$
Phospholipase A2: ng/dl				
Gallbladder (range)	888,758 (0–5,927,000) $n = 226$	283,650 (100–4,470,000) $n = 14$	431,000 (0–4,150,000) $n = 87$	747,200 (0–5,250,000) $n = 40$
Bile duct (range)	255,419 (0–1,000,897,000) $n = 166$	1,159,000 (698,000–1,620,000) $n = 2$	620,000 (0–5,630,000) $n = 97$	43,650 (0–2,110,000) $n = 18$

*$p < 0.001$ vs. pediatric CBD, **$p < 0.0001$ vs. pediatric CBD

Table 3.3 Prevalence of associated cancer according to patient group

	Pediatric ($n = 1{,}018$)		Adult ($n = 1{,}511$)	
Factors	CBD ($n = 1{,}232$)	PBM without BD ($n = 85$)	CBD ($n = 1{,}222$)	PBM without BD ($n = 645$)
Biliary cancers	3 (0.24%)	0 (0%)	268 (21.93%)	282 (43.72%)*
Liver cancer	0 (0%)	0 (0%)	8 (0.65%)	12 (1.86%)**
Pancreatic cancer	0 (0%)	0 (0%)	10 (0.82%)	9 (1.40%)
Others	0 (0%)	0 (0%)	31 (2.54%)	18 (2.79%)

*$p < 0.0001$ vs. adult CBD, **$p < 0.05$ vs. adult CBD

3.3.3 Locations of Associated Biliary Tract Cancers

Locations of associated biliary tract cancers are summarized in Table 3.4. All three associated biliary tract cancers in children with CBD were located in a dilated bile duct, one having progressed into an intrahepatic bile duct.

Bile duct cancer was identified in 7.0% ($n = 86$) and gallbladder cancer in 13.5% ($n = 165$) of adults with CBD and in 4.0% ($n = 26$) and 37.2% ($n = 240$), respectively, of adults with PBM without BD, the difference in prevalence of bile duct cancer

Table 3.4 Locations of associated biliary cancers

Factors	Pediatric (n = 1,018) CBD (n = 1,232)	Pediatric (n = 1,018) PBM without BD (n = 85)	Adult (n = 1,511) CBD (n = 1,222)	Adult (n = 1,511) PBM without BD (n = 645)
Gallbladder	0 (0%)	0 (0%)	165 (13.50%)	240 (37.21%)
Extrahepatic bile duct	2 (0.16%)	0 (0%)	82 (6.71%)	21 (3.26%)
Intrahepatic bile duct	0 (0%)	0 (0%)	2 (0.16%)	2 (0.31%)
Extrahepatic bile duct + intrahepatic bile duct	1 (0.08%)	0 (0%)	2 (0.16%)	3 (0.47%)
Gallbladder + extrahepatic bile duct	0 (0%)	0 (0%)	11 (0.90%)	13 (2.02%)
Gallbladder + intrahepatic bile duct	0 (0%)	0 (0%)	1 (0.08%)	0 (0%)
Gallbladder + extrahepatic bile duct + intrahepatic bile duct	0 (0%)	0 (0%)	3 (0.25%)	1 (0.16%)
Unknown	0 (0%)	0 (0%)	2 (0.16%)	2 (0.31%)

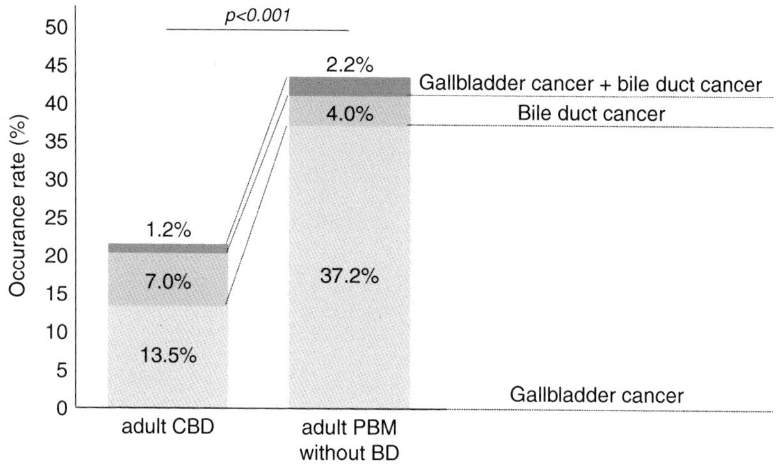

Fig. 3.3 Rates of associated biliary tract cancers in adults with PBM

being significant ($p < 0.001$) (Fig. 3.3). Additionally, the overall combined rate of bile duct and gallbladder cancers was 1.2% (n = 15) in adults with CBD and 2.2% (n = 14) in those with PBM without BD. Hence, the location of biliary tract cancers differed between adult patients with and without BD; however, gallbladder cancer was significantly predominant in both groups.

3.3.4 *Surgical Procedures for PBM without Associated Cancer*

In this study, the type of surgical procedure preferred for patients without associated cancers was also investigated (Table 3.5) because the prophylactic procedure of combined extrahepatic bile duct resection in individuals with PBM without BD is

Table 3.5 Treatment of PBM in patients without associated biliary cancer and without previous surgery (1997–2014)

	Pediatric (n = 788)		Adult (n = 741)	
Treatment	CBD (n = 734)	PBM without BD (n = 54)	CBD (n = 543)	PBM without BD (n = 198)
Cholecystectomy alone	2 (0.27%)	2 (3.70%)	17 (3.13%)	122 (61.62%)
Cholecystectomy + hepatic resection	0 (0%)	0 (0%)	0 (0%)	5 (2.53%)
Cholecystectomy + extrahepatic bile duct resection	692 (94.28%)	49 (90.74%)	473 (87.11%)	53 (26.8%)
Cholecystectomy + extrahepatic bile duct resection + hepatectomy	1 (0.13%)	0 (0%)	11 (2.03%)	3 (1.52%)
Pancreatoduodenectomy	0 (0%)	0 (0%)	14 (2.58%)	2 (1.01%)
Pancreatoduodenectomy + hepatic resection	0 (0%)	0 (0%)	1 (0.18%)	0 (0%)
Other procedures	7 (0.95%)	0 (0%)	1 (0.18%)	0 (0%)
Unknown procedure	27 (3.68%)	2 (3.70%)	7 (1.3%)	0 (0%)
No treatment	5 (0.68%)	1 (1.85%)	19 (3.50%)	13 (6.57%)

Table 3.6 Reconstruction methods after cholecystectomy + extrahepatic bile duct resection in patients without associated biliary cancer

	Pediatric (n = 741)		Adult (n = 526)	
Treatment	CBD (n = 692)	PBM without BD (n = 49)	CBD (n = 473)	PBM without BD (n = 53)
Intrahepatic hepaticojejunostomy	4 (0.57%)	1 (2.04%)	5 (1.06%)	2 (3.77%)
Hilar hepaticojejunostomy	202 (29.19%)	8 (16.32%)	164 (34.67%)	14 (26.42%)
Hepaticojejunostomy	443 (64.02%)	36 (73.47%)	262 (55.39%)	18 (33.96%)
Choledochojejunostomy	4 (0.57%)	1 (2.04%)	7 (1.48%)	4 (7.55%)
Hilar hepaticojejunostomy	11 (1.59%)	0 (0%)	0 (0%)	0 (0%)
Hepaticoduodenostomy	23 (3.32%)	2 (4.08%)	26 (5.50%)	2 (3.77%)
Choledochoduodenostomy	0 (0%)	0 (0%)	0 (0%)	9 (16.98%)
Unknown procedure	5 (0.72%)	1 (2.04%)	9 (1.91%)	4 (7.55%)

still controversial given the comparatively low risk of associated bile duct cancer. Various surgical procedures, including pancreatoduodenectomy or hepatectomy, had been performed on both pediatric and adult patients for individualized reasons.

Cholecystectomy combined with extrahepatic bile duct resection was performed on 94.3% of pediatric patients with CBD and for 90.7% of those with PBM with BD, probably because of high rate of clinical symptoms and complications. In comparison, this procedure was performed on only 29.8% of adult patients with PBM without BD but on 87.1% of those with CBD (Table 3.6). Hence, BD status made a considerable difference to the surgical procedures performed on adult patients but not to those performed on pediatric patients.

There is as yet no consensus on the optimal reconstruction procedure after extrahepatic bile duct resection. Table 3.5 shows these reconstruction procedures; hepatico- or choledochojejunostomy was performed more often than hepatico- or choledochoduodenostomy.

3.3.5 Comparison of Postoperative Complications According to Surgical Procedure Performed on Patients with PBM

Figure 3.4 shows the rates of postoperative complications after cholecystectomy alone and cholecystectomy with extrahepatic bile duct resection for both pediatric and adult patients with PBM and without associated cancers. The details of these complications are shown in Table 3.7. Ten to twenty percent of patients who had undergone cholecystectomy with extrahepatic bile duct resection developed postoperative complications, these rates being higher than in patients who had undergone cholecystectomy alone. In adults with PBM without BD, cholecystectomy with extrahepatic bile duct resection tended to have a higher complication rate than cholecystectomy alone; however, this difference was not significant (p = 0.068). Additionally, this rate did not differ from the rate of complications after cholecystectomy with extrahepatic bile duct resection in adults with CBD.

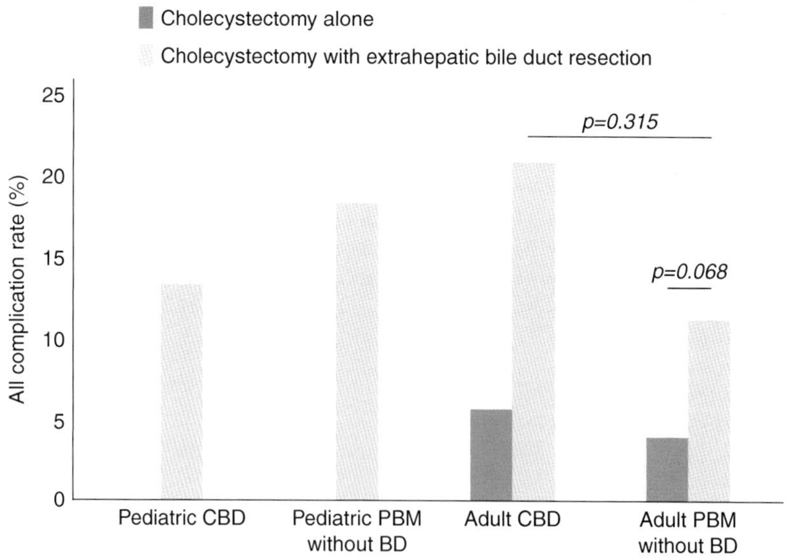

Fig. 3.4 Rates of postoperative complications in patients with PBM without associated cancers according to operative procedure and patient group

Table 3.7 Postoperative complications of cholecystectomy alone and cholecystectomy with extrahepatic bile duct resection (1997–2014)

	Pediatric (n = 4)		Adult (n = 140)	
Cholecystectomy alone	CBD (n = 2)	PBM without BD (n = 2)	CBD (n = 17)	PBM without BD (n = 123)
All complications	0 (0%)	0 (0%)	1 (5.8%)	5 (4.1%)
Cholangitis	0 (0%)	0 (0%)	0 (0%)	0 (0%)
Pancreatitis	0 (0%)	0 (0%)	0 (0%)	1 (0.81%)
Liver dysfunction	0 (0%)	0 (0%)	1 (5.8%)	1 (0.81%)
Ileus	0 (0%)	0 (0%)	0 (0%)	0 (0%)
Pancreatic fistula	0 (0%)	0 (0%)	0 (0%)	0 (0%)
Bile leakage	0 (0%)	0 (0%)	0 (0%)	2 (1.6%)
Abdominal abscess	0 (0%)	0 (0%)	0 (0%)	0 (0%)
Others	0 (0%)	0 (0%)	0 (0%)	2 (1.6%)
Cholecystectomy + extrahepatic bile duct resection	Pediatric (n = 741)		Adult (n = 526)	
	CBD (n = 692)	PBM without dilatation (n = 49)	CBD (n = 473)	PBM without dilatation (n = 53)
All complications	93 (13.4%)	9 (18.4%)	99 (20.9%)	6 (11.3%)
Cholangitis	9 (1.3%)	1 (2.0%)	15 (3.2%)	1 (1.9%)
Pancreatitis	26 (3.8%)	3 (6.1%)	14 (3.0%)	0 (0%)
Liver dysfunction	30 (4.3%)	3 (6.1%)	26 (5.5%)	2 (3.8%)
Ileus	9 (1.3%)	0 (0%)	7 (1.5%)	0 (0%)
Pancreatic fistula	5 (0.72%)	0 (0%)	15 (3.2%)	1 (1.9%)
Bile leakage	14 (2.0%)	3 (6.1%)	13 (2.6%)	1 (1.9%)
Abdominal abscess	2 (0.29%)	0 (0%)	6 (1.3%)	1 (1.9%)
Others	17 (2.5%)	1 (2.0%)	19 (4.0%)	1 (1.9%)

3.4 Discussion

In this nationwide survey, we analyzed the updated registered data of a Japanese nationwide survey of PBM, which accumulated 3,303 patients with PBM at over 100 institutions for over 25 years, and here revealed the detail of clinical features, including associated cancers. We also investigated surgical procedures performed on patients without associated cancers and their postoperative complications. We have previously published the first and second versions of this Japanese nationwide survey of PBM [6, 7]. This most recent update includes the largest cohort of individuals with PBM reported thus far and may contribute to elucidating the pathophysiology of this disease according to the presence of BD and age.

Type A confluence between the terminal common bile duct and pancreatic duct was present significantly more frequently in individuals with CBD, whereas Type B was present significantly more frequently in those with PBM without BD, regardless of age. The incidence of clinical symptoms was significantly higher in pediatric than in adult patients. However, the incidence of clinical symptoms did not differ significantly between individuals with CBD and those with PBM without BD. We identified no distinctive difference in symptoms according to BD status in either pediatric or adult patients. As to preoperative complications, acute pancreatitis and liver dysfunction tended to occur more frequently in individuals with CBD. Adult patients had a higher frequency of biliary stones, whereas pancreatic stones occurred more frequently in pediatric patients. Those findings did not differ substantially from those found at earlier stages of the Japan nationwide survey of PBM.

Our two previous Japanese nationwide surveys have highlighted the high frequency of associated biliary tract cancers and revealed that gallbladder cancer predominates regardless of the presence of BD in adults [6, 7]. We further analyzed the 3,184 eligible individuals with PBM in this study and here present the most detailed evaluation of associated biliary tract cancer distribution thus far. In this large study, we again found that the gallbladder was the most frequent site of cancer regardless of the presence of BD and that the rates of gallbladder versus bile duct cancers differed significantly between adults with CBD and those with PBM without BD. In particular, adults with PBM without BD had a much higher rate of gallbladder cancer than adults with CBD; conversely, the former's rate of bile duct cancer was lower. This cancer distribution is almost the same as that reported previously. However, the 4% rate of bile duct cancer in adults with PBM without BD found in the present study may be higher than the 3.1% of the second report. In 2009, the Japan Cancer Surveillance Research Group [14] reported the biliary tract (gallbladder and bile duct) cancer crude rates of 18.4 in male and 17.3 in female patients per 100,000 populations; thus, the overall incidence of associated bile duct cancer even in PBM without BD increased approximately 200-fold that of the general population. Additionally, we have reported the age at which individuals with PBM become susceptible to associated biliary tract cancers and suggested that they develop associated biliary tract cancers 15 or 20 years earlier than the general population. These data should be considered when making decisions on surgical strategy for individuals with PBM without BD and no associated biliary tract cancer. Additionally, our registry includes three pediatric patients with CBD and associated biliary tract cancer. Nine patients in Japan have reportedly developed associated biliary tract cancers as a complication of PBM, seven being bile duct cancers and two gallbladder cancers [5]; thus, their frequency may not be particularly high.

Given this background, we also investigated whether Japanese surgeons consider cholecystectomy combined with prophylactic extrahepatic bile duct resection a standard procedure for patients with PBM without associated biliary tract cancers. We found that this procedure is considered standard in pediatric patients. However, the treatment strategy differs considerably between adults with CBD and those with PBM without BD, cholecystectomy combined with extrahepatic bile duct resection not having been performed in the majority of adults with PBM without BD, probably because these individuals' risk of bile duct cancer is comparatively low. However, at 4.0%, this rate may be increasing, being about 200-fold that of the general population. The incidence of postoperative complications in adults with PBM without BD who had undergone cholecystectomy combined with extrahepatic bile duct resection was 11.3%, which we consider acceptable. Taken together, it may be necessary to reconsider whether this procedure should be the standard treatment.

Finally, to the best of our knowledge, over a quarter of a century, the JSPBM has registered the biggest cohort of individuals with PBM worldwide and investigated the clinical features, including associated cancers, in this study. Though it is necessary to continue to follow up these patients, data in this report could be widely used as a reference for understanding the pathophysiology and making decisions about treatment strategy for individuals with PBM.

References

1. The Japanese Study Group on Pancreaticobiliary Maljunction (JSPBM), The Committee of JSPBM for Diagnostic Criteria. Diagnostic criteria of pancreaticobiliary maljunction. J Hepatobiliary Pancreat Surg. 1994;1:219–21.
2. Kamisawa T, Ando H, Hamada Y, Fujii H, Koshinaga T, Urushihara N, Japanese Study Group on Pancreaticobiliary Maljunction, et al. Diagnostic criteria for pancreaticobiliary maljunction 2013. J Hepatobiliary Pancreat Sci. 2014;21:159–61.
3. Kamisawa T, Kaneko K, Itoi T, Ando H. Pancreaticobiliary maljunction and congenital biliary dilatation. Lancet Gastroenterol Hepatol. 2017;2:610–8.
4. Komi N, Kuwashima T, Kuramoto M, Udaka H, Ogasahara K. Anomalous arrangement of the pancreaticobiliary ductal system in choledochal cyst. Tokushima J Exp Med. 1976;23:37–48.
5. Kamisawa T, Ando H, Suyama M, Shimada M, Morine Y, Shimada H. Japanese clinical practice guidelines for pancreaticobiliary maljunction. J Gastroenterol. 2012;47:731–59.
6. Tashiro S, Imaizumi T, Ohkawa H, Okada A, Katoh T, Kawaharada Y, et al. Pancreaticobiliary maljunction: retrospective and nationwide survey in Japan. J Hepatobiliary Pancreat Surg. 2003;10:345–51.
7. Morine Y, Shimada M, Takamatsu H, Araida T, Endo I, Kubota M, et al. Clinical features of pancreaticobiliary maljunction: update analysis of 2nd Japan-nationwide survey. J Hepatobiliary Pancreat Sci. 2013;20:472–80.
8. Funabiki T. Pancreaticobiliary maljunction—focused on biliary carcinogenesis. Jpn J Gastroenterol Surg. 2000;33:261–70. (in Japanese).
9. Matsubara T, Sakurai Y, Sasayama Y, Hori H, Ochiai M, Funabiki T, et al. *K-ras* point mutations in cancerous and noncancerous biliary epithelium in patients with pancreaticobiliary maljunction. Cancer. 1996;77:1752–7.
10. Matsubara T, Sakurai Y, Zhi LZ, Miura H, Ochiai M, Funabiki T. *K-ras* and *p-53* gene mutations in noncancerous biliary lesions of patients with pancreatico biliary maljunction. J Hepato-Biliary-Pancreat Surg. 2002;9:312–21.
11. Hanada K, Itoh M, Fujii K, Tsuchida A, Hirata M, Ishimaru S, et al. Pathology and cellular kinetics of gallbladder with an anomalous junction of pancreaticobiliary duct. Am J Gastroenterol. 1996;91:1007–11.
12. Nagai M, Watanabe M, Iwase T, Yamao K, Isaji S. Clinical and genetic analysis of noncancerous and cancerous biliary epithelium in patients with pancreaticobiliary maljunction. World J Surg. 2002;26:91–8.
13. Hamada Y, Ando H, Kamisawa T, Itoi T, Urushihara N, Koshinaga T. Diagnostic criteria for congenital biliary dilatation 2015. J Hepatobiliary Pancreat Sci. 2016;23:342–6.
14. Hori M, Matsuda T, Shibata A, Katanoda K, Sobue T, Nishimoto H, Japan Cancer Surveillance Research Group. Cancer incidence and incidence rates in Japan in 2009: a study of 32 population-based cancer registries for the monitoring of cancer incidence in Japan (MCIJ) project. Jpn J Clin Oncol. 2015;45:884–91.

Chapter 4
Pancreaticobiliary Maljunction and Congenital Biliary Dilatation in Korea

Tae Jun Song and Myung-Hwan Kim

Abstract Pancreaticobiliary maljunction (PBM) is a congenital malformation in which the pancreatic duct and the bile duct join outside of the duodenal wall forming a long common channel. In patients with PBM, biliary tract cancer occurred in 11.1–37.6%, and gallbladder cancer was the most common type of cancer. PBM is frequently accompanied with congenital biliary dilatation (CBD). CBD is a congenital anomaly of the bile duct associated with varying degrees of cystic dilatation at different sites of extrahepatic and intrahepatic bile ducts. In Korea, CBD affects women about three times more frequently. In terms of CBD classification, types I and IVa CBD were the two most common types. Among patients with CBD, 9.9% presented with biliary tract cancer.

Keywords Anomalous · Biliary dilatation · Pancreaticobiliary reflux · Biliary tract cancer · Republic of Korea

4.1 Introduction

Pancreaticobiliary maljunction (PBM) is defined as a congenital malformation in which the pancreatic duct and the bile duct join outside of the duodenal wall, usually forming a long common channel [1]. Cases of PBM are classified into two categories [2, 3]: type I (biliary-pancreatic type, C-P type) and type II (pancreatic-biliary type, P-C type). In the C-P type, the bile duct joins the pancreatic duct; in the P-C type, the pancreatic duct joins the bile duct (Fig. 4.1).

Congenital biliary dilatation (CBD) is a congenital anomaly of the bile duct that manifests as cystic dilatation of the extrahepatic and intrahepatic bile ducts with varying degrees of dilatation at different sites [1, 4]. The classification proposed by

T. J. Song · M.-H. Kim (✉)
Division of Gastroenterology, Department of Internal Medicine, Asan Medical Center, University of Ulsan College of Medicine, Seoul, South Korea
e-mail: mhkim@amc.seoul.kr

T. Kamisawa, H. Ando (eds.), *Pancreaticobiliary Maljunction and Congenital Biliary Dilatation*, https://doi.org/10.1007/978-981-10-8654-0_4

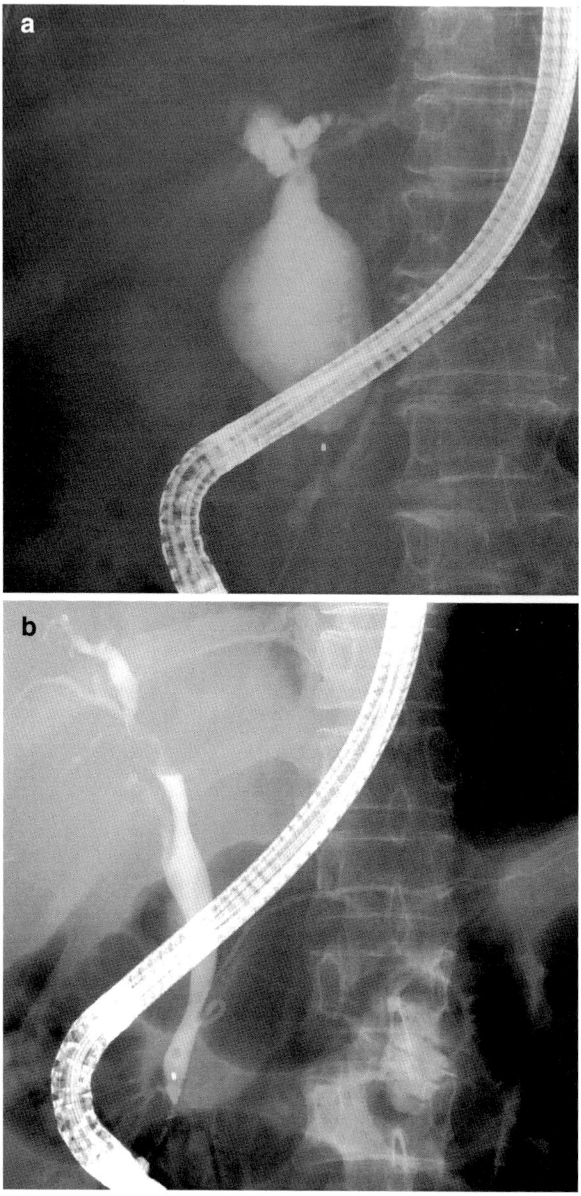

Fig. 4.1 Classification of pancreaticobiliary maljunction (PBM). (**a**) Cholangiography shows type I (biliary-pancreatic type, C-P type) PBM. (**b**) Cholangiography shows type II (pancreatic-biliary type, P-C type) PBM

Todani et al. [5] is frequently used. Type I cysts exhibit segmental or diffuse fusiform dilatation of the bile duct, and account for 80–90% of all cases (Fig. 4.2a). Type II cysts are a true choledochal diverticulum (Fig. 4.2b). Type III cysts are intraduodenal bile duct dilatations or choledochoceles (Fig. 4.2c). Type IVa cysts are multiple intrahepatic and extrahepatic bile duct cysts, and type IVb cysts are multiple extra-

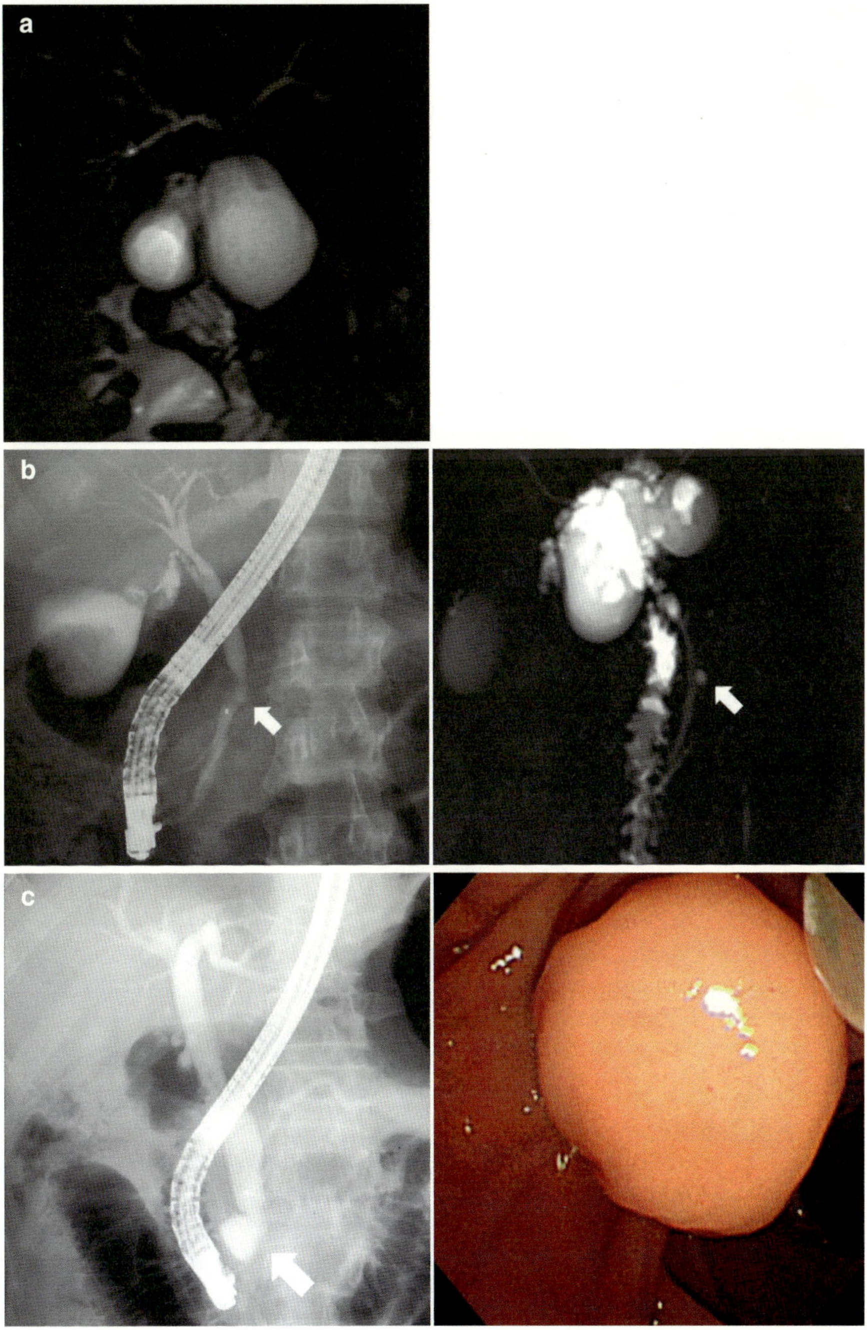

Fig. 4.2 Classification of congenital biliary dilatation. (**a**) Magnetic resonance cholangiography (MRC) shows cystic dilatation of extrahepatic bile duct. (**b**) Cholangiography and MRC show choledochal diverticulum (*arrow*). (**c**) Cholangiography and endoscopic view show intraduodenal bile duct dilatation or choledochocele (*arrow*). (**d**) MRC shows multiple intrahepatic and extrahepatic bile duct dilatations. (**e**) MRC shows multiple intrahepatic bile duct dilatations

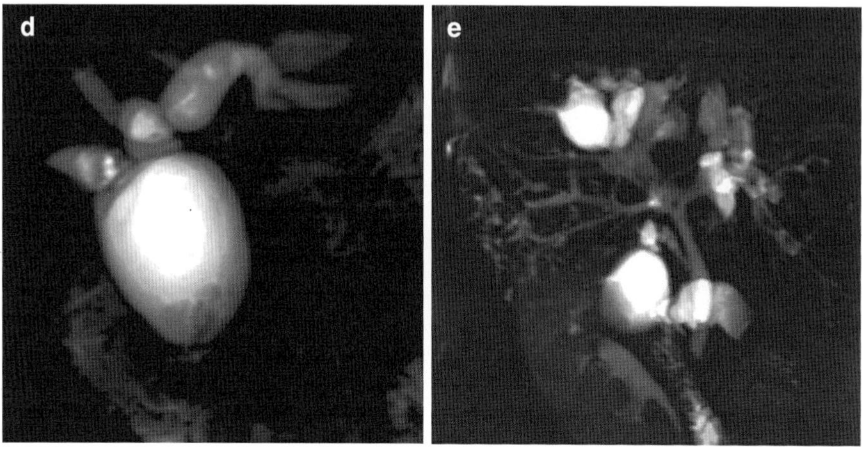

Fig 4.2 (continued)

hepatic bile duct cysts (Fig. 4.2d). Type V cysts or Caroli's disease consist of single or multiple dilatations of the intrahepatic ductal system (Fig. 4.2e) [6].

A high frequency of PBM accompanied with CBD, which may allow reflux of pancreatic juices into the biliary system, has been described [7]. CBD may also be associated with other developmental anomalies, including colonic atresia, duodenal atresia, imperforate anus, pancreatic arteriovenous malformation, multiseptate gallbladder, ventricular septal defect, aortic hypoplasia, pancreatic divisum, pancreatic aplasia, focal nodular hyperplasia of the liver, and congenital absence of the portal vein.

About two thirds of patients with PBM and CBD have been known to come to medical attention before 10 years old [8–10]. However, the diagnosis of PBM and CBD in adults has become more frequent than ever before because of the popularity of routine checkups and advances in imaging technologies [11–13]. Many patients may have long-standing disease that is not diagnosed until adulthood. Adults with CBD are being increasingly encountered, and recently up to 70% of all reported patients with CBD are adults [9, 14–17].

4.2 Epidemiology of CBD in Korea

In a nationwide multicenter study in Korea [18], 10,243 patients underwent endoscopic retrograde cholangiopancreatography (ERCP) for suspected pancreatic or biliary problems between March 1997 and June 1999. Among them, 8194 patients underwent bile duct opacification, and 26 patients (0.32%) were eventually proven to have CBD. In 17 of 26 patients (65%), CBD was associated with PBM. According to the classification of Todani et al., type I (classic CBD) was found in 18 of 26 cases (69%). In this classification, type I CBD is subclassified as Ia, Ib, and Ic, which were noted in ten, three, and five cases, respectively. Type II (localized diverticulum) and type III (choledochocele) were each present in one patient (4%). Type IV (multiple communicating intrahepatic and extrahepatic duct cysts) was present in five patients (19%). Finally, there was one case of type V CBD (Caroli's disease, cystic dilatation of intrahepatic ducts).

Another multicenter study in Korea evaluated 808 patients aged 18 years or older who underwent surgery for CBD [19]. The mean age of the patients was 42 ± 14 years and the male-to-female ratio was 1:3.8. Of the patients, 74.9% presented with abdominal pain and 12.4% had no symptoms. Type I was the most common type (68.2%), followed by type IVa (28.4%), type IVb (1.2%), type II (0.9%), type V (0.7%), and type III (0.5%).

At our institution, 204 adult patients (age >18 years) were primarily treated for CBD in the surgery department from July 1995 to June 2009 [20]. The median age of the 204 adult patients with CBD was 40.2 years (range, 18–67 years), and 157 patients (77%) among them were women. Type I was the most common type (56.9%), followed by type IVa (42.2%), type II (0.5%), and type V (0.5%). Of the 204 patients, 128 (62.7%) had PBM. Most patients (99%) had either type I or type IVa. Type III was absent because it was not indicated for surgical treatment at our institution.

In a study for infants or children under the age of 18 years old, 113 patients had CBD [21]. 70.8% were females (80/113). The 31.9% of patients were asymptomatic, while the 68.1% manifested symptoms of hepatitis, cholecystitis, pancreatitis, or an incidence of two or more of these diseases. More than half (76.6%) of symptomatic patients had hepatitis. There were 76 cases (67.2%) of type I, with type Ic of 44.2%, and the second most common type was type IVa with 24.8%.

4.3 Epidemiology of PBM in Korea

In a multicenter survey in Korea, pancreaticobiliary union was well visualized and could be analyzed in 740 cases. Among them, PBM was found in 30 patients (4.1%), 13 (43.3%) of whom had PBM alone and 17 (56.7%) had both PBM and CBD. According to the classification by Kimura et al. [3], 43.3% had the C-P type and 56.7% had the P-C type.

In another multicenter study in Korea [19], PBM was an accompanying disorder in 71.4% (467/654) of patients with CBD in whom the pancreaticobiliary junction could be visualized with ERCP or magnetic resonance cholangiopancreatography. Among these patients, 62.3% had the C-P type, 20.6% had the P-C type, and 17.1% had the complex type.

From January 1999 to December 2013, 229 patients (0.5%) were diagnosed as having PBM of 46,049 ERCP referrals at our institution [22]. In patients with PBM, the mean age was 48.79 ± 14.08 years, and the male-to-female ratio was 2.47:1. Of them, 168 patients (73.4%) had the P-C type and 61 (26.6%) had the C-P type. In addition to the biliary tract cancers, PBM could predispose to various pancreatico-biliary diseases including acute cholecystitis (71/229, 31%), cholangitis (17/229, 7.4%), and pancreatitis (10/229, 4.4%).

According to the study with 55 patients with PBM [23], the mean age was 52.8 ± 19.0 years, and 70.9% were females. P-C type was 50.9% and C-P type was 49.1%. CBD were present in 45.5% of patients. The common initial presenting symptoms were abdominal pain (43.6%) and jaundice (30.9). Occurrence of biliary tract stones was common (40.0%) including gallbladder stone (27.3%), common bile duct stone (18.2%), and intrahepatic duct stone (7.3%). Pancreatitis occurred in 14.5% of patients, and it tended to occur more frequently in patients with C-P type.

In a study with 113 pediatric patients with CBD, 73.5% of patients (83/113) had PBM [21]. Female was 68.7%. Patients with PBM manifested pancreatitis more frequently than non-PBM patients, and the number of symptomatic patients with PBM was 74.7%, whereas the number among non-PBM patients was 50.0% ($P < 0.05$).

4.4 Risk of Biliary Tract Cancer

Adult patients with PBM and CBD raise additional considerations for the presence of associated biliary tract cancer. Biliary tract cancer is reported to occur in 2.5–26% of patients with congenital dilatation of the bile duct [23–25]. Biliary tract cancers can preferentially develop at sites where there is stasis of activated pancreatic enzymes, such as in the gallbladder or dilated bile duct [22]. The concomitance of bile and pancreatic juice and their stasis in the biliary tract can induce cellular proliferation and may stimulate genetic alterations in the biliary epithelium, which may play an important role in carcinogenesis of the biliary tract [24]. As a result, it is generally thought that the risk of both bile duct and gallbladder cancer increases in PBM patients with CBD, whereas there is a significant predilection for gallbladder cancer to occur in PBM patient without CBD [7, 23, 24, 26].

The rate of associated biliary tract cancer in CBD patients was reported to be as high as 19–50% [27]. In a multicenter study in Korea [19], 9.9% (80/808) of patients with CBD presented with biliary tract cancer. Extrahepatic cholangiocarcinoma occurred in 50% (40/80), gallbladder cancer in 43.8% (35/80), and intrahepatic cholangiocarcinoma in 1.3% (1/80). Patients with type IVa more frequently had bile duct cancer, and patients with type I more frequently had gallbladder cancer. PBM was more frequently associated with gallbladder cancer than with bile duct cancer.

At our institution, among the 229 patients with PBM, 76 patients (33.2%) had gallbladder cancer (Fig. 4.3), 7 (3%) had extrahepatic cholangiocarcinoma

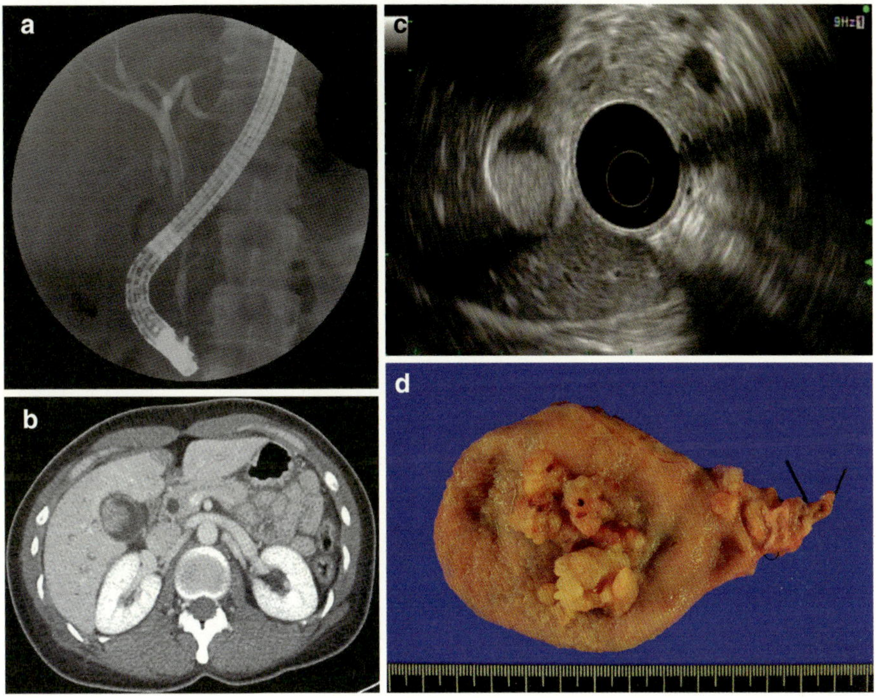

Fig. 4.3 Gallbladder cancer in a patient with pancreaticobiliary maljunction. (**a**) Cholangiography shows long common channel. (**b**) CT scan shows enhancing mass lesion at the gallbladder. (**c**) Endoscopic ultrasound shows echogenic mass lesion in the gallbladder. (**d**) Gross specimen after surgery shows lobulated mass protruding from the gallbladder

(Fig. 4.4), 7 (3%) had pancreatic cancer, and 3 (1.3%) had intrahepatic cholangiocarcinoma [22]. During the same period at our institution, a total of 1111 patients were newly diagnosed as having gallbladder cancer, 10,065 patients as having extrahepatic cholangiocarcinoma, and 3659 patients as having intrahepatic cholangiocarcinoma. Therefore, the incidence of PBM in gallbladder cancer, extrahepatic cholangiocarcinoma, and intrahepatic cholangiocarcinoma was 6.84%, 0.08%, and 0.07%, respectively. In patients aged >45 years, the rate of biliary tract cancer was significantly higher than that in patients aged <45 years (odds ratio [OR] 3.640, 95% confidence interval [CI] 2.001–6.621, $P < 0.05$). The mean age of patients with PBM with biliary tract cancer (53.8 ± 11.2 years) was significantly higher than that of patients without biliary tract cancer (45.5 ± 15.3 years) ($P < 0.05$). The P-C type was more frequently detected in patients with biliary tract cancer (42.2% vs. 24.6%; $P < 0.05$). Of the 229 patients with PBM, bile duct dilatation of >10 mm was present in 152 patients and absent in the remaining 77 patients. Among patients with PBM with bile duct dilatation, 46 (30.3%) had gallbladder cancer and 6 (3.9%) had extrahepatic cholangiocarcinoma. In patients with PBM without bile duct dilatation, gallbladder cancer occurred in 30 patients (39%) and extrahepatic cholangiocarci-

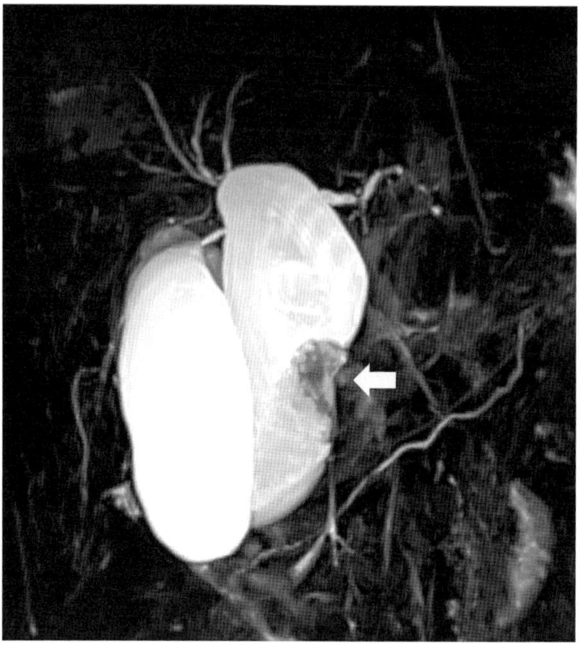

Fig. 4.4 Common bile duct cancer in a patient with congenital biliary dilatation. MRC shows marked cystic dilatation of the extrahepatic bile duct. *White arrow* indicates the mass arising from the dilated bile duct

noma in 1 patient (1.3%). Intrahepatic cholangiocarcinoma occurred in three patients with PBM, and all cases of intrahepatic cholangiocarcinoma occurred in patients without bile duct dilatation ($P < 0.014$). Although PBM is believed to increase the risk of intrahepatic cholangiocarcinoma, limited data exist in the literature concerning the association between intrahepatic cholangiocarcinoma and PBM.

In another study, 55 patients were diagnosed with PBM during 10 years [23]. Biliary tract cancers, particularly the common bile duct cancers, occurred more frequently in P-C type. In patients with PBM without bile duct dilatation, biliary tract cancer more frequently occurred (53.3% vs. 16.0%). The occurrence rate of gallbladder cancer was not significantly different between patients with PBM with/without bile duct dilatation.

In a Japanese nationwide survey [7], biliary tract cancer occurred in 22% of adult patients with PBM and bile duct dilatation and in 42% of adult patients with PBM without biliary dilatation. Biliary tract cancers in patients with CBD with bile duct dilatation developed in the gallbladder (62%) and the dilated bile duct (32%), whereas cancers associated with PBM without bile duct dilatation were located primarily in the gallbladder (88%) and rarely in the bile duct (7%).

The more frequent occurrence of bile duct cancer in Korea may be because clonorchiasis (liver fluke) and hepatolithiasis, which are known risk factors for bile duct cancer, are still endemic. It is necessary to analyze the sole contribution of PBM to the occurrence of biliary tract cancers. Otherwise, it may falsely suggest an increased risk for biliary tract cancers in patients with PBM without bile duct dilatation.

When deciding to offer surgical treatment for the prevention of biliary tract cancers, the disease morbidity, patient satisfaction, and postoperative quality of life should also be considered. Studies on factors predictive of malignancy are required to identify patients with the greatest risk of cancer in whom the risk of postoperative adverse events is outweighed by the dramatic reduction in cancer risk offered by surgery.

4.5 Conclusion

We summarize the epidemiology of PBM and CBD in Korea. PBM and CBD presented more frequently in Korea than in Western countries. Among patients with CBD, women were about three times more frequently affected than men. Types I and IVa CBD were the two most common types. PBM was frequently accompanied with CBD (71.4–73.5%). Among patients with CBD, 9.9% presented with biliary tract cancer. In patients with PBM, biliary tract cancer occurred in 11.1–37.6%, and gallbladder cancer was the most common biliary tract cancer. Associated biliary tract cancers should be considered in patients with CBD, particularly when PBM is accompanied.

References

1. Kamisawa T, Kaneko K, Itoi T, et al. Pancreaticobiliary maljunction and congenital biliary dilatation. Lancet Gastroenterol Hepatol. 2017;2:610–8.
2. Kamisawa T, Ando H, Hamada Y, et al. Diagnostic criteria for pancreaticobiliary maljunction 2013. J Hepatobiliary Pancreat Sci. 2014;21:159–61.
3. Kimura K, Ohto M, Ono T, et al. Congenital cystic dilatation of the common bile duct: relationship to anomalous pancreaticobiliary ductal union. Am J Roentgenol. 1977;128:571–7.
4. Singham J, Yoshida EM, Scudamore CH. Choledochal cysts: part 1 of 3: classification and pathogenesis. Can J Surg. 2009;52:434–40.
5. Todani T, Watanabe Y, Narusue M, et al. Congenital bile duct cysts: classification, operative procedures, and review of thirty-seven cases including cancer arising from choledochal cyst. Am J Surg. 1977;134:263–9.
6. Savader SJ, Benenati JF, Venbrux AC, et al. Choledochal cysts: classification and cholangiographic appearance. Am J Roentgenol. 1991;156:327–31.
7. Tashiro S, Imaizumi T, Ohkawa H, et al. Pancreaticobiliary maljunction: retrospective and nationwide survey in Japan. J Hepato-Biliary-Pancreat Surg. 2003;10:345–51.
8. She WH, Chung HY, Lan LC, et al. Management of choledochal cyst: 30 years of experience and results in a single center. J Pediatr Surg. 2009;44:2307–11.
9. Liu CL, Fan ST, Lo CM, et al. Choledochal cysts in adults. Arch Surg. 2002;137:465–8.
10. Kumar M, Rajagopalan S. Choledochal cyst. Med J Armed Forces India. 2012;68:296–8.
11. Jordan PH Jr, Goss JA Jr, Rosenberg WR, et al. Some considerations for management of choledochal cysts. Am J Surg. 2004;187:790–5.
12. Naga MI, Suleiman DN. Endoscopic management of choledochal cyst. Gastrointest Endosc. 2004;59:427–32.
13. Lipsett PA, Pitt HA. Surgical treatment of choledochal cysts. J Hepatobiliary Pancreat Surg. 2003;10:352–9.

14. Lipsett PA, Pitt HA, Colombani PM, et al. Choledochal cyst disease. A changing pattern of presentation. Ann Surg. 1994;220:644–52.
15. Hewitt PM, Krige JE, Bornman PC, et al. Choledochal cysts in adults. Br J Surg. 1995;82:382–5.
16. Lenriot JP, Gigot JF, Segol P, et al. Bile duct cysts in adults: a multi-institutional retrospective study. French associations for surgical research. Ann Surg. 1998;228:159–66.
17. Nicholl M, Pitt HA, Wolf P, et al. Choledochal cysts in western adults: complexities compared to children. J Gastrointest Surg. 2004;8:245–52.
18. Kim HJ, Kim MH, Lee SK, et al. Normal structure, variations, and anomalies of the pancreaticobiliary ducts of Koreans: a nationwide cooperative prospective study. Gastrointest Endosc. 2002;55:889–96.
19. Lee SE, Jang JY, Lee YJ, et al. Choledochal cyst and associated malignant tumors in adults: a multicenter survey in South Korea. Arch Surg. 2011;146:1178–84.
20. Cho MJ, Hwang S, Lee YJ, et al. Surgical experience of 204 cases of adult choledochal cyst disease over 14 years. World J Surg. 2011;35:1094–102.
21. Park SW, Koh H, Oh JT, et al. Relationship between anomalous pancreaticobiliary ductal union and pathologic inflammation of bile duct in choledochal cyst. Pediatr Gastroenterol Hepatol Nutr. 2014;17:170–7.
22. Park JS, Song TJ, Park TY, et al. Predictive factors of biliary tract cancer in anomalous union of the pancreaticobiliary duct. Medicine (Baltimore). 2016;95:e3526.
23. Kim Y, Hyun JJ, Lee JM, et al. Anomalous union of the pancreaticobiliary duct without choledochal cyst: is cholecystectomy alone sufficient? Langenbecks Arch Surg. 2014;399:1071–6.
24. Kimura W. Congenital dilatation of the common bile duct and pancreaticobiliary maljunction: clinical implications. Langenbecks Arch Surg. 2009;394:209–13.
25. Stain SC, Guthrie CR, Yellin AE, et al. Choledochal cyst in the adult. Ann Surg. 1995;222:128–33.
26. Kamisawa T, Ando H, Shimada M, et al. Recent advances and problems in the management of pancreaticobiliary maljunction: feedback from the guidelines committee. J Hepatobiliary Pancreat Sci. 2014;21:87–92.
27. Kim JW, Moon SH, Park DH, et al. Course of choledochal cysts according to the type of treatment. Scand J Gastroenterol. 2010;45:739–45.

Chapter 5
Pancreaticobiliary Maljunction and Common Bile Duct in Taiwan

Wei-Chih Liao and Hsiu-Po Wang

Abstract Pancreaticobiliary maljunction (PBM), a congenital anomaly in which the junction of the biliary and pancreatic ducts lies outside of the duodenal wall, has been associated with various biliary diseases, including choledochal cyst, gallbladder carcinoma, and gallbladder adenomyomatosis. In our study of patients undergoing ERCP for pancreaticobiliary conditions in Taiwan, the prevalence of PBM was 8.7%. PBM can be further classified into the B-P type (i.e., the common bile duct joins the pancreatic duct) and P-B type (i.e., the pancreatic duct joins the common bile duct). Choledochal cyst is the most commonly reported biliary disease associated with PBM. In our study, the prevalence of PBM in patients with choledochal cyst and gallbladder cancer were 93.8% and 62.5%, respectively. Notably, PBMs in patients with choledochal cyst were mostly of the B-P type, whereas PBMs in patients with gallbladder carcinoma were mostly of the P-B type. This chapter summarizes the literature on PBM from Taiwan.

Keywords Pancreaticobiliary maljunction · Biliary · Gallbladder · Pancreas Choledochal cyst · Cancer · Adenomyomatosis

5.1 Introduction

Pancreaticobiliary maljunction (PBM), also called anomalous pancreaticobiliary ductal union (APBDU), is a rare congenital anomaly in which the junction of the common bile duct (CBD) and pancreatic duct lies outside of the duodenal wall, with a long common ductal channel leading to the duodenal lumen [1]. Because the junction of the ducts is not encircled by the sphincter of Oddi, PBM may predispose to reflux of pancreatic juice into the bile duct, leading to changes in bile composition

W.-C. Liao · H.-P. Wang (✉)
Department of Internal Medicine, National Taiwan University Hospital, National Taiwan University College of Medicine, Taipei, Taiwan
e-mail: wanghp@ntu.edu.tw

T. Kamisawa, H. Ando (eds.), *Pancreaticobiliary Maljunction and Congenital Biliary Dilatation*, https://doi.org/10.1007/978-981-10-8654-0_5

and possibly intraductal activation of proteolytic enzymes [2]. An association between PBM and various biliary disorders and malignancies has been reported [3, 4]. This chapter reviews the literature of PBM from Taiwan.

5.2 Epidemiology

In a study that reviewed 680 patients who underwent ERCP with clearly visualized pancreaticobiliary junction in Taiwan [5], we noted that 59 (8.7%) patients had PBM, as defined by a common channel longer than 12 mm [6] and/or one duct (CBD or pancreatic) joining the other perpendicularly [7]. It should be noted that this study was conducted among patients who underwent ERCP for various biliary and pancreatic diseases; therefore, the prevalence obtained was among symptomatic patients. Another review of ERCPs performed in our center showed that PBM was present in 1.2% of consecutive patients undergoing ERCP [8]. The prevalence of PBM among subjects seen in clinical practice may lie within those ranges and may vary depending on patient mix. The prevalence of PBM in asymptomatic general population in Taiwan is not clear.

5.3 Imaging Features

PBM is characterized by a common channel longer than 12 mm [6] (corrected according to the magnification of film) and/or one duct (CBD or pancreatic) joining the other perpendicularly [7]. PBM can be further classified into two types. In the B-P-type PBM, the CBD joins the pancreatic duct. In the P-B type, the pancreatic duct joins the CBD (Fig. 5.1).

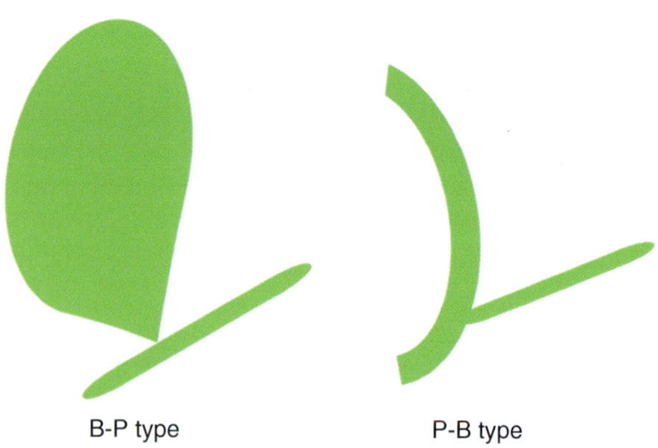

Fig. 5.1 Subtypes of pancreaticobiliary maljunction (PBM)

Among the 59 subjects with PBM in our study [5], 25 (42.4%) were of the B-P type, and the remaining 34 patients (57.6%) were of the P-B type. It is worth noting that patients with choledochal cyst tended to be with the B-P-type PBM and less with P-B type (Fig. 5.2). By contrast, gallbladder cancer (Fig. 5.3), adenomyomatosis (Fig. 5.4), and biliary pancreatitis frequently coexisted with the P-B-type PBM. Three patients with PBM had no other abnormality, consistent with other reports that a portion of subjects with PBM do not have apparent pancreaticobiliary diseases.

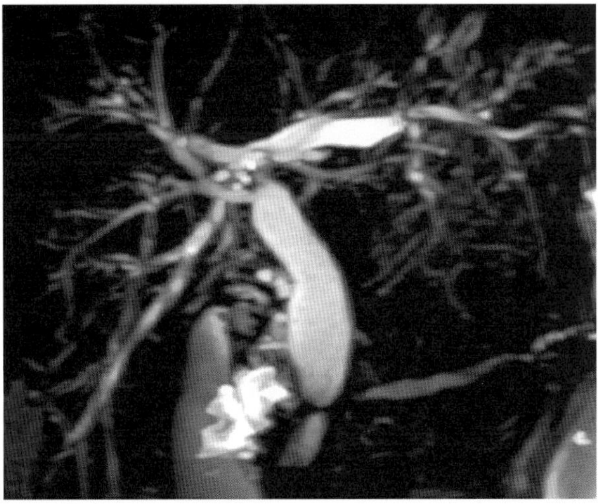

Fig. 5.2 Pancreaticobiliary maljunction (PBM), B-P type, with coexisting choledochal cyst. In our study, the B-P type occurred more than the P-B type in choledochal cysts [5]

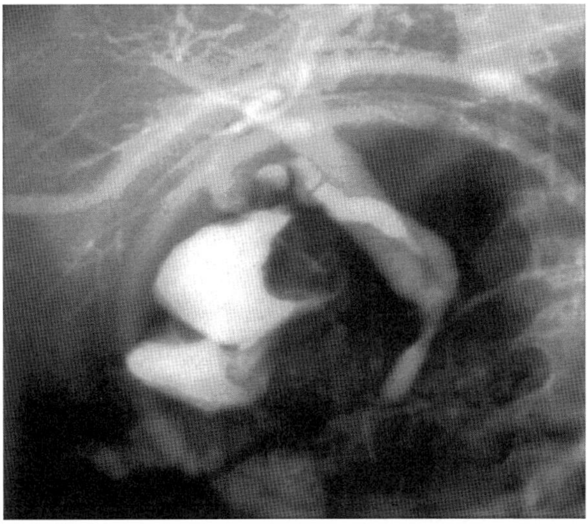

Fig. 5.3 Pancreaticobiliary maljunction (PBM), P-B type, with coexisting carcinoma of the gallbladder. In our study, the P-B type occurred more than the B-P type in gallbladder carcinoma [5]

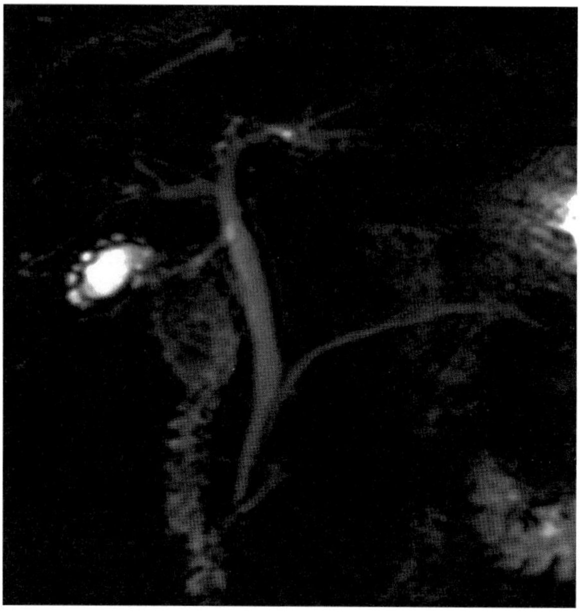

Fig. 5.4 Pancreaticobiliary maljunction (PBM), B-P type, with coexisting adenomyomatosis of the gallbladder. In our study, the P-B type occurred more than the B-P type in gallbladder adenomyomatosis [5]

5.4 Associations with Biliary Diseases

Biliary diseases including congenital cystic dilation of the bile duct, gallbladder carcinoma, and adenomyomatosis have been associated with PBM [6].

Choledochal cyst, or congenital cystic dilation of the bile duct, is the most commonly reported biliary disease associated with PBM. The incidence of choledochal cyst in patients with PBM ranged from 33% to 82.8% in the literature [9, 10]. In our previous study [5], PBM was noted in 93.8% of patients (15 of 16) with choledochal cyst. Among the 15 patients with PBM and choledochal cyst, 13 (86.7%) were of the B-P-type PBM (i.e., CBD joins the pancreatic duct) and 2 (13.3%) were of the P-B type (i.e., the pancreatic duct joins CBD). Ono et al. [11] also reported that PBMs associated with choledochal cyst were more often of the B-P type (60%), whereas Arima et al. [12] reported that 66% were of the P-B type.

Gallbladder carcinoma has also been associated with PBM. The prevalence of gallbladder carcinoma among subjects with PBM ranged between 57 and 77% [6]. In our study [5], 62.5% (5 of 8) of patients with gallbladder cancer had PBM, mostly of the P-B type.

In addition to the more commonly known association between PBM and choledochal cyst or gallbladder carcinoma, we have also observed the coexistence of PBM with other biliary diseases, including cancer of CBD, gallbladder adenomyomatosis, etc. (Table 5.1). The gallbladder adenomyomatosis has been reported to occur with gallbladder cancer [13].

In summary, the prevalence of PBM among Taiwanese patients undergoing ERCP has been reported to be 8.7%. Consistent with the literature, we noted a high

Table 5.1 Association between pancreaticobiliary maljunction (PBM) and biliary diseases in 680 Taiwanese patients undergoing ERCP [5]

	With PBM		
	B-P type	P-B type	Without PBM
Choledochal cyst	13	2	1
Alone	8	1	0
With GB cancer	0	1	0
With CBD cancer	2	0	0
GB cancer	1	3	3
CBD cancer	3	4	18
GB adenomyomatosis	1	5	6

prevalence of PBM in patients with choledochal cyst and gallbladder carcinoma, supporting that PBM might play a causative role in the pathogenesis of these diseases. PBM should be carefully sought when evaluating pancreaticobiliary imaging studies including ERCP and MRCP, and the associations with various biliary pathologies should be considered in patient management and follow-up.

References

1. Misra SP, Gulati P, Thorat VK, et al. Pancreaticobiliary ductal union in biliary diseases. An endoscopic retrograde cholangiopancreatographic study. Gastroenterology. 1989;96:907–12.
2. Kato T, Hebiguchi T, Matsuda K, et al. Action of pancreatic juice on the bile duct: pathogenesis of congenital choledochal cyst. J Pediatr Surg. 1981;16:146–51.
3. Song HK, Kim MH, Myung SJ, et al. Choledochal cyst associated the with anomalous union of pancreaticobiliary duct (AUPBD) has a more grave clinical course than choledochal cyst alone. Korean J Intern Med. 1999;14:1–8.
4. Ragot E, Mabrut JY, Ouaissi M, et al. Pancreaticobiliary maljunctions in European patients with bile duct cysts: results of the multicenter study of the French surgical association (AFC). World J Surg. 2017;41:538–45.
5. Wang HP, Wu MS, Lin CC, et al. Pancreaticobiliary diseases associated with anomalous pancreaticobiliary ductal union. Gastrointest Endosc. 1998;48:184–9.
6. Misra SP, Dwivedi M. Pancreaticobiliary ductal union. Gut. 1990;31:1144–9.
7. Kimura K, Ohto M, Saisho H, et al. Association of gallbladder carcinoma and anomalous pancreaticobiliary ductal union. Gastroenterology. 1985;89:1258–65.
8. Wu MS, Wang HP, Shun CT, et al. Coexistence of anomalous pancreaticobiliary ductal union with adenomyomatosis of the gallbladder. Gastrointest Endosc. 1995;42:265–9.
9. Sameshima Y, Uchimura M, Muto Y, et al. Coexistent carcinoma in congenital dilatation of the bile duct and anomalous arrangement of the pancreatico-bile duct. Carcinogenesis of coexistent gall bladder carcinoma. Cancer. 1987;60:1883–90.
10. Kato O, Hattori K, Suzuki T, et al. Clinical significance of anomalous pancreaticobiliary union. Gastrointest Endosc. 1983;29:94–8.
11. Ono J, Sakoda K, Akita H. Surgical aspect of cystic dilatation of the bile duct. An anomalous junction of the pancreaticobiliary tract in adults. Ann Surg. 1982;195:203–8.
12. Arima E, Akita H. Congenital biliary tract dilatation and anomalous junction of the pancreaticobiliary ductal system. J Pediatr Surg. 1979;14:9–15.
13. Morikawa T, Okabayashi T, Shima Y, et al. Adenomyomatosis concomitant with primary gallbladder carcinoma. Acta Med Okayama. 2017;71(2):113–8.

Part III
Concept and Pathophysiology

Chapter 6
Definition of PBM and CBD

Akira Toki

Abstract The criteria defined PBM as "a congenital malformation in which the pancreatic and bile ducts join anatomically outside the duodenal wall". This definition was formulated from an anatomical perspective and does not include functional elements.

The diagnostic criteria for CBD defined CBD as a "congenital malformation involving localized dilatation of the extrahepatic bile duct, including the common bile duct, and PBM."

Keywords PBM · CBD · Definition

6.1 Definition of Pancreaticobiliary Maljunction (PBM)

The revised Japanese diagnostic criteria for PBM were established in 2013, 23 years after the previous version. The revised criteria defined PBM as "a congenital malformation in which the pancreatic and bile ducts join anatomically outside the duodenal wall" [1] (Fig. 6.1). This definition was formulated from an anatomical perspective and does not include functional elements.

In the normal duodenal papilla region, the papillary sphincter surrounds the area extending from the distal portion of the bile duct to the pancreaticobiliary junction. It regulates bile flow and prevents pancreatic juice reflux into the bile duct. On the other hand, the common channel in PBM is long and surrounded by the sphincter after the pancreaticobiliary junction (Fig. 6.2). Therefore, the papillary sphincter performance does not affect the pancreaticobiliary junction area, resulting in alternate pancreatic juice and bile reflux. In general, the internal pressure of the pancreatic duct exceeds that of the bile duct, and therefore, pancreatic juice reflux into the

A. Toki
Division of Pediatric Surgery, Department of Surgery, Showa University School of Medicine, Tokyo, Japan
e-mail: atoki@med.showa-u.ac.jp

T. Kamisawa, H. Ando (eds.), *Pancreaticobiliary Maljunction and Congenital Biliary Dilatation*, https://doi.org/10.1007/978-981-10-8654-0_6

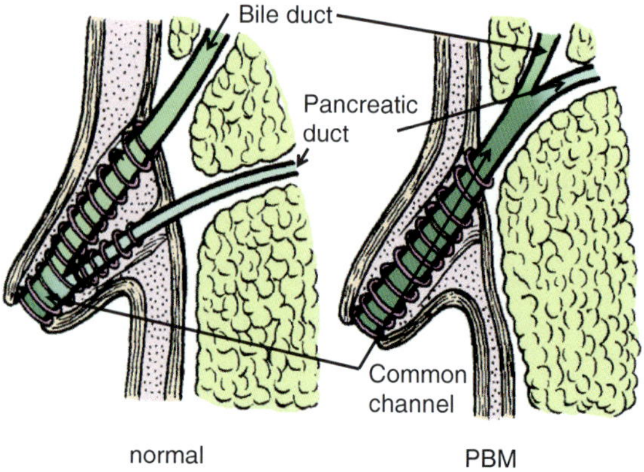

Fig. 6.1 Schema of PBM. The junction between the pancreatic duct and the biliary duct is located outside of the sphincter

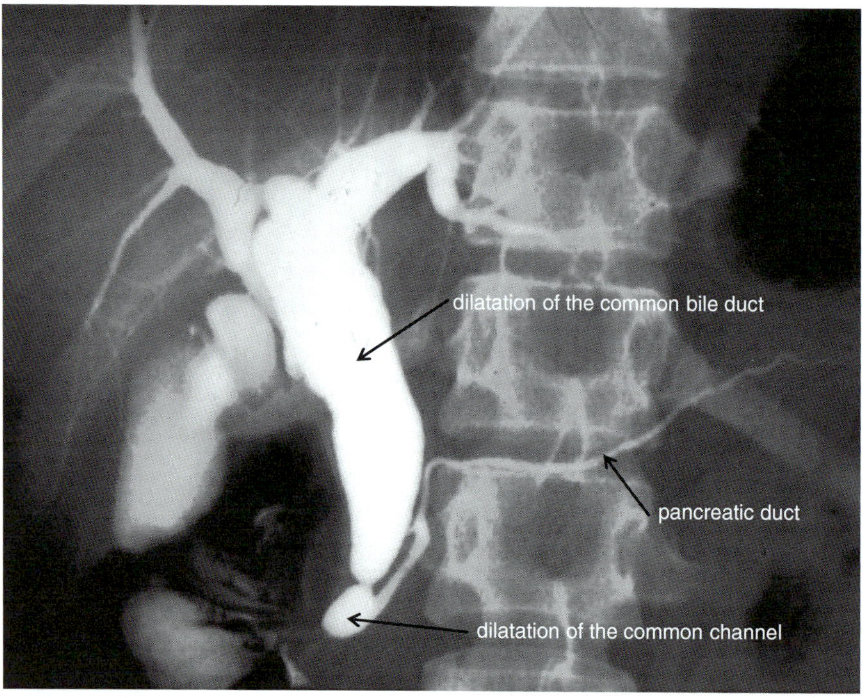

Fig. 6.2 Congenital biliary dilatation (Todani Ic) and pancreaticobiliary maljunction

bile duct readily occurs in PBM. In certain conditions, however, bile reflux into the pancreatic duct also occurs. This reflux causes pancreatic juice and bile to mix and become congestive in the gallbladder, dilated bile duct, or dilated common channel, consequently increasing the incidence of bile duct cancer and pancreatitis.

PBM can occur with or without biliary dilatation, and PBM with biliary dilatation has started being diagnosed as CBD in a more restricted sense.

6.2 Definition of Congenital Biliary Dilatation (CBD)

The diagnostic criteria for CBD were established in 2015, which defined CBD as a "congenital malformation involving localized dilatation of the extrahepatic bile duct, including the common bile duct, and PBM" [2].

In particular, CBD includes types Ia, Ic, and IV-A of the Todani classification proposed in 1995 (Fig. 6.3). Definitive diagnosis depends on the presence of localized dilatation of the extrahepatic and common bile ducts as well as PBM.

The process by which this definition was reached is described as follows. In the past, CBD had been defined in the West as congenital choledochal cyst. In 1959, Alonso-Lej classified congenital choledochal cysts into three types: type I denotes congenital cystic dilatation of the common bile duct, type II refers to congenital diverticulum of the common bile duct, and type III indicates a choledochocele [3]. In 1977, Todani et al. proposed a new five-type classification based on that of Alonso-Lej, and this became widely cited in the West. It was later found that CBD and PBM coexisted at a high rate; thus, in 1995, the Todani classification that included the concept of PBM was announced [4]. Thereafter, the incidence of type I choledochal cysts presenting with localized dilatation of the common bile duct and of type IV-A choledochal cysts presenting with dilatation of intrahepatic bile duct in addition to the localized dilatation of the common bile duct was found to be extremely high. Furthermore, in types Ia, Ic, and IV-A, most cases presented with concurrent PBM, whereas in types Ib, II, III, IV-B, and V, concurrent PBM was rarely observed.

For most current cases, CBD often implies type Ia, Ic, or IV-A of the Todani classification with PBM and is defined as such in the Japanese clinical practice

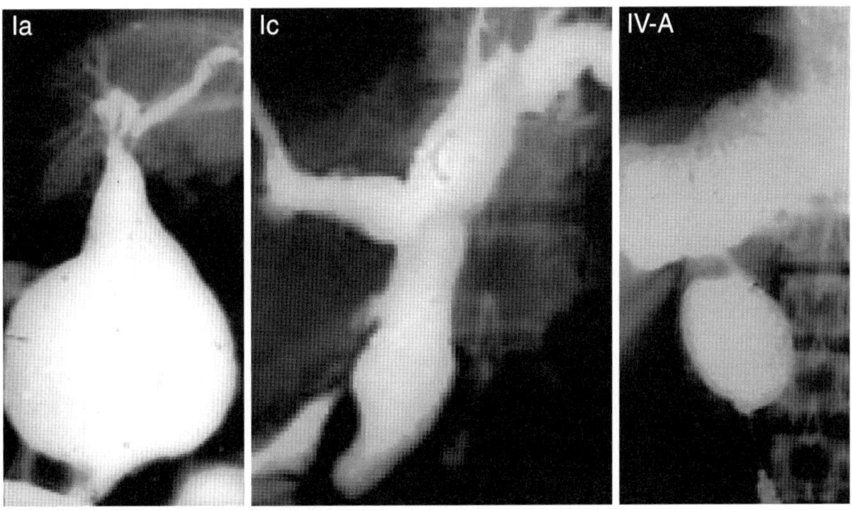

Fig. 6.3 Todani classification

guidelines for PBM. Therefore, in the diagnostic criteria for CBD in 2015, CBD has been narrowly defined as a localized dilatation of the extrahepatic and common bile ducts classified into Todani types Ia, Ic, or IV-A with concurrent PBM2 [5].

Furthermore, in reference to other chapters covering the diagnosis of bile duct dilatation, the conventional reference value for the common bile duct diameter is 10 mm in patients aged ≥15 years. However, using abdominal ultrasonography, it was found that bile duct diameter in both children and adults increases with age. Therefore, it is recommended that the reference value for the common bile duct diameter should correspond to age [6].

CBD causes various impairments due to the coexistence of PBM with impaired bile outflow. This is caused by strictured area of the duodenal side of the common bile duct and is often found concurrent with bile duct dilatation. In the event of PBM diagnosis, surgery is recommended to prevent the onset of bile duct cancer.

References

1. The Japanese Study Group on Pancreaticobiliary Maljunction. Diagnostic criteria for pancreaticobiliary maljunction. JJBA. 2013;27:785–7.
2. The Japanese Study Group on Pancreaticobiliary Maljunction. Diagnostic criteria for congenital biliary dilatation. JJBA. 2015;29:870–3.
3. Alonso-Lej F, Rever WB Jr, Pessagno DJ. Congenital choledochal cyst with a report of 2 and analysis of 94 cases. Int Abstr Surg. 1959;108:1–30.
4. Todani T. Definition and classification of congenital bile duct dilatation. J Biliary Tract Pancreas. 1995;16:715–7.
5. Kamisawa T, Kuruma S, Chiba K. Congenital biliary dilatation and pancreaticobiliary maljunction. JJpn Soc Gastroenterol. 2016;113:1991–7.
6. Hamada Y, Ando H, Kamisawa T, et al. Diagnostic criteria for congenital biliary dilatation 2015. J Hepatobiliary Pancreat Sci. 2016;23:342–6.

Chapter 7
Classification of Pancreaticobiliary Maljunction and Congenital Biliary Dilatation

Naoto Urushihara

Abstract The Committee on Diagnostic Criteria of the Japanese Study Group on Pancreaticobiliary Maljunction (PBM) proposed a PBM classification that was simple to use in clinical practice in 2015. The Committee's classification divided PBM into the following four types: (a) stenotic type, (b) non-stenotic type, (c) dilated channel type, and (d) complex type.

The classification of congenital choledochal cysts proposed by Alonso-Lej in 1959 classified cysts into three types. After the recognition of intrahepatic involvement, Todani refined this classification into five types with subtypes in 1977. This classification has been the most widely used. However, this classification did not include the concept of PBM. Type Ia, Ic, and IV-A (intrahepatic involvement) cysts are generally accompanied by PBM. Todani revised his classification to include a concept of PBM in 1997.

Keywords Pancreaticobiliary maljunction · Congenital biliary dilatation · Classification · Choledochal cyst

7.1 Pancreaticobiliary Maljunction

Pancreaticobiliary maljunction (PBM) is a congenital anomaly defined as a junction of the pancreatic and bile ducts located outside the duodenal wall, forming a long common channel [1]. As a result, regurgitation between the bile and pancreatic ducts occurs freely, causing hepatobiliary and pancreatic disorders such as cholangitis, pancreatitis, and biliary cancer. PBM is found in almost all patients with Todani type Ia, Ic, and IV-A choledochal cysts and also in cases without biliary dilatation. Gallbladder cancer frequently occurs in patients with PBM with slight or no biliary dilatation [2–4]. Excision of the extrahepatic duct with hepaticojejunostomy is a standard operation for PBM with biliary dilatation, while treatment strategies

N. Urushihara
Department of Pediatric Surgery, Shizuoka Children's Hospital, Aoi-ku, Shizuoka, Japan
e-mail: n-urushihara@i.shizuoka-pho.jp

T. Kamisawa, H. Ando (eds.), *Pancreaticobiliary Maljunction and Congenital Biliary Dilatation*, https://doi.org/10.1007/978-981-10-8654-0_7

for PBM without biliary dilatation remain controversial. In a Japanese nationwide survey, cholecystectomy alone was performed in 70% of adults with PBM without biliary dilatation [5], because gallbladder cancer usually develops in cases with PBM without biliary dilatation and the incidence of bile duct cancer is low. On the other hand, excision of the extrahepatic duct is preferred in children with PBM without biliary dilatation.

Various classifications of PBM have been reported on the basis of the types of confluence between the distal common bile duct and pancreatic duct and the morphology of the common channel [6–9]. In 1977, Komi [7] proposed a classification in which PBM was divided into three types of pancreaticobiliary junction: (a) a narrow common bile duct joining the pancreatic duct (right angle type), (b) pancreatic duct joining the common bile duct (acute angle type), and (c) complex type. Furthermore, Komi [8] proposed a new classification of PBM as a modification of the previous classification; in the new system, PBM was divided into three types, with subtypes according to the presence of common channel dilatation. However, this classification is complicated and has not been widely accepted. In 2015, the Committee on Diagnostic Criteria of the Japanese Study Group on Pancreaticobiliary Maljunction (JSGPM) proposed a PBM classification that was simple to use in clinical practice [10]. The Committee's classification divided PBM into the following four types: (a) stenotic type, (b) non-stenotic type, (c) dilated channel type, and (d) complex type.

7.1.1 Classification of PBM (Figs. 7.1, and 7.2)

PBM is generally divided into three main types (types A–C) and a rare complex type (type D):

- Type A (stenotic type)
  The stenotic or narrow segment of the distal common bile duct joins the common channel, and dilatation of the common bile duct is evident. This type is frequently seen in neonates and infants, and the incidence of cystic dilatation is high.

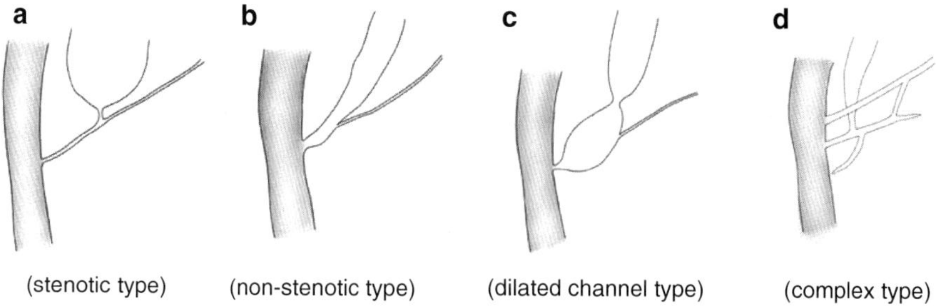

Fig. 7.1 Classification of pancreaticobiliary maljunction. (**a**) Stenotic type. (**b**) Non-stenotic type. (**c**) Dilated channel type. (**d**) Complex type

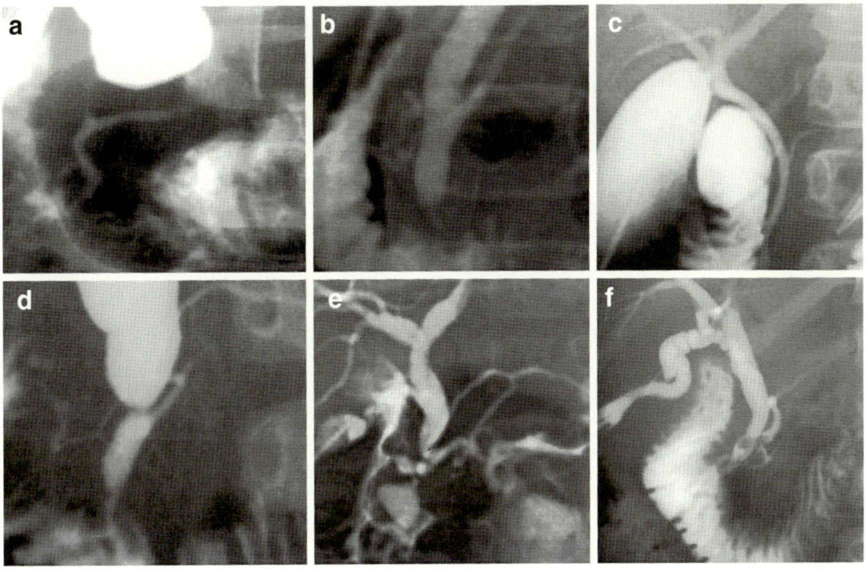

Fig. 7.2 Cholangiograms of pancreaticobiliary maljunction. (**a**) Type A (stenotic type), (**b**) type B (non-stenotic type), (**c**) type B without biliary dilatation (non-stenotic type), (**d**) type C (dilated channel type), (**e**) type D with annular pancreas (complex type), and (**f**) type D with incomplete pancreas divisum (complex type)

- Type B (non-stenotic type)
  The distal common bile duct without any stenotic or narrow segment smoothly joins the common channel. Localized dilatation of the common channel is not seen. This type shows diffuse dilatation or non-dilatation of the common bile duct, and the incidence of gallbladder cancer is high in adults.
- Type C (dilated channel type)
  The common channel is dilated. The narrow segment of the distal common bile duct joins the common channel, and abrupt dilatation of the common channel is seen. This type is frequently seen in younger children, and the incidences of protein plugs and biliary perforation are high.
- Type D (complex type)
  Complicated union of the pancreaticobiliary ductal system is seen in the form of PBM associated with annular pancreas, pancreas divisum, or other complicated duct systems. This complex type is rare. Acute or chronic pancreatitis often develops due to associated pancreatic anomalies.

7.2 Congenital Biliary Dilatation

The classification of congenital choledochal cysts proposed by Alonso-Lej [11] in 1959 classified cysts into three types. After the recognition of intrahepatic involvement, Todani [12] refined this classification into five types with subtypes in 1977.

This classification has been the most widely used and is simple to apply in clinical practice. However, this classification did not include the concept of PBM. Type Ia, Ic, and IV-A (intrahepatic involvement) cysts are generally accompanied by PBM. Todani [9] revised his classification to include a concept of PBM in 1997.

Type Ia, Ic, and IV-A cysts are often observed, and cyst excision is a standard treatment to prevent cholangitis and biliary cancer. On the other hand, type Ic, II (diverticulum), III (choledochocele), IV-B, and V (including Caroli's disease) cysts are rare and are usually not associated with PBM. The term "congenital choledochal cysts" has been used to refer to various biliary dilatations with different pathogeneses. The Japanese Study Group on Pancreaticobiliary Maljunction (JSGPM) therefore published "diagnostic criteria for congenital biliary dilatation 2015," in which congenital biliary dilatation was defined as a congenital malformation involving both dilatation of the bile duct and pancreaticobiliary maljunction (type Ia, Ic, and IV-A cysts) [12].

7.2.1 Classification of Choledochal Cyst (Figs. 7.3, and 7.4)

- Type I
  Type I shows dilatation of the common bile duct with normal intrahepatic duct. Three subtypes have been defined, with Type Ia and Ic accompanied by pancreaticobiliary maljunction.
  - Type Ia: cystic dilatation with pancreaticobiliary maljunction
  - This type is often found in neonates and infants.
  - Type Ib: dilatation with normal pancreaticobiliary union
  - Type Ic: diffuse or fusiform dilatation with pancreaticobiliary maljunction
- Type II (diverticulum)
  Type II is a diverticulum from the extrahepatic bile duct.
- Type III (choledochocele)
  Type III is known as a choledochocele (focal dilatation of the duodenal segment of the common bile duct).
- Type IV-A
  Type IV-A shows dilatations of both intra- and extrahepatic bile ducts. Dilatation of the intrahepatic bile duct is usually around the hepatic hilum and rarely in the more upstream intrahepatic bile duct. Congenital stricture of the hepatic duct is frequently seen in patients with type IV-A [9, 13].
- Type IV-B
  Type IV-B is extremely rare and has multiple cystic dilatations involving only the extrahepatic bile duct.
- Type V
  Type V involves single or multiple cystic dilatations of intrahepatic bile ducts. Multiple cystic dilatations of the intrahepatic ducts are also seen in Caroli's disease.

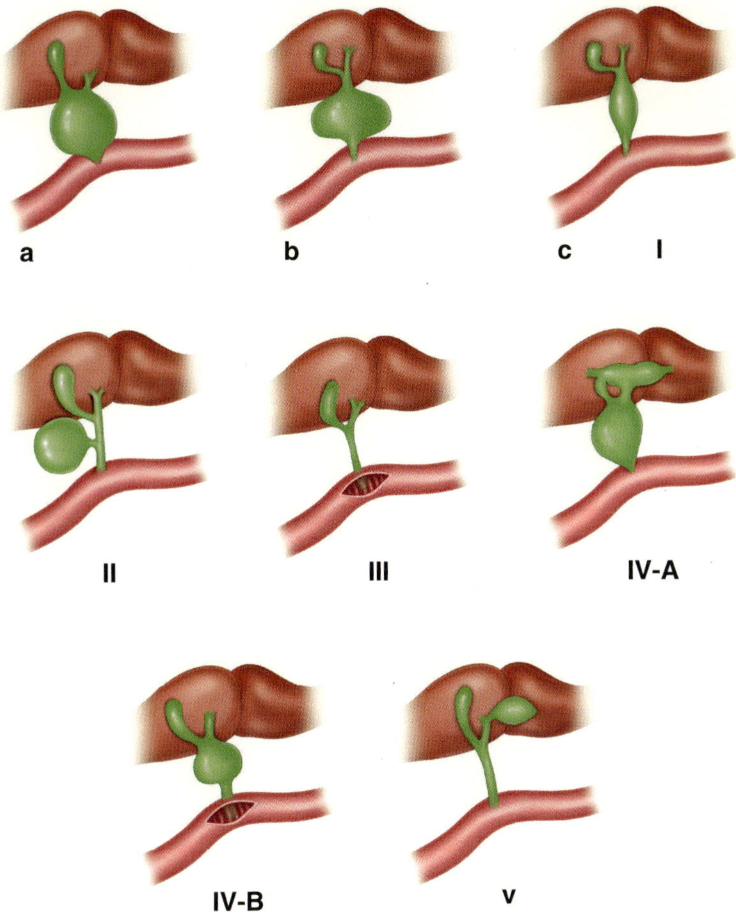

Fig. 7.3 Todani classification of choledochal cyst

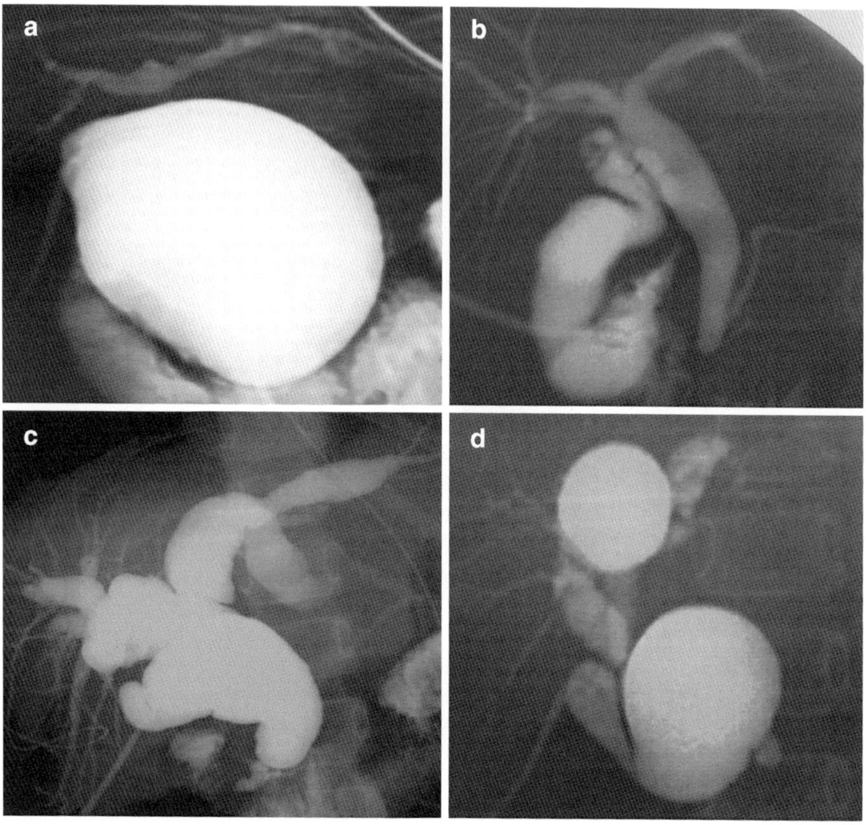

Fig. 7.4 Cholangiogram of type Ia, Ic, and IV-A choledochal cysts (congenital biliary dilatation). (**a**) Type Ia with large cystic dilatation, (**b**) type Ic with a diffuse dilatation, (**c**) type IV-A with dilatations of the extra- and intrahepatic bile ducts, and (**d**) type IV-A with cystic dilatation of the intrahepatic duct

References

1. Kamisawa T, Ando H, Hamada Y, Fujii H, Koshinaga T, Urushihara N, et al. Diagnostic criteria for pancreaticobiliary maljunction 2013. J Hepatobiliary Pancreat Sci. 2014;21:159–61.
2. Tanaka K, Nishijima A, Yamada K. Cancer of the gallbladder associated with anomalous junction of the pancreatobiliary duct system without bile duct dilatation. Br J Surg. 1993;80:622–4.
3. Chijiiwa K, Kimura H, Tanaka M. Malignant potential of the gallbladder in patients with anomalous pancreaticobiliary ductal junction. The difference in risk between patients with and without choledochal cyst. Int Surg. 1995;80:61–4.
4. Todani T, Watanabe Y, Urushihara N, Morotomi Y, Maeba T. Choledochal cyst, pancreatobiliary malunion, and cancer. J Hep Bil Pancr Surg. 1994;1:247–51.
5. Morine Y, Shimada M, Takamatsu H, Araida T, Endo I, Kubota M, et al. Clinical features of pancreaticobiliary maljunction: update analysis of 2nd Japan-nationwide survey. J Hepatobiliary Pancreat Sci. 2013;20:472–80.

6. Kimura K, Ohto M, Ono T, Tsuchiya Y, Saisho H, Kawamura K, et al. Congenital cystic dilatation of the common bile duct: relationship to anomalous pancreaticobiliary ductal union. Am J Roentgenol. 1977;128:571–7.
7. Komi N, Udaka H, Ikeda N, Kashiwagi Y. Congenital dilatation of the biliary tract: new classification and study with particular reference to anomalous arrangement of the pancreaticobiliary ducts. Gastroenterol Jpn. 1977;12:293–304.
8. Komi N, Takehara H, Kunitomo K, Miyoshi Y, Yagi T. Does the type of anomalous arrangement of pancreaticobiliary ducts influence the surgery and prognosis of choledochal cyst? J Pediatr Surg. 1992;27:728–31.
9. Todani T. Congenital choledochal dilatation: classification, clinical features, and long-term results. J Hepato-Biliary-Pancreat Surg. 1997;4:276–82.
10. Urushihara N, Hamada Y, Kamisawa T, Fujii H, Koshinaga T, Morotomi Y, et al. Classification of pancreaticobiliary maljunction and clinical features in children. J Hepatobiliary Pancreat Sci. 2017;24:449–55.
11. Alonso-Lej F, Reverx WB Jr, Pessagno DJ. Congenital choledochal cyst with a report of 2, and an analysis of 94, cases. Int Abstr Surg. 1959;108:1–30.
12. Hamada Y, Ando H, Kamisawa T, Itoi T, Urushihara N, Koshinaga T, et al. Diagnostic criteria for congenital biliary dilatation 2015. J Hepatobiliary Pancreat Sci. 2016;23:342–6.
13. Ando H, Ito T, Kaneko K, Seo T. Congenital stenosis of the intrahepatic bile duct associated with choledochal cysts. J Am Coll Surg. 1995;181:426–30.

Chapter 8
Pathophysiology of Pancreaticobiliary Maljunction and Congenital Biliary Dilatation

Kenitiro Kaneko

Abstract Pancreaticobiliary maljunction (PBM) causes pancreaticobiliary reflux. Regurgitated pancreatic juice contains trypsinogen and lithostathine. Activated trypsin cleaves soluble lithostathine into insoluble forms, which aggregate to protein plugs. Protein plugs obstruct the common channel or the narrow segment and produce characteristically intermittent symptoms and signs in most of pediatric patients. These include abdominal pain, vomiting, jaundice, and elevated levels of serum transaminases and amylase. Most plugs are fragile and disappear spontaneously; however, plugs are produced repeatedly, which explains why symptoms are usually mild and self-limiting but also why they recur. Exceptions to this protein plug theory include congenital biliary dilatation with neonatal and early infant onset. In these neonates and infants, the extremely narrow segment causes obstructive cholangiopathy independent of reflux. The mixture of bile and regurgitated pancreatic juice produces substances hazardous to the biliary epithelium. The resulting chronic inflammation causes multistep carcinogenesis through a hyperplasia-dysplasia-carcinoma sequence.

Keywords Pancreaticobiliary maljunction · Congenital biliary dilatation Pathophysiology · Protein plug · Lithostathine · Symptom · Carcinogenesis

8.1 Regurgitation

Pancreaticobiliary maljunction (PBM) causes two-way regurgitations (pancreaticobiliary and biliopancreatic reflux) because the sphincter function does not affect the junction. Because the pressure in the pancreatic duct is usually higher than that in

---

K. Kaneko
Division of Pediatric Surgery, Department of Surgery, Aichi Medical University, Nagakute, Aichi, Japan
e-mail: kkaneko@aichi-med-u.ac.jp

T. Kamisawa, H. Ando (eds.), *Pancreaticobiliary Maljunction and Congenital Biliary Dilatation*, https://doi.org/10.1007/978-981-10-8654-0_8

the bile duct [1], pancreatic juice frequently refluxes into the biliary tract. High levels of pancreatic enzymes in the bile have proved this pancreaticobiliary reflux [2]. Secretin-stimulated dynamic magnetic resonance cholangiography has also demonstrated the pancreaticobiliary reflux [3]. The biliopancreatic reflux has been confirmed by drip infusion cholangiography-computed tomography (DIC-CT), but is not seen in all cases [4]. Pancreaticobiliary reflux is continuous, but biliopancreatic reflux seems to occur sporadically.

8.2 Symptomatology

The regurgitations damage pancreaticobiliary systems. During childhood, regurgitation produces characteristically intermittent symptoms and signs, including abdominal pain, vomiting, jaundice, and elevated levels of serum transaminases and amylase. However, regurgitation is continuous and does not cause symptoms on its own. The pancreas secretes trypsinogen and a protein called lithostathine, which are regurgitated into the biliary tract [2] (Fig. 8.1). Lithostathine, previously referred to as pancreatic stone protein, is a 16-kDa soluble 144-amino acid glycoprotein, which accounts for 5–10% of the secreted proteins in the pancreatic juice. Lithostathine in secretory form is soluble but highly susceptible to trypsin cleavage. A cleaved 14-kDa carboxyl-terminus with 133 amino acids is insoluble and readily polymerizes. Dimers of S1 evolve by lateral hydrophobic interactions into tetramers. The tetramer has acidic residues on one side and basic residues on the other, contributing negative and positive charges, respectively, at a physiologic pH. The tetramers automatically assemble by longitudinal electrostatic interactions into protofibrils. Refluxed trypsinogen is activated to trypsin in the biliary tract, and trypsin then cleaves soluble lithostathine into insoluble forms, which aggregate to form protein plugs [5]. Protein plugs are compacted in the common channel or the narrow segment distal to the dilated bile duct, and then increase pancreaticobiliary ductal pressure, and provoke symptoms (Figs. 8.1 and 8.2). Hyperamylasemia is seen in 40% of children with PBM, but is not due to pancreatitis in most cases (see Chap. 23). Increased biliary pressure by plug obstruction causes cholangiovenous reflux at the liver, by which regurgitated amylase in the bile passes into the bloodstream (Fig. 8.1). Most protein plugs are fragile and vanish spontaneously; however, plugs are produced repeatedly, which explains why symptoms are usually mild and self-limiting but also why they recur. A few plugs become firm and cause significantly increased ductal pressure, leading to biliary perforation in 3% of pediatric patients (Fig. 8.2).

The protein plug theory mentioned above explains symptoms in most children and some adults with PBM. Symptoms of congenital biliary dilatation (CBD) are known to develop during pregnancy and may also be caused by protein plugs [6]. Exceptions to the protein plug theory in children include fatty calcium stone formation (see Chap. 23) and CBD with neonatal and early infancy onset. These neonates and infants have large cystic dilatation of the common bile duct and an extremely

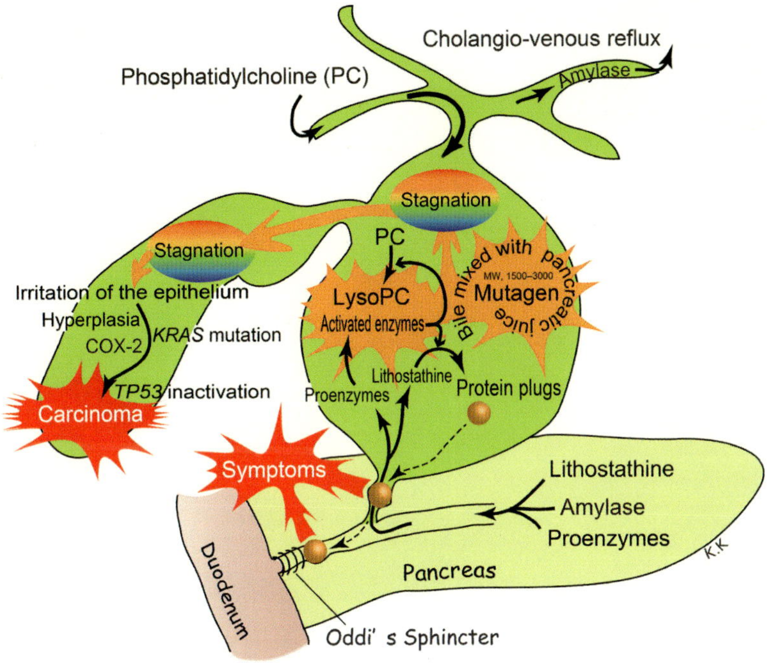

Fig. 8.1 Pathophysiology of pancreaticobiliary maljunction and congenital biliary dilatation. Regurgitated pancreatic enzymes and lithostathine produce protein plugs, which obstruct the narrow segment or common channel, causing symptoms in children. The mixture of bile and regurgitated pancreatic juice produces hazardous substances that stagnate and irritate the epithelium. The resulting chronic inflammation causes multistage carcinogenesis accompanying many molecular changes, through the hyperplasia-dysplasia-carcinoma sequence

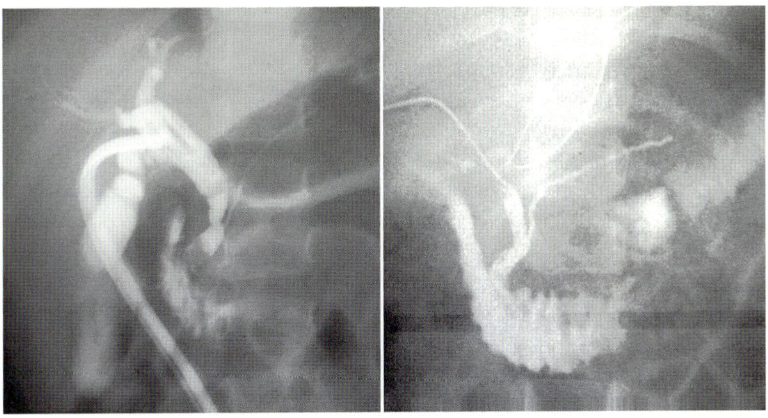

Fig. 8.2 A Case of biliary perforation. A T-tube was inserted through a perforated site of the bile duct in a 1-year-old girl. T-tube cholangiography showed a large radiolucent filling defect compacted in the common channel (*left*). Pancreaticobiliary maljunction was obvious. After 1 month, operative cholangiography showed disappearance of the filling defect in the common channel (*right*)

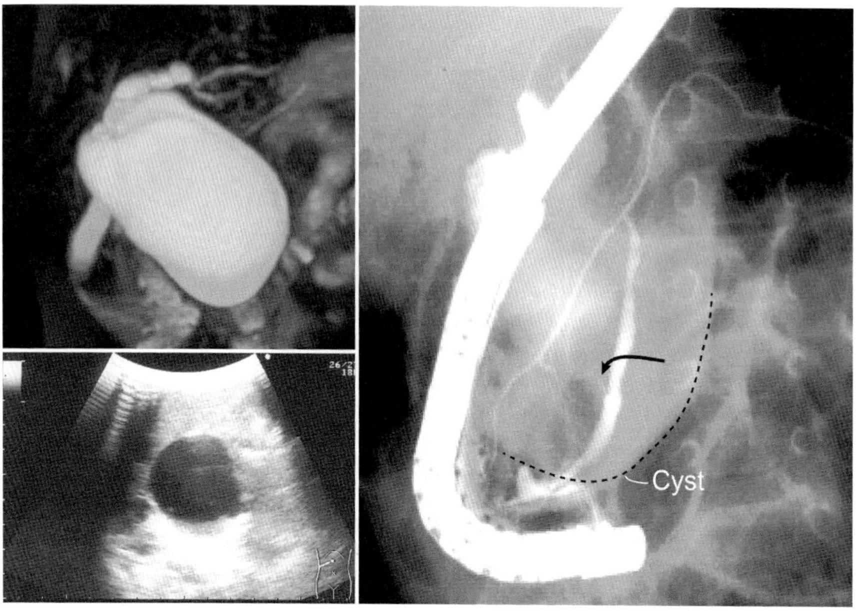

Fig. 8.3 Representative case with congenital biliary dilatation diagnosed prenatally. Magnetic resonance cholangiography after birth showed large cystic dilatation of the common bile duct, but pancreaticobiliary junction was obscure (*left upper*). One month after birth, acholic stool and mild jaundice with elevated levels of transaminase developed, when ultrasonography detected debris in the dilated bile duct (*lower left*). Serum levels of amylase and lipase were not elevated. At 5 months when symptoms subsided, endoscopic retrograde cholangiopancreatography showed pancreaticobiliary maljunction with a thin hairlike duct (*arrow*) connecting the main pancreatic duct and the cyst (*right*). The main pancreatic duct described an arc pushed by a large cyst

narrow segment distal to the cyst (Fig. 8.3). Many of these patients were identified prenatally by ultrasound [7]. Occlusion at the very narrow segment causes obstructive cholangiopathy independent of reflux [8]. Jaundice and acholic stool are the main symptoms, similar to those seen in biliary atresia. An intermediate type exists between CBD and cystic biliary atresia. Liver fibrosis frequently occurs in these CBD infants with an early onset, but the fibrosis improves after excision of the extrahepatic bile duct [9]. Irreversible fibrosis is unusual and may be present in the intermediate type but requires liver transplantation [10]. Asymptomatic children with PBM, especially those without CBD, develop biliary cancers silently as they grow older. Asymptomatic PBM was found in 30% of adult patients by ultrasonographic findings for conditions including gallstones, gallbladder polyps, dilated bile ducts, and thickened gallbladder wall [11]. The remainder of adults presented with symptoms due to biliary cancers, protein plugs, or incidental complications such as gallstones (see Chap. 23).

8.3 Carcinogenesis

There is a strong relationship between pancreaticobiliary maljunction and biliary carcinoma. Wong et al. recently demonstrated that children with CBD have de novo genetic variants that relate to both disease development and biliary carcinogenesis [12]. It is possible that the same genetic changes might cause both CBD and biliary cancers. However, other studies indicate that pancreaticobiliary reflux causes biliary carcinogenesis. First, pancreaticobiliary reflux occurs also in patients without PBM, and these patients frequently have gallbladder carcinoma (see also Chap. 10) [13]. Second, PBM with a patent accessary pancreatic duct causes less pancreaticobiliary reflux and is less frequently associated with biliary carcinoma [14].

Most cancers under the influence of PBM arise in the gallbladder or a dilated bile duct, which suggests that bile stasis is strongly related to carcinogenesis (Fig. 8.1). Bile mixed with regurgitated pancreatic juice produces substances hazardous to the biliary epithelium, including activated pancreatic enzymes, lysophosphatidylcholine (lysolecithin), and a mutagen with a molecular weight of 1500–3000 Da [15]. Secondary or free bile acids, also toxic to the cell membrane, were reported to occur in the bile in PBM, but recent reports have not confirmed the alteration. These noxious substances stagnate in the gallbladder or a dilated bile duct and irritate the epithelium. The resulting chronic inflammation causes increased cellular proliferation and subsequent epithelial hyperplasia. Hyperplasia is detected as a thickened gallbladder wall on ultrasound, by which asymptomatic PBM is found in adults undergoing medical checkups [11]. Concurrently, molecular abnormalities are induced in the biliary epithelium including the activation of the *KRAS* point mutation in the early phase and *TP53* inactivation in the late phase [16]. Biliary carcinogenesis under PBM involves the hyperplasia-dysplasia-carcinoma sequence, the details of which are described in Chaps. 20 and 21.

8.4 Relation to Biliary Dilatation

PBM is usually seen in patients with CBD. Babbitt proposed that pancreaticobiliary reflux caused biliary dilatation [17]. Refluxed and activated pancreatic enzymes weaken the bile duct wall, and pancreatic secretory pressure causes biliary dilatation. This etiology was formerly widely accepted but is now questioned. It has become to be known that there are patients with PBM but without CBD. CBD has been prenatally diagnosed at as early as 15 weeks of gestation, when no pancreatic enzymes are produced [7]. Experimental studies on PBM have failed to produce cystic dilatation in animals [18]. Currently, many researchers believe that the bile duct is dilated because of biliary ductal pressure increased by the narrow segment distal to the bile duct [19].

8.5 Activation of Regurgitated Proenzymes

Activation of pancreatic proenzymes regurgitating into the bile duct plays a key role in both symptomatology and carcinogenesis. However, there are only six studies that have demonstrated their activation in the bile under PBM [2]. The rates of activation of enzymes varied in each report. Regurgitation is certain, but activation is probable, and more evidence is required. The mechanism of activation remains a riddle. One possible explanation is the existence of enterokinase in bile, which is secreted by metaplastic biliary epithelia [20]. However, no other researchers have confirmed the presence of enterokinase in bile under PBM as yet.

References

1. Csendes A, Kruse A, Funch-Jensen P, Oster MJ, Ornsholt J, Amdrup E. Pressure measurements in the biliary and pancreatic duct systems in controls and in patients with gallstones, previous cholecystectomy, or common bile duct stones. Gastroenterology. 1979;77:1203–10.
2. Ochiai K, Kaneko K, Kitagawa M, Ando H, Hayakawa T. Activated pancreatic enzyme and pancreatic stone protein (PSP/reg) in bile of patients with pancreaticobiliary maljunction/choledochal cysts. Dig Dis Sci. 2004;49:1953–6.
3. Hosoki T, Hasuike Y, Takeda Y, Michita T, Watanabe Y, Sakamori R, Tokuda Y, Yutani K, Sai C, Mitomo M. Visualization of pancreaticobiliary reflux in anomalous pancreaticobiliary junction by secretin-stimulated dynamic magnetic resonance cholangiopancreatography. Acta Radiol. 2004;45:375–82.
4. Fumino S, Tokiwa K, Katoh T, Ono S, Iwai N. New insight into bile flow dynamics in anomalous arrangement of the pancreaticobiliary duct. Br J Surg. 2002;89:865–9.
5. Kaneko K, Ando H, Seo T, Ono Y, Tainaka T, Sumida W. Proteomic analysis of protein plugs: causative agent of symptoms in patients with choledochal cyst. Dig Dis Sci. 2007;52:1979–86.
6. Beattie GJ, Keay S, Muir BB, Boddy K. Acute pancreatitis with pseudocyst formation complicating pregnancy in a patient with a co-existent choledochal cyst. Br J Obstet Gynaecol. 1993;100:957–9.
7. Mackenzie TC, Howell LJ, Flake AW, Adzick NS. The management of prenatally diagnosed choledochal cysts. J Pediatr Surg. 2001;36:1241–3.
8. Todani T, Urushihara N, Morotomi Y, Watanabe Y, Uemura S, Noda T, Sasaki K, Yoshikawa M. Characteristics of choledochal cysts in neonates and early infants. Eur J Pediatr Surg. 1995;5:143–5.
9. Ishimaru T, Kitano Y, Uchida H, Kawashima H, Gotoh C, Satoh K, Yoshida M, Kishimoto H, Iwanaka T. Histopathologic improvement in biliary cirrhosis after definitive surgery for choledochal cyst. J Pediatr Surg. 2010;45(5):e11–4. https://doi.org/10.1016/j.jpedsurg.2010.01.030.
10. Fumino S, Higuchi K, Aoi S, Furukawa T, Kimura O, Tajiri T. Clinical analysis of liver fibrosis in choledochal cyst. Pediatr Surg Int. 2013;29:1097–102.
11. Yamao K, Mizutani S, Nakazawa S, Inui K, Kanemaki N, Miyoshi H, Segawa K, Zenda H, Kato T. Prospective study of the detection of anomalous connections of pancreatobiliary ducts during routine medical examinations. Hepato-Gastroenterology. 1996;43:1238–45.
12. Wong JK, Campbell D, Ngo ND, Yeung F, Cheng G, Tang CS, Chung PH, Tran NS, So MT, Cherny SS, Sham PC, Tam PK, Garcia-Barcelo MM. Genetic study of congenital bile-duct dilatation identifies de novo and inherited variants in functionally related genes. BMC Med Genet. 2016;9:75.

13. Horaguchi J, Fujita N, Kamisawa T, Honda G, Chijiiwa K, Maguchi H, Tanaka M, Shimada M, Igarashi Y, Inui K, Hanada K, Itoi T, Hamada Y, Koshinaga T, Fujii H, Urushihara N, Ando H, The committee of Diagnostic Criteria of The Japanese Study Group on Pancreaticobiliary Maljunction. Pancreatobiliary reflux in individuals with a normal pancreaticobiliary junction: a prospective multicenter study. J Gastroenterol. 2014;49:875–81.
14. Kamisawa T, Egawa N, Nakajima H, Matsukawa M. Dorsal pancreatic duct dominance in pancreaticobiliary maljunction. Pancreas. 2005;30:e60–3.
15. Mizuno M, Kato T, Koyama K. An analysis of mutagens in the contents of the biliary tract in pancreaticobiliary maljunction. Surg Today. 1996;26:597–602.
16. Wistuba II, Gazdar AF. Gallbladder cancer: lessons from a rare tumour. Nat Rev Cancer. 2004;4:695–706.
17. Babbitt DP. Congenital choledochal cysts: new etiological concept based on anomalous relationships of the common bile duct and pancreatic bulb. Ann Radiol (Paris). 1969;12:231–40.
18. Kaneko K, Ando H, Umeda T, Murahashi O, Hiraiwa K, Niimi N, Hossain M, Ito T. A new model for pancreaticobiliary maljunction without bile duct dilatation: demonstration of cell proliferation in the gallbladder epithelium. J Surg Res. 1996;60:115–21.
19. Turowski C, Knisely AS, Davenport M. Role of pressure and pancreatic reflux in the aetiology of choledochal malformation. Br J Surg. 2011;98:1319–26.
20. Yamasaki S, Miyoshi Y, Komi N. Immunohistochemical studies on enterokinase producing cells in the biliary tract. Jpn J Surg. 1991;21:600–5.

Chapter 9
Choledochal Malformations and Pancreaticobiliary Maljunction: A European Perspective

Filippo Parolini and Mark Davenport

Abstract Choledochal malformation (CM) may be defined as morphological abnormality of the biliary tract characterised by dilatation in the absence of acute mechanical obstruction. Bile duct maljunction with the incoming pancreatic duct and formation of a long common channel is a recognised element of CM. This allows free intermixing of pancreatic juice and bile, although the how dynamic this relationship is remains unknown. We have established that there is an inverse relationship of choledochal pressure and bile amylase (as a surrogate of reflux) and that the key component of damage to the biliary epithelium is pressure generated.

This chapter explores choledochal malformation from the European perspective where much less has been published.

Keywords Congenital choledochal malformation · Biliary amylase · Intrabiliary pressure

9.1 Introduction

Choledochal malformation (CM) may be defined as morphological abnormality of the biliary tract characterised by dilatation in the absence of acute mechanical obstruction [1, 2]. Typically there is in addition distal bile duct maljunction with the pancreatic duct ensuring a variable length of common channel (CC) prior to traversing the wall of the duodenum. This CC may or may not be dilated and contain proteinaceous debris. In the absence of a CC, the diagnosis of CM would be felt to be contentious.

CMs are relatively uncommon in Western Europe and North America but appreciably more common in Asia [3]. We have based this review principally on

F. Parolini
Kings College Hospital, London, UK

M. Davenport (✉)
Department of Paediatric Surgery, Kings College Hospital, London, UK

T. Kamisawa, H. Ando (eds.), *Pancreaticobiliary Maljunction and Congenital Biliary Dilatation*, https://doi.org/10.1007/978-981-10-8654-0_9

clinical experience derived from a large tertiary referral practice at King's College Hospital, London, the largest of the three centres for paediatric hepatobiliary disease in England and Wales [2, 4–7]. Consistency in diagnostic assessment, in surgical approach and technique throughout a 25-year period has enabled examination of key classification and pathophysiological relationship not previously described.

9.2 Incidence in Western Countries

The actual prevalence of CM in either North America or Europe is actually unknown but has been estimated in about 1 in 100,000–150,000 births [5–14]. Nevertheless, if biliary atresia is used as a guide for a condition where the incidence is known (1 in 17,000) and the ratio of the two conditions presenting in infancy is taken from our specialist hepatobiliary unit in the UK, then an approximate figure of about 1 in 53,000 live births seems a reasonable estimate (Table 9.1). Part of the problem is that CMs can present at any point in the life cycle from an antenatal scan to the postmortem table making their true incidence hard to define [4, 13]. The incidence is higher in Asian populations with old studies reporting an incidence of 1 in 13,000 individuals [3, 4]. More than two-thirds of cases are diagnosed in children less than 10 years of age, and girls outnumber boys by about 4:1. A few studies have suggested that the diagnosis of CMs in adulthood is increasing in frequency [4, 12, 15]. Whether this finding is due to higher index of suspicion and improved imaging techniques (such as ultrasound and magnetic resonance cholangiopancreatography) or, much less probably, that CMs could develop later in life is still not known [8]. The largest Western cohort derived from an international multi-institutional database of eight hepatobiliary centres predominantly from North America but also European centres such as Lisbon and Milan

Table 9.1 King's College Hospital prospective database from 1999 to 2014

Summary of database (1999–2014)	BA	CM
Patients, *n*	353	113
Female, *n* (%)	191 (54%)	84 (74%)
Ethnicity, *n* (%)		
– White	250 (70.8%)	72 (63.7%)
– Asia	78 (22.1%)	33 (29.2%)
– Afro- Caribbean	18 (5.1%)	8 (7.1%)
– Other	7 (2%)	
Incidence	1:17,000[a]	1:53,000 (estimated)

[a]Livesey E, Cortina Borja M, Sharif K, et al. Epidemiology of biliary atresia in England and Wales (1999–2006). Arch Dis Child Fetal Neonatal Ed. 2009; 94: F451–5

Table 9.2 Recent European and North American experience

Author	Setting	Population	CM classification	Incidence of PBM[a]	Incidence of biliary cancer
Soares [8]	Multicentre retrospective study (North America and Europe), (1972–2014)	394 pts	Type I–70%	48 (12.3%)	3.3%
		249 (67%) adults, median age 45 year			
		135 (34%) children median age 15 year			
Ragot [19]	Multicentre retrospective study (France, Switzerland, Italy) (1975–2012)	263 pts	Type I–70%	190 (72.2%)	8.7% of CMs, 11.1% of PBM
		126 adults (66.8%)	Type II–5%		
			Type III–3%		
		63 children (33.2%)	Type IVa–21%		
Hukkinen [14]	Retrospective study, Helsinki, Finland (1976–2013)	38 pts. (all children)	Type IC–45%	28 (61%)	0%
			Type IF–51%		

[a]*PBM* pancreaticobiliary maljunction

encompasses 394 patients accrued between 1972 and 2014 [8] and is predominantly adults (66%). A selective review of some recent large published Western studies on CMs is reiterated in Table 9.2.

9.3 Classification

We believe that there are two principle extrahepatic phenotypes: the classical cystic malformation (type 1C) and the more recently defined fusiform malformation (type 1F) [3–5]. This is at variance with Todani's original classification which recognised three [15], although the distinction seems to escape more recent authors [8, 9]. Some recent studies from China also favour this simpler cystic/fusiform distinction [16]. Todani's classification is complex, and many authors continue to misquote the original, particularly confusing cystic and fusiform [15]. Our King's College Hospital classification (Fig. 9.1) retains the structure of the original (types 1–5) but uses the non-judgemental "choledochal malformation" with whatever descriptive epithet best suits the nature of the dilatation [2, 11, 17]. Type 4 is simply defined as the combination of intra- and extrahepatic dilatation and may be the natural history of untreated type 1F and 1C. The evidence for this is that there is an increasing proportion of type 4 lesions in adult series or those where there is a combination of adults and children. For instance, in the large multicentre experience reported by

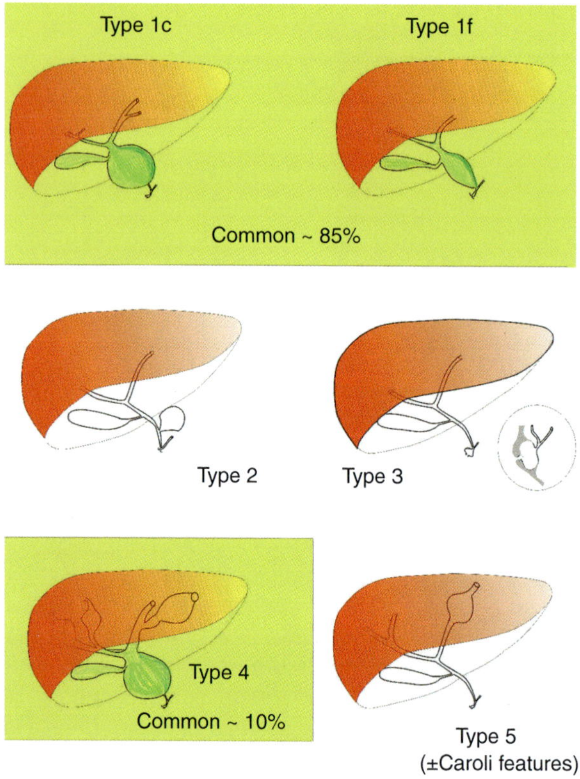

Fig. 9.1 Classification. King's College Hospital classification of CMs: type 1C, cystic malformation; type 1F, fusiform malformation (type 1F). Type 4: the combination of intra- and extrahepatic dilatation

Soares et al. [8], type IV predominated in the adult population (23.9% vs 12.0%) and type IC lesions were more often seen in children (79.7% vs 64.9%).

Type 1 and 4 account together up to 95% of cases of CMs.

9.4 Choledochal Malformations and Pancreaticobiliary Maljunction (PBM)

An intrinsic part of the CM complex is pancreaticobiliary malunion (PMU) leading to a common channel [2, 13, 18]. It is evident that this can be regarded as a spectrum with "common channel" (i.e. ductal fusion outside the ampulla) being seen in about 85% of individuals but it not being longer than 1 cm (adult criteria). Only in about 15% of cases do the bile and pancreatic ducts open either separately (9%) into the ampulla or as a V junction with the duodenal mucosa (5%) [13, 18]. Thus, in patients with PBM, early confluence occurs within the head of pancreas, resulting in a long common channel (>1 cm), usually with an abnormal angle of insertion of common bile duct and a variable degree of proximal bile duct stenosis [2]. This arrangement may be seen in <2% of the population but is characteristic of CMs [9].

Using a definition of abnormality as "a common channel >15 mm in length", one large (n = 2885) albeit retrospective series from India identified 46 (1.6%) as abnormal, and almost 90% of these had an additional CM [18]. In a series a little closer to home, a French multicentre study of 263 patients with CM found that the median length of the CC (defined as >8 mm) in patients with PBM was 15.8 (range 5–40) mm [19]. In addition there was clear evidence of pancreatic juice reflux as the median intrabiliary amylase and lipase levels were 65,249 and 172,104 UI/L, respectively. For the diagnostic of PBM, a common channel length of more than 8 mm and an intrabiliary amylase level >8000 UI/L were associated with a predictive positive value and a specificity of more than 90%.

9.5 Aetiology

In the embryo, the ventral pancreatic anlage's duct arises as a branch of the bile duct outpouching from duodenum. Following rotation around the axis of duodenum, this ventral portion merges with the dorsal anlage with resorption of the common channel into duodenum. Interruption of that process therefore leaves a long CC as the default [1, 19–21].

The pathophysiology of CM is still incompletely understood, and there are two principle hypotheses [2, 4]. The older and simplest hypothesis postulated that there is a congenital distal stenotic segment in the bile duct which partially obstructed bile flow, leading to increased proximal bile duct pressure and wall tension, with subsequent duct dilatation [21]. Initially, this occurs in the unsupported extrahepatic biliary tree, then later within the liver.

A more complex hypothesis was first suggested in 1969 by Donald Babbitt, an American radiologist [22]. He showed simply that at on-table cholangiography of a type1C CM, there was free reflux via the common channel into the pancreatic duct. He then *speculated* that if the reverse was possible, then pancreatic proteolytic enzymes might weaken the wall of the bile duct sufficiently to cause dilatation, presumably at normal choledochal pressure. Clearly the Babbitt *observation* is correct, that bile or pancreatic juice can freely reflux, but it is highly contentious that any real epithelial damage never mind structural weakness occurs. In our experience, antenatally detected lesions are almost invariably shown to be type 1C CM with low bile amylase levels and high intracystic pressure. Furthermore, pancreatic acini during the first year of life are not capable of secreting sufficient pancreatic enzymes [2, 11].

We have published a series of studies trying to determine functional difference between the two phenotypes [4–7]. Firstly, we began by measuring levels of amylase (as a surrogate of pancreatic reflux) in the bile within the CM at the time of surgery [4–6]. This showed an age-dependent range of values with the highest almost invariably having a clinical background of pancreatitis. Secondly, we began measuring actual pressures within the CM and showed an inverse relationship between this and their levels of bile amylase and a stepwise variation and increase according to the bile duct phenotype (from type 1F through type 1C to type 4) (Fig. 9.2) [4–6]. Finally, we related these variables to a histological score reflecting biliary epithelial change from normal to very abnormal including sloughing and dysplasia [4]. Our results clearly showed that those with the most abnormal histological appearance were those with the highest pressures and therefore the lowest amylase levels [4]. These findings clearly challenge the relevance of the Babbitt *speculation* (Fig. 9.3).

We recently investigated the role of CA19-9 in bile and the MIB-1 (Ki-67) epithelial proliferation index as markers of an at risk choledochal epithelium at the time of definitive surgery in 43 children with CMs. Biliary CA19-9 levels were grossly and unexpectedly raised in CM and appear to arise from biliary rather than

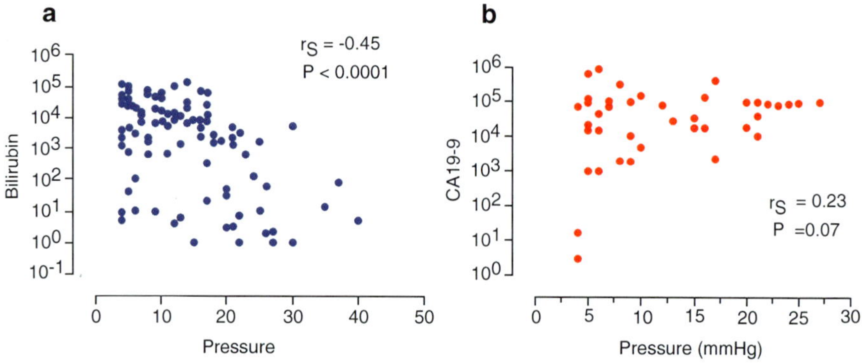

Fig. 9.2 Choledochal pressure and bile constituents. Updated relationship between choledochal pressure and (**a**) bile amylase ($r_S = -0.45$; $P < 0.0001$) ($n = 94$ pairs) and (**b**) bile CA19-9 ($r_S = 0.23$; $P = 0.07$) ($n = 40$ pairs). Note that the Y axis is logarithmic

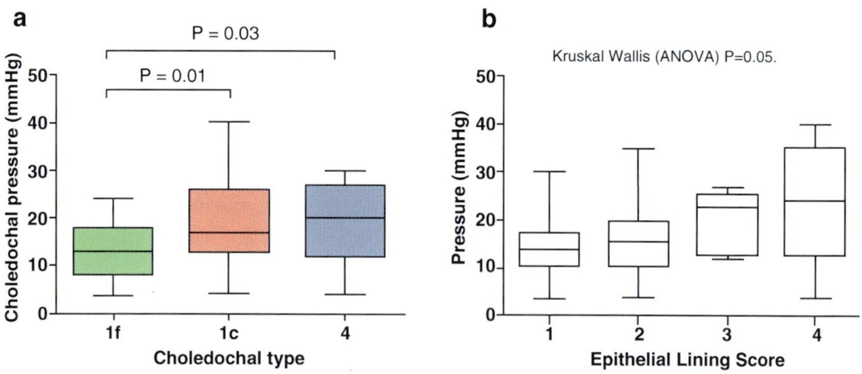

Fig. 9.3 Choledochal pressure: morphology and epithelial consequences. (**a**) Choledochal pressure (mm Hg) in relation to type of choledochal malformation in 47 patients (20 type 1f, 20 type 1c and 7 type 4). (**b**) Choledochal pressure (mm Hg) vs epithelial lining score where 1 = normal and 4 = epithelial necrosis and bile impregnation. Modified from reference #3

pancreatic epithelium. MIB-1 confirms that a small proportion (19%) has marked epithelial proliferation, but no correlation was found with choledochal pressure, CA19-9 or bile amylase [7].

9.6 Clinical Features

There are distinct differences to the pattern of presentation in adults and children [1]. Antenatal presentation makes up about 15–20% of large clinical series, and typically the cyst is detected from around 20 to 22 weeks' gestation and usually grows in line with foetal growth [1, 23]. Many reports on Eastern paediatric populations have described the classical presentation triad with abdominal pain, jaundice and an upper quadrant mass, but actually it was not recorded in the largest Western series [8]. The clinical presentation of the disease in Eastern and Western populations shows several similarities [8, 19]. Most infants tend to present with obstructive jaundice, while adolescents and adults are more likely to present with biliary or pancreatic symptoms and abdominal pain. If untreated or disregarded, biliary cirrhosis is a possible sequel, and in adulthood a small proportion will present with malignant transformation. Choledochal morphology may favour some features over others, as fusiform lesions are never large enough to be palpated, while multiple intrahepatic type 4 lesions predispose to stone formation and sepsis [8]. Moreover, both in Western than Eastern series, type I CMs were predominant in the paediatric population, while adults had significantly more type 4 CMs [4, 18, 19].

9.7 Management and Outcome

Regardless of the time of presentation, surgical intervention is indicated to mitigate potential damage to the liver, prevent jaundice and pancreatitis and (at least in adults) prevent cancer [1, 2]. Complete excision of CM and biliary reconstruction using a jejunal Roux-en-Y loop as an open operation is still the standard to compare to [17]. Laparoscopic excision begins with the reports of Farello et al. from Italy in 1995 [24] and certainly in high-volume Asian centres such as Beijing [25] and Hanoi [26]; there is now a huge experience with this technique and much more so than surgeons have in the West where single-figure experience is the norm. Although this approach is clearly feasible and safe, care should be taken before dispensing with standard open techniques, which have minimal complications and proven long-term benefit. Regardless the surgical approach, the risk of long-term problems post-surgery is significant, and whether this is due to recurrent pancreatitis secondary to the retained common channel and/or a distal stump or due to the development of biliary tract, malignancy is still a cause for concern [17].

9.8 Risk of Malignancy in Choledochal Malformations

After the first report of the association of CM with cancer from Kasai et al. in 1970 [27], many Eastern and Western series have investigated the risk of malignancy, even if it remains unknown what proportion of biliary cancers arise in cysts [8, 19, 28]. An old multicentre study from Watanabe et al. identified 154 cases of malignancy from 881 CMs (mainly adenocarcinomas of the bile ducts or gallbladder), suggesting an incidence of malignant change of 17% [28], but most of the series stated a lower incidence [8, 11, 19]. Patients with common channel alone have a higher risk of developing biliary tract malignancies than the general population (11% vs less than 0.01%, respectively) [11]. The etiopathogenesis of biliary malignancy is still unclear, even if chronic reflux of activated pancreatic enzymes (leading to ulceration and increasing epithelial turnover), recurrent cholangitis and the irritant effect of biliary tract stones might contribute to epithelial damage [8, 11]. Malignancy usually onsets in the third decade, 10–20 years sooner than bile duct cancer without cyst, but, fortunately, it appears that no child younger than 10 years of age having surgery has developed later malignancy. Biliary malignancies have been occasionally reported even after appropriate surgical treatment of CMs [14]. The risk of subsequent biliary malignancy in patients undergoing cyst excision for CMs seems to be relatively high in the long-term, suggesting that an adequate and prolonged follow-up throughout adulthood should thereby be mandatory for children affected by CMs [2, 18].

References

1. Soares KC, Arnaoutakis DJ, Kamel I, et al. Choledochal cysts: presentation, clinical differentiation, and management. J Am Coll Surg. 2014;219(6):1167–80.
2. Atkinson JJ, Davenport M. Controversies in choledochal malformation. S Afr Med J. 2014;104(11 Pt 2):816–9.
3. Takeshita N, Ota T, Yamamoto M. Forty-year experience with flow-diversion surgery for patients with congenital choledochal cysts with pancreaticobiliary maljunction at a single institution. Ann Surg. 2011;254(6):1050–3.
4. Turowski C, Knisely AS, Davenport M. Role of pressure and pancreatic reflux in the aetiology of choledochal malformation. Br J Surg. 2011;98:1319–26.
5. Davenport M, Basu R. Under pressure: choledochal malformation manometry. J Pediatr Surg. 2005;40(2):331–5.
6. Davenport M, Stringer MD, Howard ER. Biliary amylase and congenital choledochal dilatation. J Pediatr Surg. 1995;30(3):474–7.
7. La Pergola E, Zen Y, Davenport M. Congenital choledochal malformation: search for a marker of epithelial instability. J Pediatr Surg. 2016;51(9):1445.
8. Soares KC, Kim Y, Spolverato G, et al. Presentation and clinical outcomes of choledochal cysts in children and adults: a multi-institutional analysis. JAMA Surg. 2015;150(6):577–84.
9. Soares KC, Goldstein SD, Ghaseb MA, Kamel I, et al. Pediatric choledochal cysts: diagnosis and current management. Pediatr Surg Int. 2017;33(6):637–50. https://doi.org/10.1007/s00383-017-4083-6.

10. Wiseman K, Buczkowski AK, Chung SW, et al. Epidemiology, presentation, diagnosis, and outcomes of choledochal cysts in adults in an urban environment. Am J Surg. 2005;189:527–31.
11. Dabbas N, Davenport M. Congenital choledochal malformation: not just a problem for children. Ann R Coll Surg Engl. 2009;91:100–5.
12. Moslim MA, Takahashi H, Seifarth FG, et al. Choledochal cyst disease in a western center: a 30-year experience. J Gastrointest Surg. 2016;20:1453–63.
13. Nicholl M, Pitt HA, Wolf P, Cooney J, et al. Choledochal cysts in western adults: complexities compared to children. J Gastrointest Surg. 2004;8:245–52.
14. Hukkinen M, Koivusalo A, Lindahl H, et al. Increasing occurrence of choledochal malformations in children: a single-center 37-year experience from Finland. Scand J Gastroenterol. 2014;49(10):1255–60.
15. Todani T, Watanabe Y, Fujii T, et al. Cylindrical dilatation of the choledochus: a special type of congenital bile duct dilatation. Surgery. 1985;98:964–9.
16. Diao M, Li L, Cheng W. Congenital biliary dilatation may consist of 2 disease entities. J Pediatr Surg. 2011;46(8):1503–9.
17. Makin E, Davenport M. Understanding choledochal malformation. Arch Dis Child. 2012;97(1):69–72.
18. Nagi B, Kochhar R, Bhasin D, et al. Endoscopic retrograde cholangiopancreatography in the evaluation of anomalous junction of the pancreaticobiliary duct and related disorders. Abdom Imaging. 2003;28:847–52.
19. Ragot E, Mabrut JY, Ouaïssi M, Working Group of the French Surgical Association, et al. Pancreaticobiliary maljunctions in European patients with bile duct cysts: results of the multicenter study of the French Surgical Association (AFC). World J Surg. 2017;41(2):538–45.
20. Wong KC, Lister J. Human fetal development of the hepato-pancreatic duct junction--a possible explanation of congenital dilatation of the biliary tract. J Pediatr Surg. 1981;16:139–45.
21. Ito T, Ando H, Nagaya M, et al. Congenital dilatation of the common bile duct in children. The etiologic significance of the narrow segment distal to the dilated common bile duct. Z Kinderchir. 1984;39:40–5.
22. Babbit DP. Congenital choldeocal cyst: new etiological concept based on anomalous relationships of common bile duct and pancreatic bulb. Ann Radiol. 1969;12:231–41.
23. Weng R, Hu W, Cai S, et al. Prenatal diagnosis and prognosis assessment of congenital choledochal cyst in 21 cases. J Obstet Gynaecol. 2016;36(3):324–7.
24. Farello GA, Cerofolini A, Rebonato M, et al. Congenital choledochal cyst: video-guided laparoscopic treatment. Surg Laparosc Endosc. 1995;5:354–8.
25. Diao M, Li L, Cheng W. Laparoscopic versus open roux-en-Y hepatojejunostomy for children with choledochal cysts: intermediate-term follow-up results. Surg Endosc. 2011;25:1567–73.
26. Liem NT, Pham HD, Dung le A, et al. Early and intermediate outcomes of laparoscopic surgery for choledochal cysts with 400 patients. J Laparoendosc Adv Surg Tech A. 2012;22:599–603.
27. Kasai M, Asakura Y, Taira Y. Surgical treatment of choledochal cyst. Ann Surg. 1970;172:844–51.
28. Watanabe Y, Toki A, Todani T. Bile duct cancer developed after cyst excision for choledochal cyst. J Hepato-Biliary-Pancreat Surg. 1999;6:207–12.

Chapter 10
Pancreaticobiliary Reflux

Terumi Kamisawa, Sawako Kuruma, Kazuro Chiba, and Masataka Kikuyama

Abstract The sphincter of Oddi regulates the outflow of bile and pancreatic juice. In pancreaticobiliary maljunction, the junction of the pancreatic and bile ducts is located outside of the duodenal wall, and the action of the sphincter does not functionally affect the pancreaticobiliary junction. Since the hydropressure is normally higher within the pancreatic duct than within the bile duct, reflux of pancreatic juice into the biliary duct frequently occurs in PBM, resulting in carcinogenesis in the biliary tract. Diagnosis of pancreaticobiliary reflux can be diagnosed from elevated amylase levels in the bile, secretin-stimulated dynamic magnetic resonance cholangiopancreatography, and pancreatography via the minor duodenal papilla. Pancreaticobiliary reflux also occurs in high confluence of the pancreaticobiliary ducts which is defined as a common channel length of ≥6 mm, with occlusion of communication when the sphincter contracts. It can occur even in some individuals with normal pancreaticobiliary junction. Although pancreaticobiliary reflux might be related to carcinogenesis of the gallbladder, the clinical relevance of pancreaticobiliary reflux in individuals with normal pancreaticobiliary junctions is unknown. Further prospective clinical studies are needed in order to clarify the clinical implications, including appropriate management, in pancreaticobiliary reflux of individuals without PBM.

Keywords Pancreaticobiliary reflux · Pancreaticobiliary maljunction · Gallbladder cancer High confluence of pancreaticobiliary ducts

---

T. Kamisawa (✉) · S. Kuruma · K. Chiba · M. Kikuyama
Department of Internal Medicine, Tokyo Metropolitan Komagome Hospital, Bunkyo-ku, Tokyo, Japan
e-mail: kamisawa@cick.jp

T. Kamisawa, H. Ando (eds.), *Pancreaticobiliary Maljunction and Congenital Biliary Dilatation*, https://doi.org/10.1007/978-981-10-8654-0_10

10.1 Introduction

The main pancreatic duct and the common bile duct open into the duodenum separately or at one opening with or without a common channel. Common channel formation is reported to occur in 55% [1] to 82% [2] of cases. The sphincter of Oddi, which can be found at the distal end of the pancreatic and bile ducts, consists of the sphincter choledochus, the sphincter pancreaticus, and the sphincter ampullae and regulates the outflow of bile and pancreatic juice [3].

In pancreaticobiliary maljunction (PBM), the junction of the pancreatic and bile ducts is located outside of the duodenal wall, forming a very long common channel. Then, since the action of the sphincter does not functionally affect the pancreaticobiliary junction, two-way regurgitation can occur, with pancreatic juice regurgitating into the common bile duct (pancreaticobiliary reflux) and bile regurgitating into the pancreatic duct (biliopancreatic reflux). Since the hydropressure is normally higher within the pancreatic duct than within the bile duct, there is frequent reflux of pancreatic juice into the biliary duct in PBM [3, 4].

Pancreaticobiliary reflux can be evaluated by several methods, and it has become obvious that this reflux can occur in individuals without PBM. This chapter describes conditions that induce pancreaticobiliary reflux and their clinical implications.

10.2 Diagnosis of Pancreaticobiliary Reflux

Patients with PBM typically exhibit extremely high levels of pancreatic enzymes, especially amylase, in the bile within the bile duct and gallbladder, when obtained percutaneously or immediately after laparotomy [3, 4]. According to a nationwide survey [5], in adult patients with congenital biliary dilatation, the amylase level was 98,650 KIU/L in the bile of the gallbladder and 78,875 KIU/L was 98,650 KIU/L in the bile of the bile duct. The normal upper limit of the bile amylase level is unknown.

Secretin-stimulated dynamic magnetic resonance cholangiopancreatography (MRCP) can be used to visualize pancreaticobiliary reflux in patients with PBM [6, 7]. Under normal circumstances, secretin injection causes no change in the extrahepatic and intrahepatic bile ducts. However, following secretin injection in PBM patients, extrahepatic bile duct and gallbladder volumes increase due to regurgitation of secreted pancreatic fluid into the bile duct. However, since bile is also secreted after secretin stimulation, enlargement of the gallbladder may imply pancreaticobiliary reflux, bile secretion, or both [7]. It has recently been reported that time-spatial labeling inversion pulse MRI may be a useful technique for detecting pancreaticobiliary reflux, because it allows direct visualization of pancreaticobiliary flow [8].

Pancreaticobiliary reflux in PBM patients can also be shown by pancreatography via the minor duodenal papilla. When contrast medium is injected endoscopically through the minor duodenal papilla, it then refluxes into the bile duct through a long common channel without flowing out into the duodenum [9].

10.3 Pancreaticobiliary Maljunction

In PBM, the anatomic junction of the pancreatic and bile ducts occurs outside the duodenal wall. PBM is divided into PBM with biliary dilatation (congenital biliary dilatation) and PBM without biliary dilatation.

Since the pancreaticobiliary junction is not directly affected by sphincter action, and hydropressure is higher within the pancreatic duct than within the bile duct, there is consistent reflux of pancreatic juice into the biliary tract in PBM, resulting in a high incidence of carcinogenesis in the biliary tract [3, 4]. According to a nationwide survey [5], biliary tract cancers were observed in 21.6% of adult patients with congenital biliary dilatation and 42.4% of patients with PBM without biliary dilatation. The main lesions in patients with congenital biliary dilatation were gallbladder cancer in 62.3% and bile duct cancer in 32.1%, and in patients with PBM without biliary dilatation, the main lesions were gallbladder cancer in 88.1% and bile duct cancer in 7.3%. Biliary tract cancers develop about 15–20 years earlier in patients with PBM than in individuals without, and double cancers sometimes develop [3].

Stasis of bile intermingled with refluxed pancreatic juice appears to have a strong association with carcinogenesis. Activated pancreatic enzymes, increased secondary bile acids, or other mutagens constantly attack the biliary tract epithelial cells of PBM patients, which can cause hyperplastic change and increased cell proliferation. This can then lead to biliary tract carcinogenesis through oncogene and/or tumor suppressor gene mutations in the epithelia. The etiology of biliary tract cancer in patients with PBM is thought to be related to the hyperplasia-dysplasia-carcinoma sequence that is induced by chronic inflammation caused by pancreatic juice reflux into the biliary tract, and this mechanism is different from the de novo carcinogenesis or the adenoma-carcinoma sequence that is associated with biliary tract cancers in persons without PBM.

When the diagnosis of PBM is made, prophylactic resection of the biliary tract is recommended before cancer develops [10, 11].

10.4 High Confluence of Pancreaticobiliary Ducts

In some cases, there is a relatively long common channel that is not considered to be PBM because the sphincter of Oddi in such cases does include the pancreaticobiliary ductal junction.

The average length of the common channel has been reported to be 4.4 mm, with a range of 1–12 mm [12]. In another report, the average length was also 4.4 mm, while the range went from 1.2 to 8.4 mm [1]. Rienhoff and Pickrell [13] reported a common channel length within 2 mm in 92 (53%) of 173 cases, ranging from 3 to 5 mm in 62 (36%) and >6 mm in 19 (11%). Given the above findings, to investigate the clinical significance of a relatively long common channel, high confluence of the pancreaticobiliary ducts (HCPBD) was defined as a common channel length of ≥6 mm, with occlusion of communication when the sphincter contracts (Fig. 10.1a, b) [14].

In our previous data, of 3459 patients who underwent endoscopic retrograde cholangiopancreatography (ERCP) in our hospital, 74 patients (2.1%) had PBM, including 33 without biliary dilatation and 65 (1.9%) with HCPBD. In comparing clinical data between 95 patients with HCPBD and 66 patients with PBM without biliary dilatation, there was no difference between the sexes in patients with HCPBD, although PBM occurred predominantly in females. The average age at the time of diagnosis was significantly younger in PBM patients with biliary dilatation. Of 19 patients with HCPBD who underwent postoperative T- or C-tube cholangiography, 17 (89%) showed reflux of contrast medium into the pancreatic duct (Fig. 10.2). In HCPBD patients, the average bile amylase level was increased to 28,564 ± 58,760 IU/L, but it was lower than that of PBM patients. The rate of gallbladder cancer was 12% (11/95) in HCPBD patients, which was significantly lower than that in PBM patients without biliary dilatation but higher than that in controls (Table 10.1).

The average age at the time of diagnosis of gallbladder cancer in patients with HCPBD (64.8 years old) was between that of PBM patients without biliary dilatation (56.5 years old) and patients without these maljunctions (69.5 years old). The rate of gallbladder stones was significantly lower in conjunction with gallbladder cancer associated with HCPBD (21%) or PBM (5%) than in those with gallbladder cancers without these maljunctions (62%). Similar to PBM patients without biliary dilatation, hyperplastic change of the gallbladder mucosa with increased epithelial cell proliferative activity was detected in cases of HCPBD. Furthermore, K-ras mutations of the non-cancerous epithelium of the gallbladder were detected in 5 (28%) of 18 HCPBD cases. A relatively long common channel, as well as a long common channel with PBM, appears to be an important risk factor for the develop-

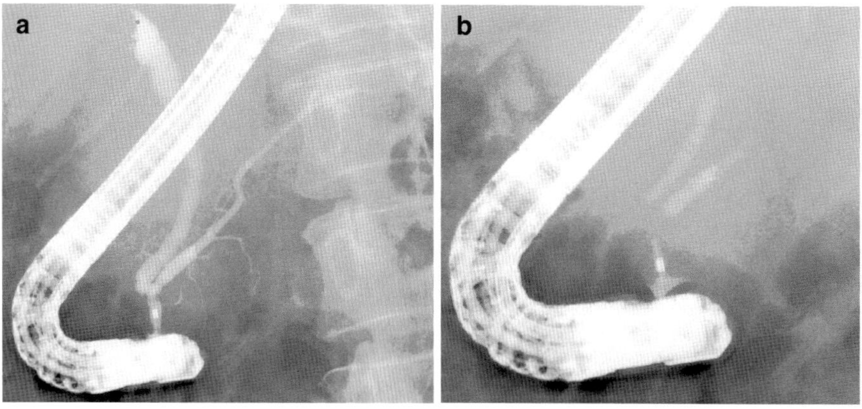

Fig. 10.1 (**a**) Endoscopic retrograde cholangiopancreatogram of a patient with high confluence of pancreaticobiliary ducts, showing a common channel length of 8 mm. (**b**) The communication between the pancreatic and bile ducts is obliterated with sphincter contraction

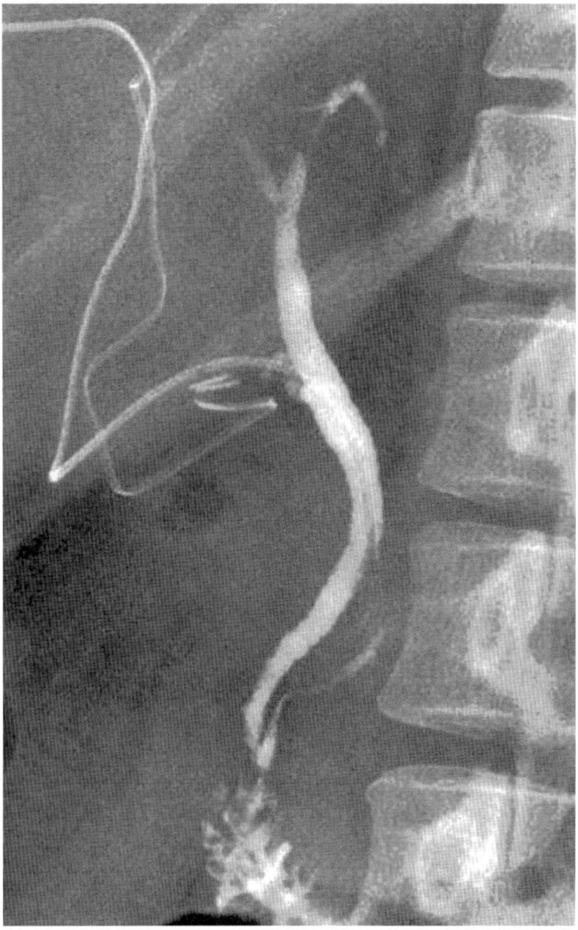

Fig. 10.2 Postoperative C-tube cholangiography of a patient with high confluence of pancreaticobiliary ducts showing the pancreatic duct through the common channel when the sphincter is relaxed

Table 10.1 Clinical difference between high confluence of pancreaticobiliary ducts and pancreaticobiliary maljunction without biliary dilatation

	HCPBD	PBM without BD	*P* value
Number of cases	95	66	
Age at diagnosis	63.0 ± 12.4[a]	57.5 ± 11.5	<0.01
Male/female	1:0.8	1:3.7	<0.01
Gallbladder cancer	11 (12%)	44 (67%)	<0.01
Bile duct cancer	0 (0%)	2 (3%)	
Chronic cholecystitis	7 (7%)	3 (5%)	
Gallbladder hyperplastic polyp	3 (3%)	2 (3%)	
Gallbladder adenomyomatosis	0 (0%)	3 (5%)	
Gall stone	28 (30%)	6 (9%)	<0.01
Amylase levels in bile			
Elevated cases	20/23 (86%)	22/22 (100%)	
Levels (IU/L)	28,564 ± 58,760[a]	186,590 ± 160,330	<0.01
Biliopancreatic reflux	17/19 (89%)	22/22 (100%)	

[a]Mean ± SD

ment of gallbladder cancer. However, since there are several differences in sex, age at diagnosis, bile amylase level, and incidence of associated gallbladder cancer between HCPBD and PBM patients, HCPBM now should be treated as an entity separate from PBM. Although further research is necessary to determine the appropriate management, including prophylactic cholecystectomy, of patients with HCPBD, clinicians should be vigilant regarding the development of gallbladder cancer in such patients [3, 9, 10, 14].

10.5 Pancreaticobiliary Reflux in Individuals with a Normal Pancreaticobiliary Junction

High bile amylase levels are found in some patients without PBM or HCPBD. The bile amylase level obtained through an indwelling T-tube has been reported to be higher than the serum amylase level in 21 (81%) of 26 patients with biliary tract disease, with considerable fluctuation of the bile amylase level in the same patient [15]. Itokawa et al. [16] reported that the amylase level in the bile obtained during ERCP was higher than the serum amylase level in 22 (26%) of 86 patients, and the rate of a high amylase level in the bile was significantly higher in patients who were elderly, in those who had a dilated common bile duct, and in those who had choledocholithiasis.

Occult pancreaticobiliary reflux, which is characterized by functional pancreaticobiliary reflux despite a normal pancreaticobiliary junction, was first proposed by Sai et al. [17]. They demonstrated enhanced visualization of the intrahepatic and extrahepatic bile ducts and gallbladder with increased maximal diameter of the extrahepatic bile duct and short axis of the gallbladder on secretin-stimulated dynamic MRCP in four patients who had a normal pancreaticobiliary junction on ERCP. The bile amylase level was markedly elevated in all four patients, and three of these four patients had gallbladder cancer. In the study by Fujimoto et al. [18], occult pancreaticobiliary reflux was detected in 22 of 31 patients with gallbladder tumors and normal pancreaticobiliary junctions, and 9 of them had gallbladder cancer. This would suggest that there is a relationship between pancreaticobiliary reflux in individuals with a normal pancreaticobiliary junction and gallbladder cancer.

Pancreaticobiliary reflux can also occur in cases of sphincter dysfunction [19], periampullary diverticula [20], and after endoscopic sphincterotomy. Pancreaticobiliary reflux in many cases with normal pancreaticobiliary junctions seems to be caused by sphincter of Oddi dysfunction. Furthermore, unlike in PBM, pancreaticobiliary reflux in individuals with a normal pancreaticobiliary junction does not occur continuously, but transiently. Carcinogenesis in the biliary tract is strongly related to stagnation of bile intermingled with refluxed pancreatic juice. Since pancreatic juice refluxes into the common bile duct and is cleared rapidly without stasis in individuals with a normal pancreaticobiliary maljunction, the occurrence of gallbladder cancer poses a problem in such cases. Although pancreaticobiliary reflux might be related to carcinogenesis of the gallbladder, the clinical relevance of pancreaticobiliary reflux in individuals with normal pancreaticobiliary junctions is unknown. Further prospective clinical studies including appropriate management are needed.

10.6 Conclusion

Pancreaticobiliary reflux can be evaluated using various methods, and it has become clear that reflux can occur in some individuals without PBM. Although the true prevalence and the mechanism of pancreaticobiliary reflux in individuals without PBM are unclear, the reflux might be related to carcinogenesis in the gallbladder even in individuals with a normal pancreaticobiliary junction. More cases need to be studied in order to determine the clinical implications, including appropriate management.

Acknowledgments This work was supported by a grant from the Ministry of Health, Labor, and Welfare of Japan (H28-nanchitou(nan)-ippan-021, research on rare and intractable diseases, and Health and Labor Sciences Research Grants.

References

1. Sterling JA. The common channel for bile and pancreatic ducts. Surg Gynecol Obstet. 1954;98:420–4.
2. Suda K, Miyano T, Konuma I, Matsumoto M. An abnormal pancreatico-choledocho-ductal junction in cases of biliary tract carcinoma. Cancer. 1983;52:2086–8.
3. Kamisawa T, Ando H, Suyama M, Shimada M, Morine Y, Shimada H, et al. Japanese clinical practice guidelines for pancreaticobiliary maljunction. J Gastroenterol. 2012;47:731–59.
4. Kamisawa T, Ando H, Hamada Y, Fujii H, Koshinaga T, Urushihara N, et al. Diagnostic criteria for pancreaticobiliary maljunction 2013. J Hepatobiliary Pancreat Sci. 2014;21:159–61.
5. Morine Y, Shimada M, Takamatsu H, Araida T, Endo I, Kubota M, et al. Clinical features of pancreaticobiliary maljunction: update analysis of 2nd Japan-nationwide survey. J Hepatobiliary Pancreat Sci. 2013;20:472–80.
6. Hosoki T, Hasuike Y, Takeda Y, Michita T, Watanabe Y, Sakamori R, et al. Visualization of pancreaticobiliary reflux in anomalous pancreaticobiliary junction by secretin-stimulated dynamic magnetic resonance cholangiopancreatography. Acta Radiol. 2004;45:375–82.
7. Motosugi U, Ichikawa T, Araki T, Kitahara F, Sato T, Itakura J, et al. Secretin-stimulating MRCP in patients with pancreatobiliary maljunction and occult pancreatobiliary reflux: direct demonstration of pancreatobiliary reflux. Eur Radiol. 2007;17:2262–7.
8. Sugita R, Furuta A, yamazaki T, Ito K, Noda Y. Pancreaticobiliary juice reflux in patients with a morphologically normal ductal system: assessment using unenhanced MRI with spin labeling. Am J Roentgenol. 2017;208:322–7.
9. Kamisawa T, Okamoto A. Biliopancreatic and pancreatobiliary refluxes in cases with and without pancreaticobiliary maljunction: diagnosis and clinical implications. Digestion. 2006;73:228–36.
10. Kamisawa T, Kuruma S, Chiba K, Tabata T, Koizumi S, Kikuyama M. Biliary carcinogenesis in pancreaticobiliary maljunction. J Gastroenterol. 2017;52:158–63.
11. Kamisawa T, Kaneko K, Itoi T, Ando H. Pancreaticobiliary maljunction and congenital biliary dilatation. Lancet Gastroenterol Hepatol. 2017;2:610–8.

12. Dowdy GS, Waldron GW, Brown WG. Surgical anatomy of the pancreatobiliary ductal system. Observations. Arch Surg. 1962;84:229–46.
13. Rienhoff WF, Pickrell KL. Pancreatitis: an anatomic study of the pancreatic and extrahepatic biliary systems. Arch Surg. 1945;51:205–19.
14. Kamisawa T, Amemiya K, Tu Y, Egawa N, Sakaki N, Tsuruta K, et al. Clinical significance of a long common channel. Pancreatology. 2002;2:122–8.
15. Anderson MC, Hauman RL, Suriyapa C, Schiller WR. Pancreatic enzyme levels in bile of patients with extrahepatic biliary tract disease. Am J Surg. 1979;137:301–6.
16. Itokawa F, Itoi T, Nakamura K, Sofuni A, Kakimi K, Moriyasu F, et al. Assessment of occult pancreatobiliary reflux in patients with pancreaticobiliary disease by ERCP. J Gastroenterol. 2004;39:988–94.
17. Sai JK, Suyama M, Kubokawa Y, Tadokoro H, Sato N, Maehara T, et al. Occult pancreatobiliary reflux in patients with a normal pancreaticobiliary junction. Gastrointest Endosc. 2003;57:364–8.
18. Fujimoto T, Ohtsuka T, Nakashima Y, Gotoh Y, Date K, Mori Y, et al. Elevated bile amylase level without pancreaticobiliary maljunction is a risk factor for gallbladder carcinoma. J Hepatobiliary Pancreat Sci. 2017;24:103–8.
19. Peveretos P, Polydorou A, Golematis P, Golematis B. The role of the pancreatic enzymes in the pathogenesis of cholelithiasis. Mt Sinai J Med. 1988;55:369–73.
20. Sugiyama M, Atomi Y. Periampullary diverticula cause pancreatobiliary reflux. Scand J Gastroenterol. 2001;36:994–7.

Part IV
Diagnosis

Chapter 11
Diagnostic Criteria of Pancreaticobiliary Maljunction and Congenital Biliary Dilatation

Yoshinori Hamada

Abstract *Diagnostic Criteria of Pancreaticobiliary Maljunction*: Pancreaticobiliary maljunction is a congenital malformation in which the pancreatic and bile ducts join anatomically outside the duodenal wall. Pancreaticobiliary maljunction is diagnosed by either imaging test or anatomical examination. An abnormally long common channel and/or an abnormal union between the pancreatic and bile ducts must be evident on direct cholangiography such as ERCP, PTC, or intraoperative cholangiography, MRCP, or 3D-DIC-CT. The elevated amylase levels in bile and extrahepatic bile duct dilatation strongly suggest the existence of pancreaticobiliary maljunction.

Diagnostic Criteria of Congenital Biliary Dilatation: Congenital biliary dilatation is a congenital malformation involving both local dilatation of the extrahepatic bile duct, including the common bile duct, and pancreaticobiliary maljunction. However, cases associated with intrahepatic bile duct dilatation can be included in this entity. For a diagnosis of congenital biliary dilatation, both abnormal dilatation of the bile duct and pancreaticobiliary maljunction must be evident by either imaging or anatomical examination. Diagnosis of biliary dilatation must be established by using the diameter, site, and characteristic form of dilatation of the bile duct. Acquired or secondary dilatation of the bile duct, which is caused by obstruction due to biliary stones or malignancy, is strictly excluded.

Keywords Diagnostic criteria · Pancreaticobiliary maljunction · Congenital biliary dilatation · Choledochal cyst · Congenital malformation · Dilatation of the extrahepatic bile duct

---

Y. Hamada
Division of Pediatric Surgery, Department of Surgery, Kansai Medical University, Hirakata City, Osaka, Japan
e-mail: hamaday@hirakata.kmu.ac.jp

T. Kamisawa, H. Ando (eds.), *Pancreaticobiliary Maljunction and Congenital Biliary Dilatation*, https://doi.org/10.1007/978-981-10-8654-0_11

11.1 Introduction

Pancreaticobiliary maljunction is a congenital malformation in which the pancreatic and bile ducts join anatomically outside the duodenal wall. The diagnostic criteria for pancreaticobiliary maljunction [1] were proposed in Japanese in 1987, and the slightly revised English version [2] was published in 1994. The committee of The Japanese Study Group on Pancreaticobiliary Maljunction (JSGPM) for diagnostic criteria for pancreaticobiliary maljunction began to revise the diagnostic criteria in 2011, taking recently advanced diagnostic imaging techniques into consideration. The Japanese clinical practice guidelines for pancreaticobiliary maljunction [3] were published by JSGPM with the support of the Japan Biliary Association (JBA) in 2012. The final revised version of the diagnostic criteria for pancreaticobiliary maljunction was approved at the 36th Annual Meeting of JSGPM in 2013, and the diagnostic criteria for pancreaticobiliary maljunction 2013 [4] were published in 2014. In the diagnostic criteria, pancreaticobiliary maljunction was defined to include one type that is associated with bile duct dilatation (congenital biliary dilatation) and another that is not associated with bile duct dilatation (pancreaticobiliary maljunction without biliary dilatation).

However, definition of bile duct dilatation remained unclear. Thus, the committee of JSGPM for diagnostic criteria for pancreaticobiliary maljunction started to collect data about the mean diameter of the bile duct using ultrasonography (US) beginning in 2006 and established the standard diameter of the bile duct first in children in 2010 [5] and subsequently in adults in 2013 [6, 7]. Based on the standard bile duct diameter, a definition of dilatation of the bile duct was proposed in 2014 [8], and as a next step, the diagnostic criteria for congenital biliary dilatation was prepared by the committee of JSGPM in 2014. The final revised version was approved at the 38th Annual Meeting of JSGPM in 2015, and the diagnostic criteria for congenital biliary dilatation 2015 [9] were published in 2016. The Japanese clinical practice guidelines for congenital biliary dilatation [10] were published by JSGPM in 2017.

In this book, the original descriptions were referenced mostly to introduce both the diagnostic criteria of pancreaticobiliary maljunction [4] and the diagnostic criteria of congenital biliary dilatation [9], because each term and expression used in these diagnostic criteria express the exact meaning based on anatomical knowledge and long-standing clinical experiences.

11.2 Diagnostic Criteria of Pancreaticobiliary Maljunction [4]

11.2.1 Definition

Pancreaticobiliary maljunction is a congenital malformation in which the pancreatic and bile ducts join anatomically outside the duodenal wall.

11.2.2 Pathophysiology

In pancreaticobiliary maljunction, the duodenal papillary sphincter (sphincter of Oddi) fails to exert any influence on the pancreaticobiliary junction due to the abnormally long common channel. Therefore, reciprocal reflux between pancreatic juice and bile occurs, resulting in various pathologic conditions, such as inhibiting the excretion of bile and pancreatic juice and biliary cancer, in the biliary tract and pancreas.

Pancreaticobiliary maljunction is defined as a congenital malformation in which pancreatic and bile ducts meet anatomically outside the duodenal wall. Normally, at the duodenal papilla, the duodenal papillary sphincter surrounds the pancreaticobiliary junction from the end of the bile duct, and it regulates the flow of bile while preventing the reflux of pancreatic juices into the bile duct. However, in pancreaticobiliary maljunction, the common channel is longer than normal, which debilitates the effect of the sphincter on the pancreaticobiliary junction, allowing the reciprocal reflux of pancreatic juices and bile. The reflux of pancreatic juices into the biliary tract (pancreaticobiliary reflux) provokes higher rates of biliary tract cancer, and reflux of bile into the pancreatic duct (biliopancreatic reflux) may sometimes cause pancreatitis [1–3].

11.2.3 Diagnostic Criteria

Pancreaticobiliary maljunction is diagnosed by either imaging test or anatomical examination.

11.2.3.1 Imaging Diagnosis

(a) An abnormally long common channel and/or an abnormal union between the pancreatic and bile ducts must be evident on direct cholangiography, such as endoscopic retrograde cholangiopancreatography (ERCP), percutaneous transhepatic cholangiography (PTC), or intraoperative cholangiography; magnetic resonance cholangiopancreatography (MRCP); or three-dimensional drip infusion cholangiography computed tomography (3D-DIC-CT). However, in cases with a relatively short common channel, it is necessary to confirm that the effect of the papillary sphincter does not extend to the junction by direct cholangiography.

(b) Pancreaticobiliary maljunction can be diagnosed if the pancreaticobiliary junction outside the wall can be depicted by endoscopic ultrasonography (EUS) or multi-planar reconstruction (MPR) images provided by multi-detector row computed tomography (MD-CT).

11.2.3.2 Anatomical Diagnosis

It should be confirmed by surgery or autopsy that the pancreaticobiliary junction lies outside the duodenal wall or pancreatic and bile ducts unite abnormally.

11.2.4 Supplementary Diagnosis

The following findings strongly suggest the existence of pancreaticobiliary maljunction.

11.2.4.1 Elevated Amylase Levels in Bile

Pancreatic enzymes, especially amylase, in the bile within the bile duct and gallbladder obtained immediately after laparotomy, endoscopically or percutaneously are generally at extremely high levels. However, levels close to or below the normal serum value are occasionally observed in patients with pancreaticobiliary maljunction. Clinical features similar to pancreaticobiliary maljunction, including elevation of pancreatic enzymes in bile, are observed in some cases with a relatively long common channel, showing the effect of the sphincter on the pancreaticobiliary junction.

11.2.4.2 Extrahepatic Bile Duct Dilatation

Pancreaticobiliary maljunction includes one type that is associated with bile duct dilatation (congenital biliary dilatation) and another that is not (pancreaticobiliary maljunction without biliary dilatation). When cystic, fusiform, or cylindrical dilatation is detected in the extrahepatic bile duct, careful investigations are needed to determine whether pancreaticobiliary maljunction is present. Standard values for the maximum diameter of the common bile duct at each age are useful for diagnosing pancreaticobiliary maljunction with or without biliary dilatation.

11.3 Diagnostic Criteria of Congenital Biliary Dilatation [9]

11.3.1 Definition

Congenital biliary dilatation is a congenital malformation involving both local dilatation of the extrahepatic bile duct, including the common bile duct, and pancreaticobiliary maljunction. However, cases associated with intrahepatic bile duct dilatation can be included in this entity.

Congenital biliary dilatation has long been called "congenital choledochal cyst," which was classified into the three types by Alonso-Lej et al. [11] in 1959. Later, in 1977, Todani et al. [12] reported a new classification based on the Alonso-Lej's classification, and thus the new classification has been used worldwide. As congenital biliary dilatation has been widely known to be extremely highly associated with pancreaticobiliary maljunction, Todani [13, 14] remade his classification to include a concept of pancreaticobiliary maljunction in 1995. According to the accumulation of case reports on congenital biliary dilatation from around the world, it has been understood that most cases are classified as either type I with local dilatation of the common bile duct or as type IV-A, which is associated with involvement of the intrahepatic bile duct. In addition, it has been clarified that pancreaticobiliary maljunction is extremely highly associated with types Ia, Ic, and IV-A; however, it is almost never associated with types Ib, II, III, IV-B, and V.

11.3.2 Pathophysiology

Various kinds of pathological conditions, such as flow disturbances of bile and pancreatic juice, reciprocal reflux between bile and pancreatic juice, and malignancy of biliary systems, can occur in the hepatobiliary system and pancreas secondary to bile duct dilatation and pancreaticobiliary maljunction.

11.3.3 Diagnostic Criteria

For a diagnosis of congenital biliary dilatation, both abnormal dilatation of the bile duct and pancreaticobiliary maljunction must be evident by either imaging or anatomical examination. Acquired or secondary dilatation of the bile duct, which is caused by obstruction due to biliary stones or malignancy, is strictly excluded.

11.3.3.1 Diagnosis of Biliary Dilatation

Diagnosis of biliary dilatation must be established by using the diameter, site, and characteristic form of dilatation of the bile duct.

(a) *Diameter of the bile duct*
Measurement of the diameter of the bile duct must be obtained by nonpressure imaging modalities on the biliary system, such as ultrasonography, magnetic resonance cholangiopancreatography (MRCP), and computed tomography (CT including multi-planar reconstruction [MPR] images provided by multi-detector row computed tomography [MD-CT], etc.). The inner diameter of the most dilated site of the common bile duct must be estimated as the maximum diameter for the patient. The standard diameter of the bile duct, measured by ultrasonography, significantly correlates with age, and diagnosis of dilatation is considered based on the upper limit of bile duct diameter in each patient (Table 11.1).

(b) *Site of bile duct dilatation*
The common bile duct must be included as the site of bile duct dilatation. In addition, cases involving intrahepatic bile duct dilatation can be included in congenital biliary dilatation.

Table 11.1 Diagnosis of dilatation of the bile duct

Age	Standard value	Upper limit	Diagnosis of dilatation
0	1.5 mm	3.0 mm	3.1 mm~
1	1.7 mm	3.2 mm	3.3 mm~
2	1.9 mm	3.3 mm	3.4 mm~
3	2.1 mm	3.5 mm	3.6 mm~
4	2.3 mm	3.7 mm	3.8 mm~
5	2.4 mm	3.9 mm	4.0 mm~
6	2.5 mm	4.0 mm	4.1 mm~
7	2.7 mm	4.2 mm	4.3 mm~
8	2.9 mm	4.3 mm	4.4 mm~
9	3.1 mm	4.4 mm	4.5 mm~
10	3.2 mm	4.5 mm	4.6 mm~
11	3.3 mm	4.6 mm	4.7 mm~
12	3.4 mm	4.7 mm	4.8 mm~
13	3.5 mm	4.8 mm	4.9 mm~
14	3.6 mm	4.9 mm	5.0 mm~
15	3.7 mm	5.0 mm	5.1 mm~
16	3.7 mm	5.1 mm	5.2 mm~
17	3.7 mm	5.2 mm	5.3 mm~
18	3.8 mm	5.3 mm	5.4 mm~
19	3.8 mm	5.4 mm	5.5 mm~
20–29	3.9 mm	5.9 mm	6.0 mm~
30–39	3.9 mm	6.3 mm	6.4 mm~
40–49	4.3 mm	6.7 mm	6.8 mm~
50–59	4.6 mm	7.2 mm	7.3 mm~
60–69	4.9 mm	7.7 mm	7.8 mm~
70~	5.3 mm	8.5 mm	8.6 mm~

(c) *Form of bile duct dilatation*

Cystic dilatation and cylindrical (fusiform) dilatation of the common bile duct can be classified subjectively. Congenital biliary dilatation is expressed as Ia, Ic, and IV-A according to Todani's classification (Fig. 11.1).

As most cases of congenital biliary dilatation show the characteristic figures, as described below, diagnosis is recommended to reference these morphological characteristics [15–20].

1. Narrow segment at the duodenal side of the dilated common bile duct
2. Local dilatation at the base of the cystic duct in cases of intrahepatic involvement

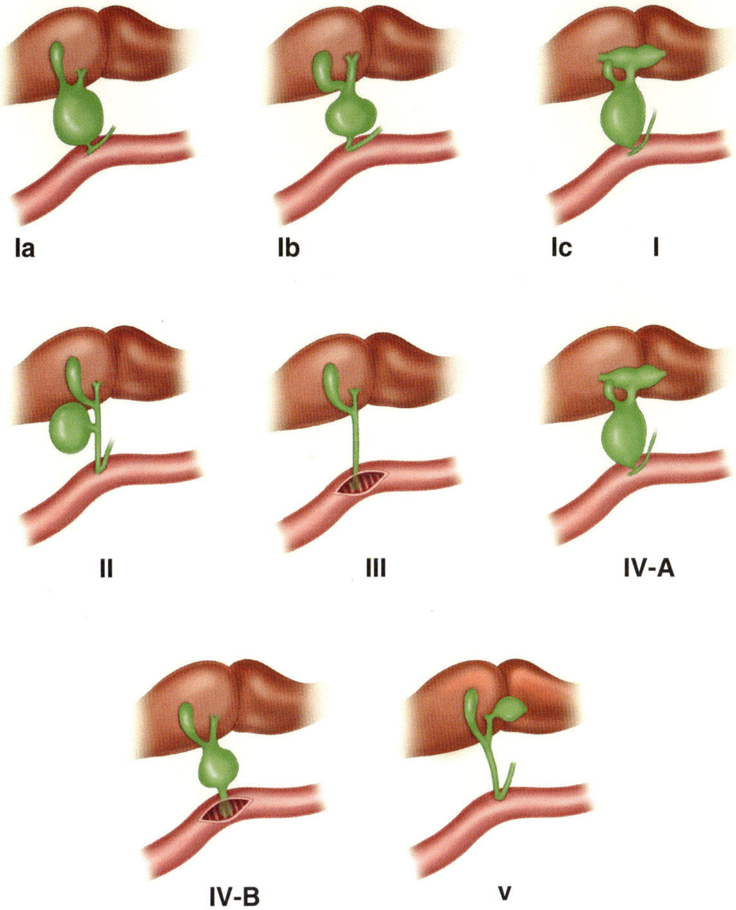

Fig. 11.1 Todani's Classification

3. Relative stenosis at the porta hepatis in cases of local intrahepatic involvement
4. Abrupt caliber change between the dilated intrahepatic bile duct and the peripheral bile duct

11.3.3.2 Diagnosis of Pancreaticobiliary Maljunction

Diagnosis of pancreaticobiliary maljunction is essential for diagnosis of congenital biliary dilatation, and it must be diagnosed strictly based on the diagnostic criteria for pancreaticobiliary maljunction 2013 [4].

11.3.4 Reference to Diagnosis

11.3.4.1 Suspicious Findings

These findings are suspicious for congenital biliary dilatation and are helpful for diagnosis [3].

1. Cystic lesion at the porta hepatis by prenatal ultrasonography
2. Intermittent direct bilirubinemia in newborns
3. Repeated attacks of abdominal pain since childhood
4. High amylase levels in serum or urine at a time of abdominal pain in childhood
5. Bile peritonitis due to idiopathic perforation of the biliary tract in childhood

11.3.4.2 Similar Medical Terms

These similar medical terms have been used; however, we recommend the term "congenital biliary dilatation."

1. Congenital bile duct dilatation (Todani [13])
2. Congenital choledochal cyst (Alonso-Lej et al. [11])
3. Choledochal cyst [20]

11.3.4.3 Measurement of Bile Duct Diameter

Diameter of the bile duct was measured to obtain standard value of the bile duct. The maximum inner diameter (integral value) of the common bile duct was measured using transabdominal US by routine right hypochondriac oblique scan under fasting condition. The frequency of the ultrasound probe ranged from 3.5 to 5 MHz. Cases with any history of hepatobiliary-pancreatic diseases or abnormal findings in the liver, biliary tract, and pancreas on US were excluded.

In children [5], a prospective, multicenter study was carried out from October 2005 to September 2008 in the eight institutions in Japan. In children (Fig. 11.2), maximum diameter of the common bile duct correlated significantly with age in months by polynomial expression degree 2 as follows: pediatric common bile duct $= 1.64 + 0.014\ \text{Month} - (3.26\ \text{e} - 5)\ (\text{Month} - 63.0)^2$. Mean diameters of the common bile duct were 2.4 mm at 5 years, 3.2 mm at 10 years, and 3.7 mm at 15 years. Upper limits of normal for the common bile duct were further calculated as 3.9, 4.5, and 5.0 mm, respectively. Mean diameter of the common bile duct also increased significantly with height and body weight. Diameter of the common bile duct thus increases in relation to body growth and is not expressed by one value in the pediatric population.

In adults [6], a prospective, multicenter study was carried out from October 2010 to April 2011 in the five institutions in Japan. In adults (Fig. 11.3), a mean diameter for the common bile duct was 4.5 ± 1.4 mm. The relationship between maximum diameter of the common bile duct and age was as follows: adult common bile

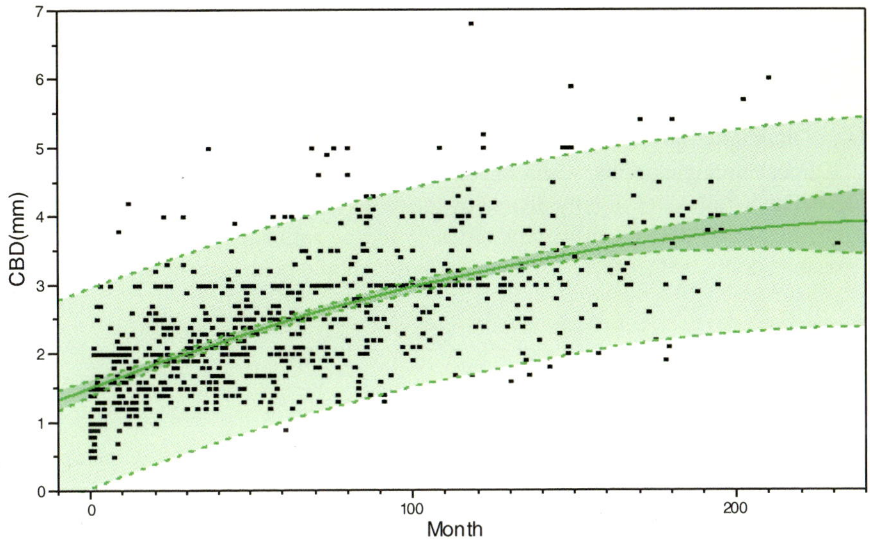

Fig. 11.2 Mean diameter of common bile duct in children

Fig. 11.3 Mean diameter of common bile duct in adults

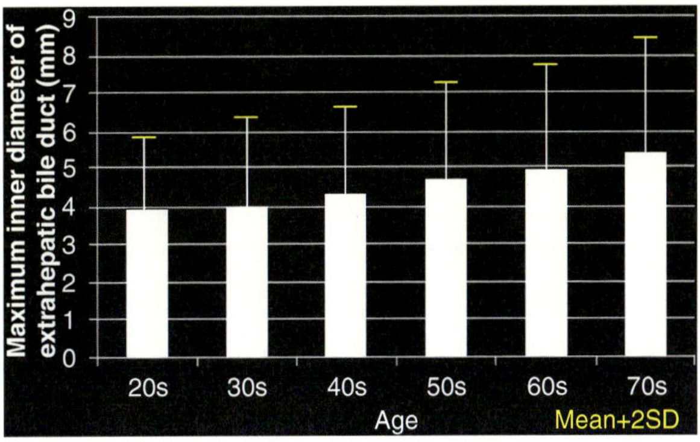

duct = 2.83 + 0.03 × age. In all age groups but the 20s and 30s, there was statistically significant maximum diameter of the common bile duct among each age group. Mean, mode value, and median diameter of the common bile duct increased with age as follows: 20s, 3.9 ± 1.0 mm; 30s, 3.9 ± 1.2 mm; 40s, 4.3 ± 1.2 mm; 50s, 4.6 ± 1.3 mm; 60s, 4.9 ± 1.4 mm; and >70s, 5.3 ± 1.6 mm.

As the standard diameter of the bile duct by US significantly correlates with age [5, 6], the standard values for maximum diameter of the common bile duct in each age will be useful for diagnosing PBM with or without biliary dilatation [7]. In children under 19 years old, upper limit of normal for the common bile duct was not calculated by standard value plus standard deviation × 2 but automatically expressed by the polynomial expression degree 2 graph [5]. In adults, upper limit was calculated by standard value plus standard deviation × 2 [6]. As a diagnosis of bile duct dilatation should be considered based on the upper limit of the bile duct diameter in each patient, diagnosis of dilatation of bile duct was defined as the value of 0.1 mm larger than upper limit in each age group [8] (Table 11.1).

Direct cholangiography, such as ERCP, PTC, and intraoperative cholangiography, can make the bile duct slightly dilated by the effect of increased intraductal pressure. Thus, measured data by these modalities would be estimated as provisional and a decision about whether there is dilatation or not should be done carefully.

References

1. The Japanese Study Group on Pancreaticobiliary Maljunction (JSGPM), Committee for Diagnostic Criteria for Pancreaticobiliary Maljunction. Diagnostic criteria of pancreaticobiliary maljunction (in Japanese). Tan to Sui. 1987;8:115–8.
2. The Japanese Study Group on Pancreaticobiliary Maljunction (JSPBM), The Committee of JSPBM for Diagnostic Criteria. Diagnostic criteria of pancreaticobiliary maljunction. J Heptobiliary Pancreat Surg. 1994;1:219–21.
3. Kamisawa T, Ando H, Suyama M, Shimada M, Morine Y, Shimada H, Working Committee of Clinical Practice Guidelines for Pancreaticobiliary Maljunction. Japanese clinical practice guidelines for pancreaticobiliary maljunction. J Gastroenterol. 2012;47:731–59.
4. Kamisawa T, Ando H, Hamada Y, Fujii H, Koshinaga T, Urushihara N, The Japanese Study Group on Pancreaticobiliary Maljunction, et al. Diagnostic criteria for pancreaticobiliary maljunction 2013. J Hepatobiliary Pancreat Sci. 2014;21:159–61.
5. Hamada Y, Takehara H, Ando H, Itoi T, Kamisawa T, Koshinaga T, et al. Definition of biliary dilatation based on the standard diameter of the bile duct in children (in Japanese). Tan to Sui. 2010;31:1269–72.
6. Itoi T, Kamisawa T, Fujii H, Inui K, Maguchi H, Hamada Y, et al. Extrahepatic bile duct measurement by using transabdominal ultrasound in Japanese adults: multi-center prospective study. J Gastroenterol. 2013;48:1045–50.
7. Kamisawa T, Ando H, Shimada M, Hamada Y, Itoi T, Takayashiki T, et al. Recent advances and problems in the management of pancreaticobiliary maljunction: feedback from the guidelines committee. J Hepatobiliary Pancreat Sci. 2014;21:87–92.
8. Hamada Y, Hamada H, Takahashi Y, Nakamura Y, Nakano T. Definition of congenital bile duct dilatation based on the standard diameter of the common bile duct (in Japanese). Tan to Sui. 2014;35:943–5.
9. Hamada Y, Ando H, Kamisawa T, Itoi T, Urushihara N, Koshinaga T, et al. Diagnostic criteria for congenital biliary dilatation 2015. J Hepatobiliary Pancreat Sci. 2016;23(6):342.
10. Ishibashi H, Shimada M, Kamisawa T, Fujii H, Hamada Y, Kubota M, et al. Japanese clinical practice guidelines for congenital biliary dilatation. J Hepatobiliary Pancreat Sci. 2017;24:1–16.
11. Alonso-Lej F, Rever WB Jr, Pessagno DJ. Congenital choledochal cyst, with a report of 2, and an analysis of 94, cases. Int Abstr Surg. 1959;108:1–30.
12. Todani T, Watanabe Y, Narusue M, Tabuchi K, Okajima K. Congenital bile duct cysts: classification, operative procedures, and review of thirty-seven cases including cancer arising from choledochal cyst. Am J Surg. 1977;134:263–9.
13. Todani T. Definition and classification of congenital bile duct dilatation (in Japanese). Tan to Sui. 1995;16:715–7.

14. Todani T. Congenital choledochal dilatation: classification, clinical features, and long-term results. J Hepato-Biliary-Pancreat Surg. 1997;4:276–82.
15. Ando H, Ito T, Sugito T. Histological study of the choledochal cyst wall (in Japanese). Nippon Shokakibyo Gakkai zasshi. 1987;84:1797–801.
16. Fujii H. Variations of the union between the terminal bile duct and the pancreatic duct in patients with pancreaticobiliary maljunction. Yamanashi Med J. 2003;18:67–75.
17. Matsumoto Y, Fujii H, Itakura J, Matsuda M, Nobukawa B, Suda K. Recent advances in pancreaticobiliary maljunction. J Hepato-Biliary-Pancreat Surg. 2002;9:45–54.
18. Hosomura N, Fujii H, Amemiya H, Kawaida H, Kohno H, Shiba S, et al. Clinical definition and diagnosis of congenital bile duct dilatation (in Japanese). Tan to Sui. 2010;31:1273–8.
19. Matsumoto Y, Fujii H, Yoshioka M, Sekikawa T, Wada T, Yamamoto M, et al. Biliary strictures as a cause of primary intrahepatic bile duct stones. World J Surg. 1986;10:867–75.
20. Ando H, Ito T, Kaneko K, Seo T. Congenital stenosis of the intrahepatic bile duct associated with choledochal cysts. J Am Coll Surg. 1995;181:426–30.

Chapter 12
Role of Ultrasonography for the Diagnosis of Pancreaticobiliary Maljunction and Congenital Biliary Dilatation

Keiji Hanada, Akinori Shimizu, and Tomoyuki Minami

Abstract PBM is one of the anomalous conditions in which the bile duct and the pancreatic duct merge outside the duodenal wall, which causes continuous pancreaticobiliary reflux (PR). PBM is classified into two groups as follows: PBM with biliary dilatation (congenital biliary dilatation, CBD) and PBM without dilatation. US must be the best method for the diagnosis of PBM associated with CBD, revealing extrahepatic or intrahepatic bile duct dilatation. In adults, the maximum inner diameter of extrahepatic bile duct (MDEBD) was recently reported. MDEBD positively correlated with age. In cases of PBM without bile duct dilatation, thickening of the gallbladder wall as a characteristic sonographic feature has been reported. Hyperplastic changes with increased cell proliferation in gallbladder mucosa induced by PR could reflect as thickening of the gallbladder. A high confluence of pancreaticobiliary ducts (HCPBD) has been defined as a disease state. In HCPBD cases, PR and hyperplastic changes in gallbladder were observed. US is an important image modality to give clues to the diagnosis in cases with PBM, CBD, and HCPBD, because it can reveal sonographic characteristics such as gallbladder wall thickening and/or mild dilatation of the extrahepatic bile duct.

Keywords Ultrasonography · Pancreaticobiliary maljunction · Congenital biliary dilatation · Biliary cancer · Wall thickness of gallbladder

12.1 Introduction

Recent advances in image diagnosis, particularly magnetic resonance cholangiopancreatography (MRCP), have increased chances of detecting pancreaticobiliary maljunction (PBM). PBM is one of the anomalous conditions in which the bile duct and the pancreatic duct merge outside the duodenal wall, which causes continuous

K. Hanada (✉) · A. Shimizu · T. Minami
Department of Gastroenterology, Onomichi General Hospital, Onomichi, Japan
e-mail: kh-ajpbd@nifty.com

T. Kamisawa, H. Ando (eds.), *Pancreaticobiliary Maljunction and Congenital Biliary Dilatation*, https://doi.org/10.1007/978-981-10-8654-0_12

pancreaticobiliary reflux (PR) [1]. PBM is classified into two groups as follows: PBM with biliary dilatation (congenital biliary dilatation, CBD) and PBM without dilatation [2].

It has been reported that refluxed pancreatic juice into the biliary tract injures the mucosal epithelium of the biliary tract and may promote the carcinogenesis of the biliary tract. In PBM, a hyperplasia-dysplasia-carcinoma sequence induced by chronic inflammation caused by PR has been suspected in the carcinogenesis of biliary tract [3]. It has been reported that thickening of the gallbladder wall reflecting epithelial hyperplasia was frequently found in cases of PBM [1]. The clinical practice guidelines for the management of biliary tract cancers edited by the Japanese Society of Hepato-Biliary-Pancreatic Surgery reported that PBM is one of the important risk factors of biliary tract carcinoma [4].

In congenital biliary dilatation (CBD), it has been known that most adult cases of CBD are associated with PBM. PBM detected in childhood in many cases is associated with bile duct dilatation; pediatric cases of PBM without biliary dilatation are rare [5]. For the diagnosis of PBM, a long common channel or an abnormal union between the bile duct and the pancreatic duct should be approved.

Ultrasonography (US) is a noninvasive imaging modality for screening of pancreaticobiliary diseases. It has been reported that US must be the best method for the diagnosis of PBM associated with CBD, revealing extrahepatic or intrahepatic bile duct dilatation [6]. However, the accurate diagnosis of PBM may be limited by only using US in cases of PBM. MRCP, endoscopic US (EUS), or endoscopic retrograde cholangiopancreatography (ERCP) should be needed to confirm diagnosis of PBM [6]. In cases of PBM without bile duct dilatation, thickening of the gallbladder wall as a characteristic sonographic feature has been reported. US could give clues to diagnosis in these cases.

In this article, we would like to review roles of US in diagnosis of PBM.

12.2 Japanese Clinical Practice Guidelines for PBM and CBD

The Japanese Study Group on Pancreaticobiliary Maljunction (JSGPM) established a PBM clinical practice guidelines on how to deal with PBM, with support of the Japan Biliary Association (JBA) in 2012 [1]. And, the Japanese Study Group on Congenital Biliary Dilatation (JSCBD) also established a CBD clinical guideline on how to deal with CBD [7]. In these guidelines, clinical questions (CQs) about effectiveness of US for diagnosis of PBM and CBD were considered. Figure 12.1 demonstrates statements for these questions. These two clinical guidelines recommend that US is a simple and noninvasive form of imaging, and it is a vital and useful screening method of the age of case [1, 7, 8]. They also indicate that the thickening of the hypoechoic inner layer of the gallbladder is one of the important image findings in the initial diagnosis of PBM or CBD (Fig. 12.2) [1, 7].

Guidelines for CBD

Is ultrasound effective in CBD screening?

- US detects the dilatation of the common bile duct, intrahepatic bile duct and the thickening of the hypoechoic inner layer of the gallbladder, presenting the first opportunity to diagnose CBD.
- It is useful to screen for CBD and implemention is recommended.

Guidelines for PBM

What is the role of US in diagnosing PBM?

- US is useful to screen for PBM.
- Detecting dilatation of the common bile duct and/or intrahepatic bile duct by US may be the first opportunity to diagnose CBD.
- A thickening of the hypoechoic inner layer of the gallbladder wall may be fundamental for the diagnosis PBM without dilatation.

Fig. 12.1 Statements of Japanese clinical practical guidelines for congenital biliary dilatation and pancreaticobiliary maljunction

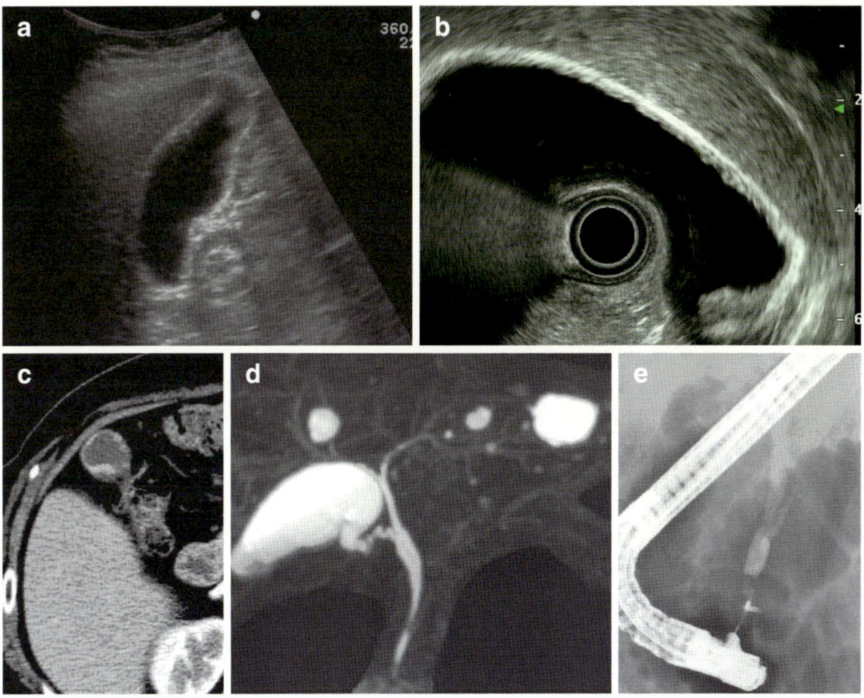

Fig. 12.2 A case of PBM without dilatation of the common bile duct (51 years old, female). The gallbladder wall thickening in the inner layer was detected in US (**a**) and EUS (**b**). Enhanced CT demonstrated the gallbladder wall thickening (**c**). MRCP suspected the presence of PBM (**d**). Finally, ERCP demonstrated the PBM without dilatation of the common bile duct (**e**)

12.3 Clues for Diagnosis of PBM and CBD

12.3.1 Dilatation of Common Bile Duct

In both adult and pediatric patients, dilatation of the common bile duct is one of the important image findings for diagnosis of PBM. US must be a simple and useful screening modality. When conducting an US on patients without jaundice, and severe cystic dilatation of the common bile duct is observed, CBD should be suspected [7]. In comparison to dilatation of the bile duct associated with biliary occlusion because of choledocholithiasis or malignant tumor, the dilatation of the bile duct in CBD is characterized with sudden transition to a normal-sized bile duct [7].

In adults, less than 10-mm bile duct has been recognized as "non-dilated bile duct" though there was no obvious evidence. Recently, Itoi et al. have reported the maximum inner diameter of extrahepatic bile duct (MDEBD) of Japanese adults by using transabdominal US in a multicenter prospective study [9]. The relationship between the MDEBD and age was as follows: MDEBD = 2.83 + 0.03 × age. Mean, mode value, and median MDEBD is increasing according to the age as follows: 20s, 3.9 ± 1.0 mm; 30s, 3.9 ± 1.2 mm; 40s, 4.3 ± 1.2 mm; 50s, 4.6 ± 1.3 mm; 60s, 4.9 ± 1.4 mm; and >70s, 5.3 ± 1.6 mm. These results suggested that MDEBD positively correlated with age. In PBM, whether the extrahepatic bile duct demonstrates dilatation or not is very important when considering prophylactic bile duct resection to avoid the acquired bile duct cancer [9]. Precise definition of "dilated bile duct" in each age may be able to lead to decrease of bile duct cancers after cholecystectomy in cases with PBM without biliary dilatation.

12.3.2 Wall Thickening of Gallbladder

According to a nationwide study in Japan, biliary cancer was found in 21.6% of adult cases with CBD and 42.4% of adult PBM cases without biliary dilatation [10]. The location ratio of cancers in bile duct and gallbladder were 32.1% and 62.3% in CBD and 7.3% and 88.1% in PBM cases without biliary dilatation.

The mechanism of carcinogenesis in PBM cases may be related to continuous PR into the biliary tract. Some activated proteolytic pancreatic enzymes in the biliary tract may produce cytotoxic substances and induce chronic inflammation leading repeated cycles of damage and regeneration in the biliary mucosa [3, 11, 12]. These observations in the biliary mucosa in conjunction with *K-ras* mutations and increased cell proliferation may promote biliary cancer. A sequence of hyperplasia-dysplasia-carcinoma is considered in the development of biliary cancers in PBM cases [12, 13]. Mutation of suppressor gene *p53* and microsatellite instability may be regarded as a late event in carcinogenesis in PBM cases [14, 15]. *Bcl-2* expression and increased telomerase activity in the gallbladder mucosa of PBM cases were also reported [16]. The gallbladder mucosa was significantly higher in PBM cases than in healthy control cases and can be considered to represent a premalignant region [3, 11] (Fig. 12.3).

Recently, a high confluence of pancreaticobiliary ducts (HCPBD) has been defined as a disease state in which the common channel length is more than 6 mm and

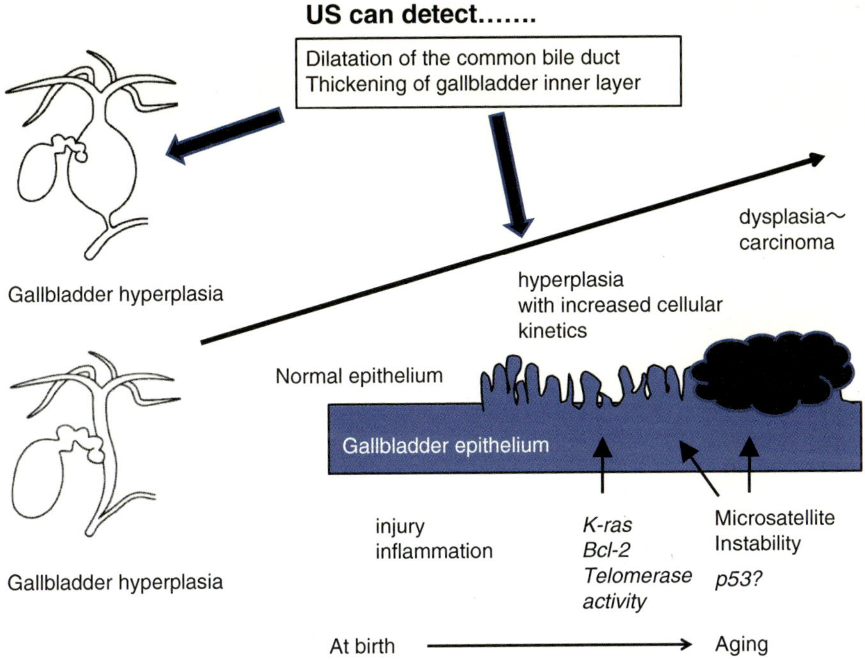

Fig. 12.3 Role of US for the diagnosis of PBM

communication is occluded during contraction of the sphincter [17]. In HCPBD cases, PR and hyperplastic changes in gallbladder mucosa cancer were also observed (Fig. 12.4). Gallbladder cancer was observed in 12% of HCPBD cases. Similar to PBM cases, *K-ras* mutation and increased cell proliferation were reported in gallbladder mucosa with HCPBD [18, 19]. Although the risk is lower than that in relation to PBM and CBD, HCPBD could be considered as an important risk factor for the development of gallbladder cancer. The hyperplastic change in gallbladder mucosa in PBM, CBD, and HCPBD reflects as a thickening of the hypoechoic inner layer by US.

These observations strongly suggest that US is an important image modality to give clues to the diagnosis in cases with PBM, CBD, and HCPBD, because it can reveal sonographic characteristics such as gallbladder wall thickening and/or mild dilatation of the extrahepatic bile duct.

12.4 Role of US for Diagnosis of PBM Cases in Routine Medical Checkup

Yamao et al. reported an interesting prospective study about the routine medical checkup for PBM cases. Of the 27,076 subjects who underwent US, gallbladder wall thickening or dilatation of the common bile duct is found in 2466 cases (9.1%). EUS and ERCP were actually performed in 333 and 22 cases; PBM was finally detected in 9 cases, yielding a detection rate of 0.03%. Gallbladder cancer was detected in one case [20].

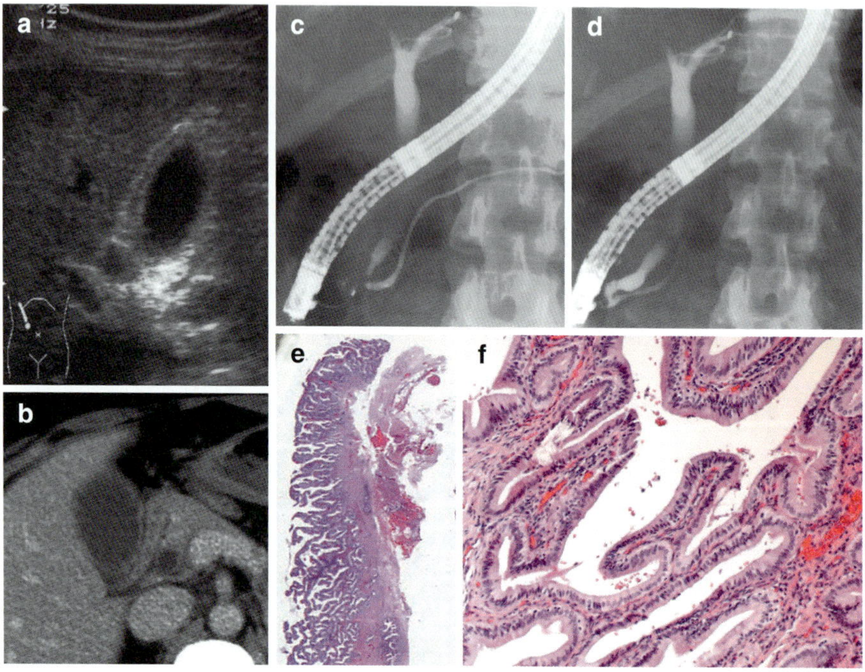

Fig. 12.4 A case of HCPBD without dilatation of the common bile duct (31 years old, female). The gallbladder wall thickening in the inner layer was detected in US (**a**) and enhanced CT (**b**). A cholangiopancreatography was obtained from a long common channel using an ERCP catheter (**c**). After removing a catheter, pancreaticobiliary reflux was detected via a long common channel during sphincter relaxation (**d**). Hyperplastic change was found in the gallbladder mucosa (**e**, **f**)

Early detection of PBM/CBD and concomitant gallbladder cancer could be achieved by a serial examination of US, EUS, MRCP, and ERCP in asymptomatic patients.

12.5 Conclusions

US is the best screening method for the diagnosis of PBM, CBD, HCPBD revealing extrahepatic and/or intrahepatic bile duct dilatation, and gallbladder wall thickening.

References

1. Kamisawa T, Ando H, Suyama M, et al. Japanese clinical practice guidelines for pancreaticobiliary maljunction. J Gastroenterol. 2012;47:731–59.
2. Kamisawa T, Ando H, Shimada M, et al. Recent advances and problems in the management of pancreaticobiliary maljunction: feedback from the guidelines committee. J Hepatobiliary Pancreat Sci. 2014;21:87–92.

3. Hanada K, Itoh M, Fujii K, et al. Pathology and cellular kinetics of gallbladder with an anomalous junction of pancreaticobiliary duct. Am J Gastroenterol. 1996;91:1007–11.
4. Miyazaki M, Yoshitomi H, Miyakawa S, et al. Clinical practice guidelines for the management of biliary tract cancers 2015: the 2nd English edition. J Hepatobiliary Pancreat Sci. 2015;22:249–73.
5. Ando H, Ito T, Nagaya M, et al. Pancreaticobiliary maljunction without choledochal cyst in infants and children: clinical features and surgical therapy. J Pediatr Surg. 1995;30:1358–663.
6. Yamao K, Nakamura T, Suzuki T, et al. The diagnosis of pancreaticobiliary maljunction. In: Koyanagi K, Aoki T, editors. Pancreaticobiliary maljunction. Tokyo: Igakutosho; 2002. p. 39–46.
7. Ishibashi H, Shimada M, Kamisawa T, et al. Japanese clinical practice guidelines for congenital biliary dilatation. J Hepatobiliary Pancreat Sci. 2017;24:1–16.
8. Sugai M, Ishido K, Endoh M, et al. Sonographic demonstration of wall thickness of the gallbladder in pediatric patients with pancreatico-biliary maljunction. J Hepatobiliary Pancreat Sci. 2010;17:345–8.
9. Itoi T, Kamisawa T, Fujii H, et al. Extrahepatic bile duct measurement by using transabdominal ultrasound in Japanese adults: multi-center prospective study. J Gastroenterol. 2013;48:1045–50.
10. Morine Y, Shimada M, Takamatsu H, et al. Clinical features of pancreaticobiliary maljunction: update analysis of 2nd Japan-nationwide survey. J Hepato-Biliary-Pancreat Surg. 2013;20:472–80.
11. Kamisawa T, Kuruma S, Tabata T, et al. Pancreaticobiliary maljunction and biliary cancer. J Gastroenterol. 2015;50:273–9.
12. Hanada K, Tsuchida A, Kajiyama G. Cellular kinetic and gene mutations in gallbladder mucosa with an anomalous junction of pancreaticobiliary duct. J Hepato-Biliary-Pancreat Surg. 1996;6:223–8.
13. Hanada K, Tsuchida A, Iwao T, et al. Gene mutations of K-ras in gallbladder mucosae and gallbladder carcinoma with an anomalous junction of the pancreaticobiliary duct. Am J Gastroenterol. 1999;94:1638–42.
14. Nagai M, Watanabe M, Iwase T, et al. Clinical and genetic analysis of noncancerous and cancerous biliary epithelium in patients with pancreaticobiliary maljunction. World J Surg. 2002;26:91–8.
15. Hanada K, Itoh M, Fujii K, et al. K-ras and p35 mutations in stage I gallbladder carcinoma with an anomalous junction of the pancreaticobiliary duct. Cancer. 1996;77:452–8.
16. Ichikawa Y, Kamiyama M, Sekido H, et al. Telomerase activity and Bcl-2 expression in gallbladder of pancreaticobiliary maljunction patients: a preliminary study. J Hepato-Biliary-Pancreat Surg. 2004;11:34–9.
17. Kamisawa T, Amemiya K, Tu Y, et al. Clinical significance of a long common channel. Pancreatology. 2002;2:122–8.
18. Itoi T, Tsuchida A, Itokawa F, et al. Histologic and genetic analysis of the gallbladder in patients with occult pancreatobiliary reflux. Int J Mol Med. 2005;15:425–30.
19. Kamisawa T, Kuruma S, Chiba K, et al. Biliary carcinogenesis in pancreaticobiliary maljunction. J Gastroenterol. 2017;52:158–63.
20. Yamao K, Mizutani S, Nakazawa S, et al. Prospective study of the detection of anomalous connection of pancreaticobiliary ducts during routine medical exanimations. Hepato-Gastroenterology. 1996;43:1238–45.

Chapter 13
Significance of ERCP for the Diagnosis and Treatment of Pancreaticobiliary Maljunction and Congenital Biliary Dilatation

Takeshi Saito and Hideo Yoshida

Abstract The advantages of performing ERCP in patients with pancreaticobiliary maljunction (PBM) or congenital biliary dilatation (CBD) lie in the clear depiction of the pancreaticobiliary junction, precise understanding of the dynamic function of the sphincter muscle, bile collection or biopsy if needed, and possible transition from the diagnostic to therapeutic approach. On the other hand, the drawbacks include its invasiveness, causing incidental pancreatitis, infection and perforation, radiation exposure, and cardiorespiratory morbidity associated with deep sedation and general anesthesia. The choice of including ERCP in the diagnostic workup greatly depends on the age of patients, along with consideration of the likelihood of occurrence of biliary carcinoma, diagnostic value of other imaging modalities, vulnerability to the invasiveness of ERCP, requirement of endoscopic therapeutic measures, and the need for sedation or general anesthesia during ERCP. Experienced endoscopists can satisfactorily perform both pediatric and adult ERCP with excellent visualization rates of the pancreaticobiliary junction, along with almost little major adverse events. However, since the combination of MRCP and intraoperative cholangiopancreatography (IOCP) can achieve superior visualization rates of the intrahepatic bile duct (IHBD) and determination of the subtype of common bile duct, and comparable results as ERCP for PBM in pediatric subjects, the indications for preoperative ERCP should be carefully considered, especially in small children.

Keywords Children · Choledochal cyst · Congenital biliary dilatation · Drip infusion cholangiography with computed tomography · Endoscopic retrograde cholangiopancreatography · Intraoperative cholangiopancreatography · Magnetic resonance cholangiopancreatography · Pancreaticobiliary maljunction · Pancreatitis Pediatric

---

T. Saito (✉) · H. Yoshida
Department of Pediatric Surgery (E6), Graduate School of Medicine, Chiba University, Chiba City, Chiba, Japan
e-mail: takk@faculty.chiba-u.jp

T. Kamisawa, H. Ando (eds.), *Pancreaticobiliary Maljunction and Congenital Biliary Dilatation*, https://doi.org/10.1007/978-981-10-8654-0_13

Abbreviations

CBD	Congenital biliary dilatation
DIC-CT	Drip infusion cholangiography with computed tomography
ERCP	Endoscopic retrograde cholangiopancreatography
HCPBD	High confluence of pancreaticobiliary ducts
IHBD	Intrahepatic bile duct
IOCP	Intraoperative cholangiopancreatography
MRCP	Magnetic resonance cholangiopancreatography
PD	Pancreatic duct
PBM	Pancreaticobiliary maljunction

13.1 Points of Focus of the Pancreaticobiliary System for the Diagnosis and Treatment of PBM or CBD

Various imaging modalities are used to assess pancreaticobiliary anatomy and identify the characteristic features of PBM or CBD. These features include intra- and extrahepatic biliary dilatations, intrahepatic biliary strictures, a narrow segment of the lower common bile duct, and extraordinarily long common channel or complicated pancreaticobiliary anatomy (Fig. 13.1). Moreover, additional valuable

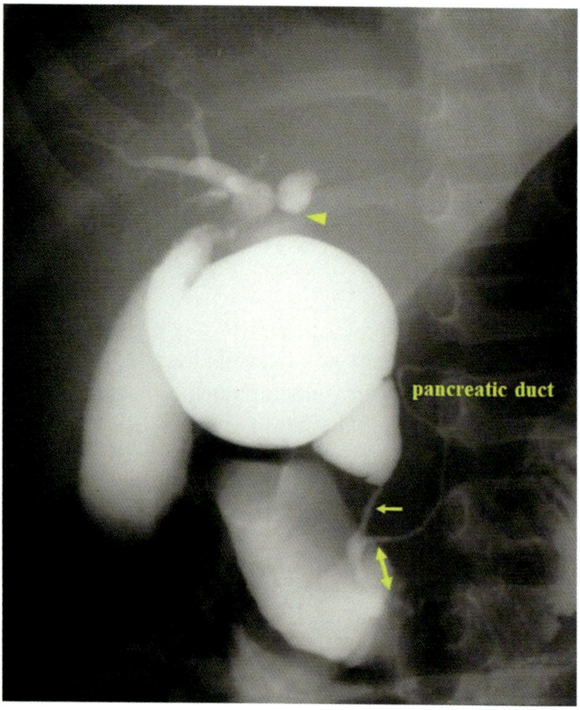

Fig. 13.1 ERCP image in a 10-year-old female with cystic-type congenital biliary dilatation (CBD) showing intrahepatic biliary dilatation associated with hepatic duct strictures (*arrow head*), a narrow segment of the lower common bile duct (*arrow*), and pancreaticobiliary maljunction (PBM) (*double arrow*)

information on coexisting biliary pathologies, including concomitant biliary cancer, pancreaticobiliary stones, and protein plugs can be obtained. The guidelines for PBM published in 2012 [1] and for CBD in 2016 [2] stressed the importance of direct cholangiography, including ERCP, to delineate details of the pancreaticobiliary junction. However, based on the fact that 1018 of 2529 patients with PBM registered in the Japanese nationwide survey from 1990 to 2007 were pediatric patients [3], the selection of diagnostic imaging modalities should consider not only the comparative advantages of each modality but also their possible age-dependent adverse events.

13.2 Significance of ERCP in the Diagnosis and Treatment of PBM or CBD

The most striking feature of ERCP is its ability to depict detailed anatomy of the pancreaticobiliary junction and to assess dynamic functioning of the sphincter muscle regulating the connection between the biliary and pancreatic ducts by its contraction and relaxation. The diagnosis of PBM requires demonstration of an abnormally long common channel between the common bile duct and pancreatic duct converging outside the duodenal wall, or their complicated communication, allowing bidirectional reflux, with flow of bile into the pancreatic duct and pancreatic juice into the bile duct. Direct cholangiography, including ERCP, was recommended for the definitive diagnosis of PBM in 2012 guideline [1]. However, in view of recent technological advances in imaging and their increasing clinical use, revised diagnostic criteria indicate several other imaging modalities that can also be used [4].

The biliary and pancreatic ducts drain into the duodenum either separately or via a common channel. Previous studies demonstrated that a common channel is present in 55–82% of the normal population [5–7], as reported in autopsy studies or using resected materials. On the other hand, a prospective ERCP study on the relationship between the formation of the common channel and the incidence of pancreaticobiliary diseases revealed that 63% of adult subjects had two separate orifices for the common bile duct and pancreatic duct, without a common channel [8]. Reportedly, the length of the common channel ranges variously from 1 mm to 12 mm (mean, 4.4 mm) [9], from 1.2 mm to 8.4 mm (4.4 mm) [5], and from 3 mm to 5 mm [10]. Even though the length of the common channel, as assessed by direct cholangiography in 184 PBM patients with an average age of 41 years, was suggested to be 16.2 ± 6.9 mm [11], questions remain regarding whether the length of the common channel, as measured on cholangiography, might be affected by the choice of diagnostic procedure, such as ERCP, percutaneous transhepatic cholangiography, intraoperative cholangiography, and T- or C-tube cholangiography, the posture of the patient, or by age in children.

Recently, the concept of high confluence of pancreaticobiliary ducts (HCPBD) was introduced in the adult setting, with subjects being found to have a relatively long common channel (defined as >6 mm in the original study [12]), where reciprocal reflux can occur during relaxation of the sphincter, while the communication is occluded during its contraction. Adult patients with HCPBD were reported to have similar potential for malignancy of the gallbladder as those with PBM but with different clinical features [1]. ERCP is considered to be the most effective way of distinguishing PBM from HCPBD. The significance of HCPBD in the pediatric population, however, remains to be investigated.

Even though the empirical definition of a dilated common bile duct, whose diameter is >10 mm in adults and >6 mm in children, was used, standard values of the diameter of the common bile duct measured by US have been established, thereby helping to diagnose CBD and PBM with and without biliary dilatation [13]. Determining the actual diameter of the biliary duct by ERCP undoubtedly causes overestimation of the dilatation due to further distension by the large volume of contrast medium injected. Although PBM without biliary dilatation is associated with a higher incidence of gallbladder cancer [1] and is a topic of interest, standardization of the choice of the imaging modality that should be used for its diagnosis has not been established.

CBD subtypes (cystic or fusiform), presence of associated intrahepatic bile duct (IHBD) stenosis or dilatation, length of the distal narrow segment, and presence of biliary variants can be confirmed by ERCP. However, filling the extra- and intrahepatic duct sufficiently with the contrast medium should be avoided because of concerns of ERCP-related adverse events, particularly among patients with huge cystic-type CBDs who require large amounts of contrast medium to depict the entire pancreaticobiliary image.

In adult patients with PBM or CBD, endoscopic ultrasonography or intraductal ultrasonography is sometimes performed following ERCP, in order to definitively diagnose PBM or biliary tract cancer [4]. Although the usefulness of these imaging modalities has been reported in previous studies, they are not performed at all centers due to the associated technical difficulties. In addition, the relatively low incidence of associated biliary cancer among pediatric populations with PBM or CBD [1, 3] does not justify the routine use of these technically advanced endoscopic procedures.

Protein plugs, which are reportedly associated with abdominal pain, vomiting, icterus, and occasionally perforation of the biliary tract among patients with PBM or CBD, are seen on ERCP as radiolucent filling defects in the dilated common channel [14]. They can be mistakenly interpreted as inadvertent air injection during ERCP or can make visualization of the PBM by ERCP via major duodenal papillae more difficult due to the protein plug preventing the contrast medium from filling the pancreaticobiliary system. In the latter situations, ERCP via minor accessory papillae can be effective in delineating detailed pancreaticobiliary anatomy, including PBM [15].

Despite its relative invasiveness, the use of ERCP in the diagnostic workup of adult PBM or CBD cases is acceptable, given the fact that the incidence of biliary tract cancer in association with CBD and PBM without biliary dilatation is reportedly 21.6% and 42.4%, respectively, in a Japanese nationwide survey [3] including 1511 adult patients. On the other hand, since only nine pediatric cases of biliary tract cancer have been reported so far in Japan [1], the acceptability of ERCP eventually depends on the age of patients with PBM or CBD.

A systematic survey of prospective studies reported the occurrence rate of ERCP-related adverse events at 6.85%, including pancreatitis in 3.47%, bleeding in 1.34%, infection in 1.44%, perforation in 0.60%, cardiovascular and/or analgesia-related complications in 1.33%, and mortality in 0.33% of cases [16]. Of note, these ERCP-related complications included those caused by both diagnostic and therapeutic ERCP. In terms of ERCP-related pancreatitis, the 2015 guidelines for acute pancreatitis indicated a complication rate of 0.4–5.6% for diagnostic ERCP and of 3.1–5.4% for therapeutic ERCP [17]. Through our experience with 235 ERCP procedures (227 diagnostic, 8 therapeutic) in 220 pediatric patients, including 92 with PBM or CBD, post-ERCP hyperamylasemia occurred in 9.4% of the patients [18], which resolved with the administration of protein synthesis inhibitors. In patients with PBM or CBD, hyperamylasemia or pancreatitis after ERCP can sometimes occur partly because of the pathophysiology of the pancreaticobiliary anomaly.

13.3 Results of ERCP for PBM or CBD

Visualization rates for each pancreaticobiliary site in adult patients with PBM or CBD have not been demonstrated in detail, perhaps because endoscopists rarely find it difficult to cannulate the papillae and obtain anatomical information regarding the different pancreaticobiliary sites.

On the other hand, several articles dealing with pediatric patients with PBM or CBD referred to the success rates of ERCP cannulation and the visualization rates of specific pancreaticobiliary features. Our group reported a 99% success rate of cannulation in 102 attempts in 92 pediatric CBD patients with a median age of 3 years (56 days to 20 years) [18]. Of note, we experienced cannulation failure in only one patient, who was a 59-day-old infant with large cystic-type CBD. We also demonstrated visualization rates of the PBM, pancreatic duct (PD), common bile duct, and IHBD of 82%, 95%, 77%, and 32%, respectively, among small children with PBM or CBD (Table 13.1) [19], while Hiramatsu et al. revealed rates of 91%, 97%, 94%, and 67%, respectively, among 63 pediatric cases [20]. These disparities could be due to the differences in catheter cannulation techniques, volume of contrast medium injected into the pancreaticobiliary system, definition of successful depiction of each site, and ratio between cystic and fusiform types of CBD in the studies.

In terms of the visualization rates according to the subtype of CBD, more satisfactory results for visualization of the PBM, PD, common bile duct, and IHBD of 90%, 100%, 97%, and 65%, respectively, are obtained in cases of fusiform CBD, as compared to visualization rates of 73%, 91%, 69%, and 16%, respectively, for

Table 13.1 Visualization rates for pancreaticobiliary sites in pediatric CBD patients by each imaging modality

	PBM (%)	PD (%)	Common bile duct (%)	IHBD (%)
ERCP	82	95	77	32
MRCP	57	64	100	100
DIC-CT	25	21	75	90
IOCP	87	87	100	100
MRCP+IOCP	89	91	100	100

CBD congenital biliary dilatation, *DIC-CT* drip infusion cholangiography with computed tomography, *ERCP* endoscopic retrograde cholangiopancreatography, *IHBD* intrahepatic bile duct, *IOCP* intraoperative cholangiopancreatography, *MRCP* magnetic resonance cholangiopancreatography, *PBM* pancreaticobiliary maljunction, *PD* pancreatic duct

cystic-type CBD [18]. It is true that in cystic-type CBD, the entire biliary tree, including the intra- and extrahepatic biliary duct, can be opacified if a large amount of contrast medium is injected, although this would increase the risk of some of the ERCP-related adverse events mentioned above.

13.4 Comparison of Visualization Rates of Specific Pancreaticobiliary Sites Between Different Imaging Modalities in Pediatric PBM or CBD

In the diagnostic workup of PBM or CBD, the ability to depict the pancreaticobiliary junction is often used to compare efficacies between different imaging modalities. Previous reports pointed out the visualization rates of PBM in adult patients at 82–100% and in pediatric ones at 40–80% by MRCP [1], showing its comparable or inferior rates to ERCP. However, based on the notable anatomical features mentioned above for the diagnosis and treatment of PBM or CBD, other pancreaticobiliary sites besides the pancreaticobiliary junction also need to be explored and compared when determining visualization by different imaging modalities. Thus, our group compared the usefulness of MRCP, ERCP, and drip infusion cholangiography with computed tomography (DIC-CT) and intraoperative cholangiopancreatography (IOCP) when visualizing not only the PBM but also the PD, common bile duct, and IHBD in pediatric CBD patients [19] (Table 13.1). In particular, since we (pediatric surgeons) routinely perform IOCP during radical surgery for PBM or CBD, it needs to be included in comparisons and evaluations. As shown in Table 13.1, ERCP and IOCP achieved significantly higher visualization rates of PBM than MRCP or DIC-CT. ERCP achieved a significantly higher visualization rate of the PD than MRCP or DIC-CT, while showing a comparable rate as IOCP. Additionally, the visualization rate of the common bile duct by MRCP or IOCP was excellent at 100%, which is higher than by ERCP or DIC-CT. Regarding the depiction of the IHBD, ERCP scored the lowest rate at 32%, which was significantly lower than with MRCP, DIC-CT, or

IOCP. Moreover, the combination of MRCP and IOCP yielded excellent results for PBM, PD, the common bile duct, and IHBD, with only visualization of the PD being inferior to ERCP.

Relying only on IOCP for investigation of anatomical morphology does not allow enough time in the operating room for thorough debate and discussion on the surgical treatment policy the team will take, while preoperative MRCP can help solve the issue. Thus, as far as pediatric patients with PBM or CBD are concerned, combination of preoperative MRCP and IOCP is the most balanced approach in terms of the quality and quantity of information obtained by the least number of assessment modalities and with lower invasiveness as compared to diagnostic ERCP.

13.5 Conclusions

1. ERCP can be adequately performed by experienced endoscopists with a high success rate across all patient age ranges, providing detailed anatomical and functional information on the pancreaticobiliary junction.
2. The indications of diagnostic ERCP in the treatment of PBM or CBD are inevitably different between adult and pediatric populations.
3. In general, ERCP is recommended for patients suspected of having a relatively long common channel (HCPBD cannot be ruled out by less invasive modalities) or associated biliary carcinoma and those expected to need an endoscopic therapeutic procedure.
4. Among pediatric patients, the need for ERCP can be reduced by using the combination of MRCP and IOCP.

References

1. Kamisawa T, Ando H, Suyama M, Shimada M, Morine Y, Shimada H, Working Committee of Clinical Practice Guidelines for Pancreaticobiliary Maljunction, Japanese Study Group on Pancreaticobiliary Maljunction. Japanese clinical practice guidelines for pancreaticobiliary maljunction. J Gastroenterol. 2012;47:731–59.
2. Hamada Y, Ando H, Kamisawa T, Itoi T, Urushihara N, Koshinaga T, Saito T, Fujii H, Morotomi Y. Diagnostic criteria for congenital biliary dilatation 2015. J Hepatobiliary Pancreat Sci. 2016;23:342.
3. Morine Y, Shimada M, Takamatsu H, Araida T, Endo I, Kubota M, Toki A, Noda T, Matsumura T, Miyakawa S, Ishibashi H, Kamisawa T, Shimada H. Clinical features of pancreaticobiliary maljunction: update analysis of 2nd Japan-nationwide survey. J Hepatobiliary Pancreat Sci. 2013;20:472–80.
4. Kamisawa T, Ando H, Hamada Y, Fujii H, Koshinaga T, Urushihara N, Itoi T, Shimada H, Japanese Study Group on Pancreaticobiliary Maljunction. Diagnostic criteria for pancreaticobiliary maljunction 2013. J Hepatobiliary Pancreat Sci. 2014;21:159–61.

5. Sterling JA. The common channel for bile and pancreatic ducts. Surg Gynecol Obstet. 1954;98:420–4.
6. Suda K, Miyano T, Hashimoto K. The choledocho-pancreatico-ductal junction in infantile obstructive jaundice diseases. Acta Pathol Jpn. 1980;30:187–94.
7. Suda K, Miyano T, Konuma I, Matsumoto M. An abnormal pancreatico-choledocho-ductal junction in cases of biliary tract carcinoma. Cancer. 1983;52:2086–8.
8. Kamisawa T, Tu Y, Nakajima H, Egawa N, Tsuruta K, Okamoto A. The presence of a common channel and associated pancreaticobiliary diseases: a prospective ERCP study. Dig Liver Dis. 2007;39:173–9.
9. Dowdy GS Jr, Waldron GW, Brown WG. Surgical anatomy of the pancreatobiliary ductal system. Observations. Arch Surg. 1962;84:229–46.
10. Rienhoff WF Jr, Pickrell KL. Pancreatitis; an anatomic study of the pancreatic and extrahepatic biliary systems. Arch Surg. 1945;51:205–19.
11. Itokawa F, Kamisawa T, Nakano T, Itoi T, Hamada Y, Ando H, Fujii H, Koshinaga T, Yoshida H, Tamoto E, Noda T, Kimura Y, Maguchi H, Urushihara N, Horaguchi J, Morotomi Y, Sato M, Hanada K, Tanaka M, Takahashi A, Yamaguchi T, Arai Y, Horiguchi A, Igarashi Y, Inui K, Committee of Diagnostic Criteria of The Japanese Study Group on Pancreaticobiliary Muljunction. Exploring the length of the common channel of pancreaticobiliary maljunction on magnetic resonance cholangiopancreatography. J Hepatobiliary Pancreat Sci. 2015;22:68–73.
12. Kamisawa T, Funata N, Hayashi Y, Egawa N, Nakajima H, Tsuruta K, Okamoto A, Yamaguchi T. Pathologic changes in the non-carcinomatous epithelium of the gallbladder in patients with a relatively long common channel. Gastrointest Endosc. 2004;60:56–60.
13. Kamisawa T, Ando H, Shimada M, Hamada Y, Itoi T, Takayashiki T, Miyazaki M. Recent advances and problems in the management of pancreaticobiliary maljunction: feedback from the guidelines committee. J Hepatobiliary Pancreat Sci. 2014;21:87–92.
14. Kaneko K, Ando H, Ito T, Watanabe Y, Seo T, Harada T, Ito F. Protein plugs cause symptoms in patients with choledochal cysts. Am J Gastroenterol. 1997;92:1018–21.
15. Kouchi K, Yoshida H, Matsunaga T, Kuroda H, Hishiki T, Saito T, Matsuura G, Komatsu S, Ohnuma N. Efficacy of ERCP via the accessory papilla in children with choledochal cysts. Gastrointest Endosc. 2004;59:119–23.
16. Andriulli A, Loperfido S, Napolitano G, Niro G, Valvano MR, Spirito F, Pilotto A, Forlano R. Incidence rates of post-ERCP complications: a systematic survey of prospective studies. Am J Gastroenterol. 2007;102:1781.
17. Yokoe M, Takada T, Mayumi T, Yoshida M, Isaji S, Wada K, Itoi T, Sata N, Gabata T, Igarashi H, Kataoka K, Hirota M, Kadoya M, Kitamura N, Kimura Y, Kiriyama S, Shirai K, Hattori T, Takeda K, Takeyama Y, Hirota M, Sekimoto M, Shikata S, Arata S, Hirata K. Japanese guidelines for the management of acute pancreatitis: Japanese guidelines 2015. J Hepatobiliary Pancreat Sci. 2015;22:405–32.
18. Saito T, Terui K, Mitsunaga T, Nakata M, Kuriyama Y, Higashimoto Y, Onuma N, Takahashi H, Yoshida H. Role of pediatric ERCP in an era stressing less-invasive imaging modalities. J Pediatr Gastroenterol Nutr. 2014;59:204–9.
19. Saito T, Terui K, Mitsunaga T, Nakata M, Yoshida H. Significance of imaging modalities for preoperative evaluation of the pancreaticobiliary system in surgery for pediatric choledochal cyst. J Hepatobiliary Pancreat Sci. 2016;23:347–52.
20. Hiramatsu T, Itoh A, Kawashima H, Ohno E, Itoh Y, Sugimoto H, Sumi H, Funasaka K, Nakamura M, Miyahara R, Katano Y, Ishigami M, Ohmiya N, Kaneko K, Ando H, Goto H, Hirooka Y. Usefulness and safety of endoscopic retrograde cholangiopancreatography in children with pancreaticobiliary maljunction. J Pediatr Surg. 2015;50:377–81.

Chapter 14
Diagnosis of PBM and CBD by MRCP

Shigehisa Fumino and Tatsuro Tajiri

Abstract A diagnostic work-up of pancreaticobiliary maljunction (PBM) and congenital biliary dilatation (CBD) depends on noninvasive imaging modalities rather than direct cholangiography. Magnetic resonance cholangiopancreatography (MRCP) is widely used for hepatobiliary and pancreatic disease and should be considered the first-line imaging test for PBM and CBD after ultrasonography in current clinical practice. The advantages of MRCP over computed tomography and endoscopic retrograde cholangiopancreatography in such cases include its excellent contrast resolution, low invasiveness, and lack of irradiation. However, it is still challenging to perform high-quality MRCP in children, especially very young children, due to these patients' small-caliber ducts, a poor signal, and unavoidable patient motion, which creates artifacts. MRCP was able to visualize PBM in only 44.4% of cases, and the minimum age for successful visualization of PBM with MRCP was 1 year and 11 months in the authors' series. Recent technical improvements in the image quality may lead to better diagnostic accuracy of MRCP in young patients in the near future.

Keywords Magnetic resonance cholangiopancreatography (MRCP) · Endoscopic retrograde cholangiopancreatography (ERCP) · Pancreaticobiliary maljunction (PBM) · Congenital biliary dilatation (CBD) · Protein plug

14.1 Perspective of MRCP

A diagnostic work-up of pancreaticobiliary maljunction (PBM) and congenital biliary dilatation (CBD) depends on noninvasive imaging modalities rather than direct cholangiography. Magnetic resonance cholangiopancreatography (MRCP) is

S. Fumino (✉) · T. Tajiri
Department of Pediatric Surgery, Graduated School of Medical Science, Kyoto Prefectural University of Medicine, Kyoto, Japan
e-mail: fumin@koto.kpu-m.ac.jp

T. Kamisawa, H. Ando (eds.), *Pancreaticobiliary Maljunction and Congenital Biliary Dilatation*, https://doi.org/10.1007/978-981-10-8654-0_14

widely used for hepatobiliary and pancreatic disease and should be considered the first-line imaging test for PBM and CBD after ultrasonography in current clinical practice [1].

Magnetic resonance imaging (MRI) depends on the detection of energy released from hydrogen protons after their forcible alignment in a strong field. The technique is safe with certain provisos (i.e., patients with claustrophobia or metal foreign bodies, such as pacemakers and stainless plates). MRI has excellent contrast resolution, better than that of computed tomography (CT), although worse spatial resolution than CT. Multiple planes (axial, coronal, sagittal) can be reconstructed as needed. For MRCP, the bile within the biliary tree is imaged with heavily T2-weighted sequences without contrast medium. The sequences are heavily T2 weighted using long echo times in the range of 300–1000 msec, so that only tissues or fluid with a prolonged transverse relaxation time (T2) retains the signal. These tissues and fluid are seen as hyperintense structures. The background soft tissues with a shorter T2 do not retain a significant signal long enough in a sequence with a prolonged echo time and are, therefore, suppressed. Blood vessels are not seen, since flowing blood does not produce any signal on these images. Therefore, MRCP can depict the overall biliary system, including the intrahepatic and extrahepatic bile ducts as well as PBM (see Fig. 14.1) [2].

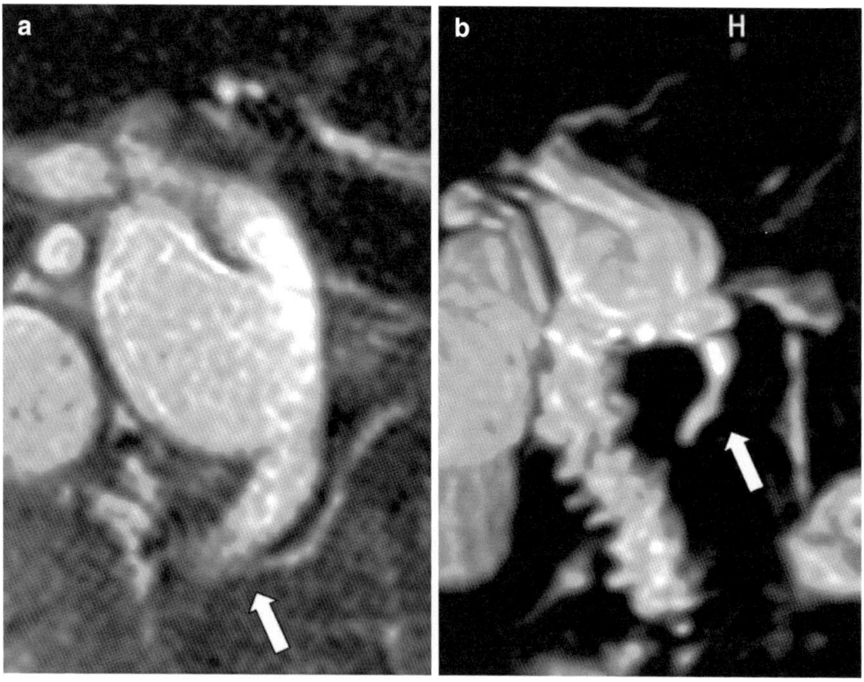

Fig. 14.1 (**a**) A 3-year-old boy with cystic-type choledochal dilatation. MRCP showed clearly PBM (arrow). (**b**) A 23-month-old girl with cystic-type choledochal dilatation. MRCP showed clearly PBM (arrow)

14.2 Diagnostic Purpose and Accuracy of MRCP for CBD and PBM

The purposes of imaging studies for PBM and CBD are principally classified into four items [3].

1. First, the most important role of imaging is the total evaluation of the biliary system. This is important because the presence of a choledochal cyst must be confirmed, and these obtained images provide a road map for surgical planning. Furthermore, the morphological changes in the intrahepatic bile duct, such as stenosis and enlargement, must be assessed simultaneously.
2. Imaging also allows for the evaluation of the pancreatic system. Using imaging, one can visualize the changes of the pancreas parenchyma, the dilatation of the pancreatic duct, and the presence of a protein plug (see Fig. 14.2). This may be accompanied by pancreas divisum or an annular pancreas.
3. Imaging also allows for the demonstration of PBM, which is necessary particularly for the diagnosis of non-dilatation-type PBM to assess surgical indications.
4. Imaging allows for functional evaluations. In PBM, two-way regurgitation can occur with pancreatic juice reflux into the bile duct or bile juice regurgitation into the pancreatic duct. Contrast material-enhanced MRCP and dynamic MRCP with secretin have been reported useful in this regard [4].

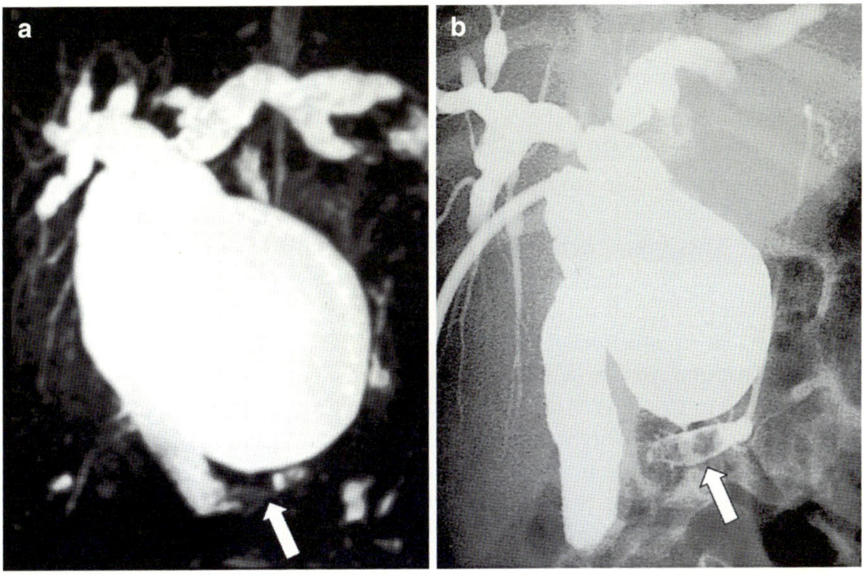

Fig. 14.2 (**a**) Pre-drainage MRCP showed a protein plug (arrow) within a common channel in a cystic-type CBD. (**b**) At percutaneous bile drainage, the protein plug was confirmed by direct cholangiography (arrow)

MRCP is suitable for the abovementioned purposes. Furthermore, a major advantage of MRCP is that it is less invasive and involves no irradiation, unlike CT and endoscopic retrograde cholangiopancreatography (ERCP). MRCP is also superior to ERCP in the depiction of the overall biliary tract including the intrahepatic and extrahepatic bile ducts. Although it is a noninvasive test, which is particularly useful for pediatric patients, the visualization of PBM is often difficult for infants and patients with a short common channel.

The rate of MRCP accurately detecting CBD is reported to be 38–100%. In addition, the diagnostic criteria of MRCP for PBM are equivalent to those with ERCP; however, the definitive detection rate thereof is reported to be 60–100%. The detection rates of PBM for adults and children are reported to be 82–100% and 40–80%, respectively. In cases where the common channel is ≥15 mm, the detection rate is reported to be 82%. The incomplete detection of PBM is often due to the overlap of the dilated bile duct and PBM. As MRCP does not possess as high a spatial resolution as X-ray examinations, it is unclear how precisely it depicts complicated junctions. Therefore, in cases with short or complicated junction, a definitive diagnosis of PBM using direct cholangiography, such as ERCP or intraoperative cholangiography, is required [5].

14.3 Practical Consideration of MRCP

In practical use, MRCP requires some consideration. It is still challenging to perform high-quality MRCP in children, especially very young children, due to these patients' small-caliber ducts, poor signal, and unavoidable patient motion, which creates artifacts.

The need for deep sedation because of the long sequence time is another major drawback of pediatric MRCP. In our institute, infants are sedated with 30–50 mg/kg of body weight oral chlorate hydrate, and children over 1 year of age who cannot tolerate the examination are administered 30–50 mg/kg thiopental sodium rectally.

Although MRCP has been shown to be almost 100% accurate in the evaluation of a choledochal cysts, the visualization rate of PBM ranges from 40% to 83% [6]. It is particularly difficult to visualize PBM in children under 2 years of age and in those with a large choledochal cyst overlapping PBM.

In our institute, routine MRCP imaging is preoperatively performed using the Intera 1.5 T (Philips, Best, Netherlands) with a body array wraparound coil without breath-holding. Patients are studied in the supine position with a thick-slab 2D turbo spin echo (TSE), obtaining coronal and oblique coronal 40 mm thick slices on a 320 × 256 matrix. These image sections are then processed by the standard maximum intensity projection (MIP) algorithm to obtain views of the entire pancreaticobiliary system.

In our series, MRCP was able to demonstrate the extrahepatic bile duct clearly in all patients. The gallbladder was visualized in 92.6%, and the main pancreatic duct was visualized in 81.5%. However, MRCP was able to visualize PBM in only 44.4%

of cases, and the minimum age for successful visualization of PBM with MRCP was 1 year and 11 months. This means that we obtained a diagnostic accuracy of almost 100% in the presence of a choledochal cyst, but the accurate diagnosis rate of PBM was under 50% in the MRCP study. Therefore, routine direct cholangiography is still mandatory, especially in non-dilatation-type PBM [7].

However, MRCP is being used increasingly frequently and has become a viable alternative to ERCP for diagnostic purposes. Furthermore, MRCP can visualize the other surrounding organs outside the pancreaticobiliary luminal structure, including hepatosplenomegaly, hepatic tumors, pancreatic masses, intestinal disease, cystic kidney, and so on. Several recent technological advances have resulted in improvements in coil technology, an increased speed of acquisition, and refinements in respiratory compensation techniques. Therefore, continuous improvements in the image quality are expected to lead to greater diagnostic accuracy of MRCP in the near future.

References

1. Kamisawa T, Tu Y, Egawa N, et al. MRCP of congenital pancreaticobiliary malformation. Abdom Imaging. 2007;32:129–33.
2. Chapter 5: Ultrasound, computed tomography and magnetic resonance imaging. In: Sherlock S, & Dooley J, editors. Disease of the liver and biliary system. 11th ed. Oxford: Blackwell Publishing; 2002.
3. Chavhan GB, Babyn PS, Manson D, et al. Pediatric MR cholangiopancreatography: principles, technique, and clinical applications. Radiographics. 2008;28:1951–62.
4. Fumino S, Ono S, Iwai N, et al. Diagnostic impact of computed tomography cholangiography and magnetic resonance cholangiopancreatography on pancreaticobiliary maljunction. J Pediatr Surg. 2011;46:1373–8.
5. Hamada Y, Tanano A, Takada K, et al. Magnetic resonance cholangiopancreatography on postoperative work-up in children with choledochal cysts. Pediatr Surg Int. 2004;20:43–6.
6. Ishibashi H, Ando H, Japanese Study Group on Congenital Biliary Dilatation (JSCBD), et al. Japanese clinical practice guidelines for congenital biliary dilatation. J Hepatobiliary Pancreat Sci. 2017;24:1–16.
7. Kim MJ, Han SJ, Yoon CS, et al. Using MR cholangiopancreatography to reveal anomalous pancreaticobiliary ductal union in infants and children with choledochal cysts. Am J Roentgenol. 2002;179:209–14.

Chapter 15
Diagnosis of PBM and CBD by EUS

Hiroyuki Maguchi, Akio Katanuma, and Kuniyuki Takahashi

Abstract PBM is a congenital anomaly in which the pancreatic duct and bile duct join anatomically outside the duodenal wall, usually forming a markedly long common channel. EUS can observe not only the pancreatic and bile ducts but also the muscularis propria of the duodenum and pancreatic parenchyma. In PBM patients, EUS can detect the confluence of the pancreatic duct and bile duct outside the muscularis propria of the duodenal wall regardless of the length of the common channel. In addition, in PBM, bile duct cancer and/or gallbladder cancer is frequently observed and more predisposed to forming biliary tract stones than individuals without the disease. EUS can evaluate not only the diagnosis of PBM but also further examine the bile duct and gallbladder in the same session. Experienced specialists must perform or assist EUS as its diagnostic accuracy is guaranteed by operator skills.

Keywords Pancreaticobiliary maljunction (PBM) · Congenital biliary dilation (CBD) · EUS · Gallbladder cancer · Bile duct cancer

15.1 Introduction

PBM can be classified into two categories, with or without biliary dilation. In PBM the common channel is longer than normal, and PBM is a congenital anomaly in which the pancreatic duct and bile duct join anatomically outside the duodenal wall. Therefore, demonstrating an extraordinarily long common channel and/or having an abnormal union between the pancreatic and bile ducts by direct cholangiopancreatography such as ERCP is regarded as a diagnostic criterion. MD-CT providing maximum intensity projection (MIP) images, MRCP, and EUS are now potential diagnostic modalities for this disease [1, 2].

H. Maguchi (✉) · A. Katanuma · K. Takahashi
Center for Gastroenterology, Teine-Keijinkai Hospital, Sapporo, Japan
e-mail: maguchi@tb3.so-ne.ne.jp

T. Kamisawa, H. Ando (eds.), *Pancreaticobiliary Maljunction and Congenital Biliary Dilatation*, https://doi.org/10.1007/978-981-10-8654-0_15

EUS has a high resolution and excellent ability of local observation. It is one of the most accurate diagnostic modalities, particularly for the pancreas and biliary regions including the pancreaticobiliary junction [3–6].

15.2 EUS Imaging of the Pancreaticobiliary Junction

EUS can observe not only the pancreatic and bile ducts but also the muscularis propria of the duodenum and pancreatic parenchyma [3–6]. In EUS examination, the muscularis propria is defined as the border between the pancreas and duodenum. In a normal healthy state, the main pancreatic duct and the common bile duct run separately in the pancreas parenchyma of the pancreas head and do not join until the major papilla (Fig. 15.1a). In PBM, the pancreatic duct and bile duct join in the pancreas parenchyma. EUS can detect the confluence of pancreatic duct and bile duct in the pancreas parenchyma outside the muscularis propria of the duodenum [1, 3, 4]. The confluence is so-called common channel (Fig. 15.1b, c). When PBM is known in advance, it may be relatively easy to depict the confluence regardless of the bile duct dilation [1]. In addition in the case of complex types, in which the pancreatic duct and the bile duct meet in a complex manner, it is possible to diagnose using EUS (Fig. 15.2).

15.3 Detectability of PBM by EUS

There were several reports on the detection rate of PBM by EUS [3, 4, 6]. According to them, the detection rates ranged from 88% to 100%. Diagnosis of PBM with biliary dilation is easier than those without biliary dilation. As the finding of biliary

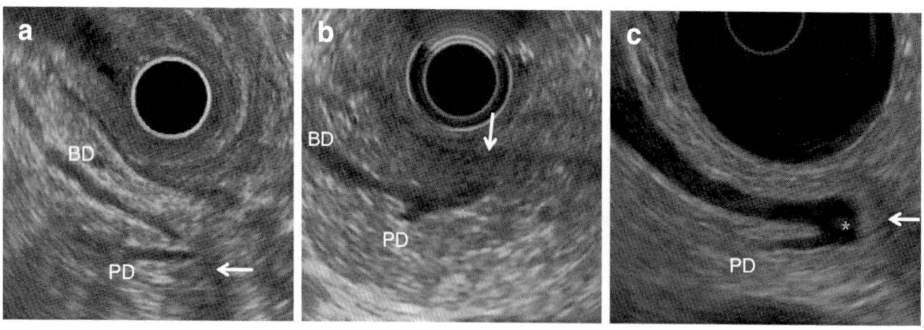

Fig. 15.1 EUS imaging. (**a**) In a normal healthy state, the main pancreatic duct (PD) and the common bile duct (BD) run separately in the pancreas parenchyma (*white arrow*, muscularis propria of the duodenum). (**b**, **c**) In PBM, EUS can detect the confluence of the pancreatic duct (PD) and bile duct (BD) in the pancreas parenchyma outside of the duodenal wall, so-called common channel (*asterisks*) (*white arrow*: muscularis propria of the duodenum)

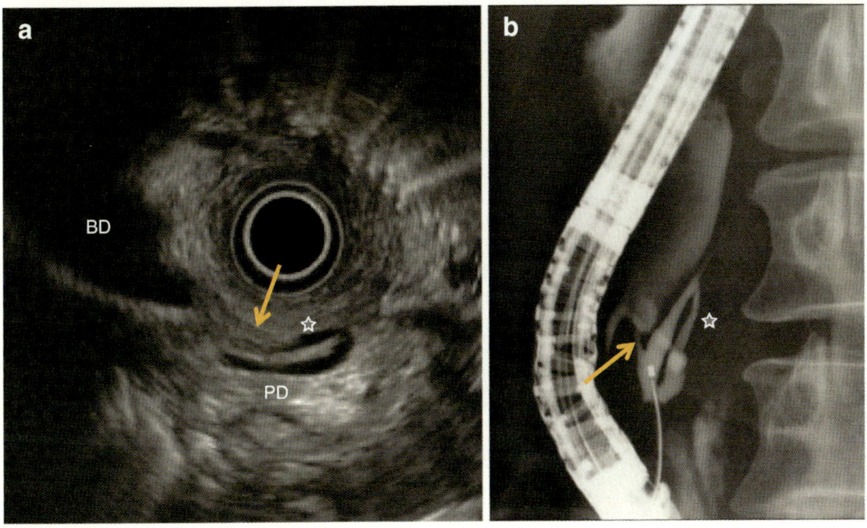

Fig. 15.2 (**a**) EUS imaging shows PD loops back on itself (*star*), and a thin duct (*yellow arrow*) is connected to BD. (**b**) ERCP confirmed PD loops back on itself (*star*), and a thin duct (*yellow arrow*) is connected to BD

dilation such as choledochal cyst is strongly suggesting PBM, EUS observation of the confluence of the pancreatic duct and bile duct in the pancreas parenchyma may be carefully performed. In addition, the majority of PBM were women younger than 30 years of age [1]. The duodenal lumen of the younger women is thinner than that in the others. In young woman, EUS evaluation of the relationship between the pancreatic duct, the bile ducts, and the muscularis propria is more difficult.

A thickening of the hypoechoic inner layer of the gallbladder on US is a supplemental finding of PBM without biliary dilation [7–9]. During EUS, careful observation of the pancreatic duct, the bile duct, and the muscularis propria of the duodenum is very important.

15.4 Advantages of EUS

EUS is positioned as the second-line modality followed by US, CT, and MRCP. However, EUS is less invasive than ERCP and is usually performed in outpatients. It has been gaining popularity around the world.

The biggest advantage of EUS is direct visualization of not only the pancreatic duct and bile duct but also the muscularis propria of the duodenum at the same time [1]. Therefore, EUS can decide whether the location of pancreaticobiliary junction is outside the duodenal wall or not, even though PBM has a short common channel. Furthermore, the bile duct and gallbladder can be studied in detail in a series of

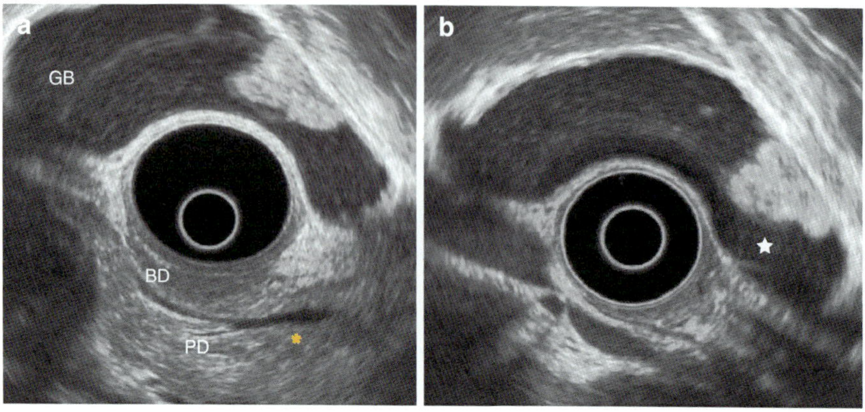

Fig. 15.3 PBM with gallbladder cancer. (**a**) EUS can detect PBM (*asterisks*) and gallbladder tumor. (**b**) EUS shows gallbladder cancer (*star*)

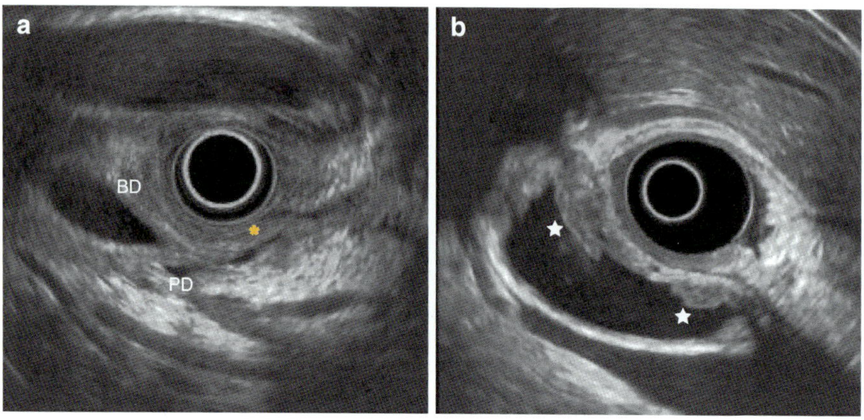

Fig. 15.4 Congenital biliary dilation with bile duct cancer. (**a**) EUS demonstrates PBM (*asterisks*) with biliary dilation. (**b**) EUS can diagnose bile duct cancer (*star*)

scans following the diagnosis of PBM. In PBM, bile duct cancer and/or gallbladder cancer are frequently observed and also more predisposed to forming biliary tract stones than individuals without the disease [1, 2, 4, 7–9]. EUS can evaluate not only the diagnosis of PBM but also further examine the bile duct and gallbladder in the same session (Figs. 15.3 and 15.4).

However, experienced skills are required for EUS evaluation; hence, EUS is sometimes called operator-dependent examination. That is a disadvantage of EUS examination. Experienced specialists must perform or assist EUS, and it is mandatory to foster a large number of future EUS experts.

References

1. Kamisawa T, Ando H, Suyama M, et al. Japanese clinical practice guidelines for pancreaticobiliary maljunction. J Gastroenterol. 2012;47:731–59.
2. Kamisawa T, Kuruma S, Tabata T, et al. Pancreaticobiliary maljunction and biliary cancer. J Gastroenterol. 2015;50:273–9.
3. Mitake M, Nakazawa S, Naitoh Y, et al. Value of endoscopic ultrasonography in the detection of anomalous connection of the pancreatobiliary duct. Endoscopy. 1991;23:117–20.
4. Sugiyama M, Atomi Y. Endoscopic ultrasonography for diagnosing anomalous pancreaticobiliary junction. Gastrointest Endosc. 1997;45:261–7.
5. EFJ working group on standardization of pancreatobiliary EUS. Standard imaging techniques in the pancreatobiliary region using radial scanning endoscopic ultrasonography. Dig Endosc. 2004;16:S118–33.
6. Yusuf TE, Bhutani MS. Role of endoscopic ultrasonography in diseases of the extrahepatic biliary system. J Gastroenterol Hepatol. 2004;19:243–50.
7. Tanno S, Obara T, Maguchi H, et al. Thickened inner hypoechoic layer of the gallbladder wall in the diagnosis of anomalous pancreaticobiliary ductal union with endosonography. Gastrointest Endosc. 1997;46:520–6.
8. Kamisawa T, Takuma K, Itokawa F, et al. Endoscopic diagnosis of pancreaticobiliary maljunction. World J Gastrointest Endosc. 2011;3:1–5.
9. Takuma K, Kamisawa T, Tabata T, et al. Importance of early diagnosis of pancreaticobiliary maljunction without biliary dilation. World J Gastroenterol. 2012;18:3409–14.

Chapter 16
Diagnosis of PBM by MD-CT and DIC-CT

Shin Ishihara, Masahiro Ito, Yukio Asano, and Akihiko Horiguchi

Abstract Pancreaticobiliary maljunction (PBM) is a congenital malformation in which the pancreatic and bile ducts join anatomically outside the duodenal wall. PBM can be diagnosed if the pancreaticobiliary junction outside the wall is shown in multi-planar reconstruction images provided by multidetector row computed tomography (MD-CT). A total of 29 cases were diagnosed with PBM by MD-CT. Three studies have investigated the capability of MD-CT to diagnose PBM, including the present study. These studies reported only a few cases ranging from 9 to 46 cases. The detection rate for PBM lesion is 100% in adults and 19.5% in children.

A major advantage of drip infusion cholangiography with CT (DIC-CT) is that it can detect more dynamic and physiological bile flows. In addition, using DIC-CT, it is possible to detect biliopancreatic reflux, which is physiologically correlated with PBM. For biliopancreatic reflux, the detection rates of DIC-CT in children are 40.0% and 63.6%. This rate was not reported in adults. Investigation involving adults is still anticipated.

Keywords Pancreaticobiliary maljunction · MD-CT · DIC-CT · Diagnosis

16.1 Introduction

Pancreaticobiliary maljunction (PBM) is a congenital malformation in which the pancreatic and bile ducts join anatomically outside the duodenal wall [1]. PBM can be diagnosed if the pancreaticobiliary junction outside the wall is depicted by endoscopic ultrasonography (EUS) or multi-planar reconstruction (MPR) images provided by multidetector row computed tomography (MD-CT) [1]. However, the diagnostic capability of EUS varies depending on the operator; therefore, it is

S. Ishihara (✉) · M. Ito · Y. Asano · A. Horiguchi
Department of Surgery, Fujita Health University, Toyoake City, Aichi, Japan
e-mail: ishin@fujita-hu.ac.jp; akihori@fujita-hu.ac.jp

T. Kamisawa, H. Ando (eds.), *Pancreaticobiliary Maljunction and Congenital Biliary Dilatation*, https://doi.org/10.1007/978-981-10-8654-0_16

necessary that a specialist performs EUS. Therefore, it is MD-CT that there is no difference in diagnostic ability in any facility.

Drip infusion cholangiography with CT (DIC-CT) provides clear three-dimensional images of the intra- and extrahepatic ducts of patients with PBM [2]. In addition, using DIC-CT, it is possible to detect biliopancreatic reflux, which is physiologically correlated with PBM [2].

We describe our diagnostic experience using MD-CT and literature considerations of DIC-CT.

16.2 MD-CT

Recent advances in helical CT technology, such as multidetector and subsecond rotation, have enabled scanning of the pancreatic and biliary systems [3]. This results in further improvement in the quality of MPR images because of the superior resolution in the Z-axis. Subsequently, MPR images enable us to select the optimal sectional planes for evaluation of the pancreatic and bile ducts and their confluence [3]. We described the diagnosis of PBM using MD-CT based on the results of our case.

16.2.1 Patients

From 2006 to 2016, a total of 29 patients with PBM were consecutively diagnosed and treated at our institute. Of these patients, five were males and 24 were females; their median age at diagnosis was 52 (range, 18–73) years.

16.2.2 CT Image Acquisition

Specific scan protocols varied depending on the CT scanner available at the time of examination. Between January 2006 and August 2009, CT scanning was performed using a 64-detector-row helical CT (Aquilion 64; Toshiba Medical, Tokyo, Japan). From September 2009, it was performed using 80-detector-row helical CT (Aquilion PRIME; Toshiba Medical, Tokyo, Japan). Nonionic contrast material with an iodine concentration of 370 mgIg/mL was injected at 1.8 mg/kg of body weight per second over 20 s. For the three-phase contrast-enhanced CT studies of patients, arterial phase scanning was initiated as soon as possible after the attenuation values in the aorta, whose level is similar to that at the start of scanning, reached 200 HU using the automatic bolus tracking method (SureStart; Toshiba Medical, Japan).

16.2.3 Results

Overall, 29 patients were diagnosed with PBM. According to the classification of The Japanese Study Group on Pancreaticobiliary Maljunction [2], 13 cases were of the bile duct (junction) type (Fig. 16.1), 15 cases of pancreatic duct type (Fig. 16.2), and one case of complex type (Fig. 16.3). Choledochal dilatation

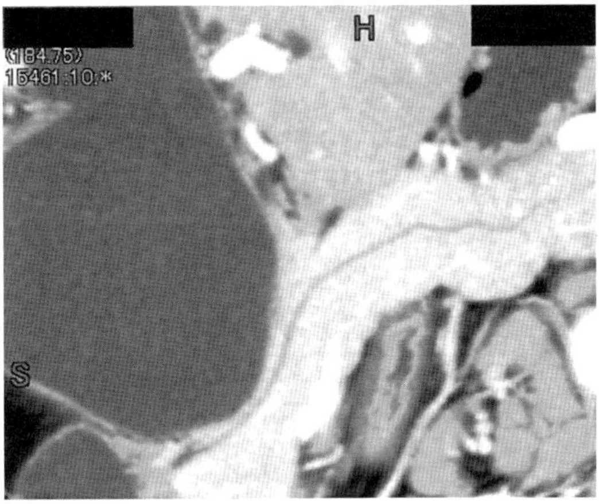

Fig. 16.1 MD-CT image of bile duct (junction) type

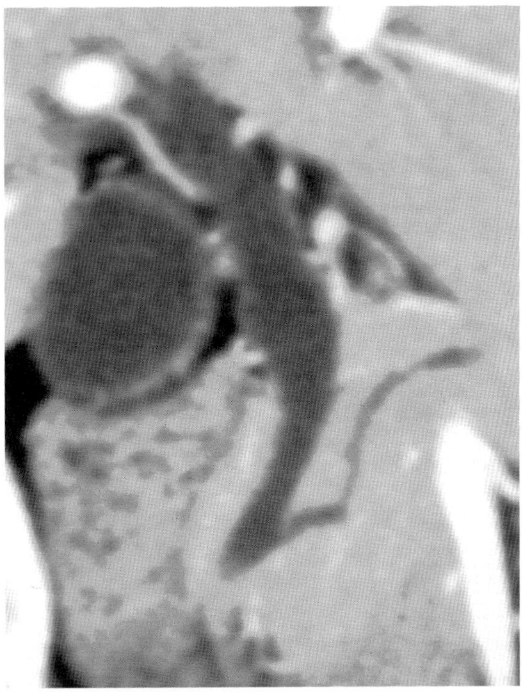

Fig. 16.2 MD-CT image of pancreatic duct type

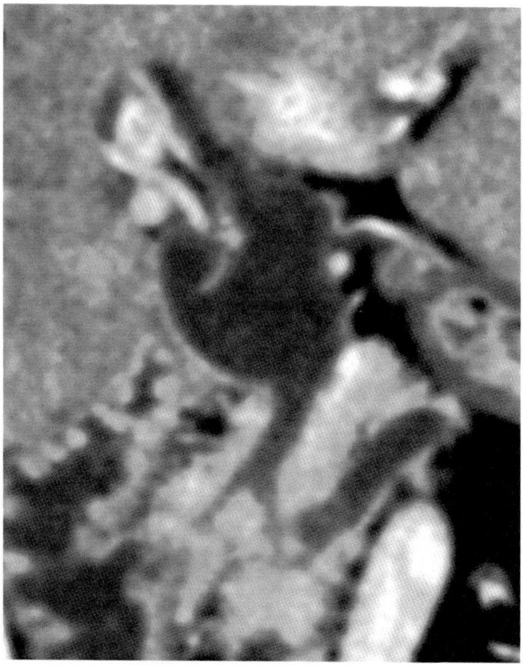

Fig. 16.3 MD-CT image of complex type

Table 16.1 Summary of literature on the detection rates of MD-CT

Year	Author	Period (year)	Age (y.o)	Number of cases	Detected rate (%)
2006	Itoh	2001–2003	24–67	9	100.0
2012	Guo	2002–2011	0–13	46	19.6
2014	Our cases	2006–2013	18–73	27	100.0

types were cystic (n = 16), fusiform (n = 7), and nondilated (n = 6). Among 23 patients with choledochal cysts, nine are of Todani IA, seven of Ic, and seven of IV-A types [4].

16.2.4 Diagnostic Capability of MD-CT

Only three studies, including the present study, have investigated the capability of MD-CT to diagnose PBM. These studies reported only a few cases, ranging from 9 to 46 cases. The detection rate for PBM lesion is 100% in adults and 19.5% in children (Table 16.1) [3, 5]. In adult patients, the diagnostic capability of MD-CT is satisfactory, although only a small number of studies exist, including the present study. The diagnosis rate in children is 19.6%, which is not satisfactory. However, Okada et al. reported that 3 of the 18 childhood cases, which could not be diagnosed with magnetic resonance cholangiopancreatography and endoscopic retrograde cholangiopancreatography, could be diagnosed with MD-CT alone [6]. Therefore, although the diagnosis rate is low in children, some cases can be diagnosed with MD-CT only, and it is useful as a diagnostic tool, even in children.

16.3 DIC-CT

DIC-CT is also a conventional and noninvasive method for evaluation of the biliary system besides radiation therapy [7]. The reported visualization rates of PBM by DIC-CT have been low, ranging from 25% to 38.2% [7, 8]. From this result, the significance of using DIC-CT to diagnose PBM is low. The main advantage of this modality is that it can depict more dynamic and physiological bile flows [9]. In addition, biliopancreatic reflux detection is possible, which is physiologically correlated with PBM [9]. For biliopancreatic reflux, the detection rates of DIC-CT in children are 40.0% and 63.6% [9, 10]. This rate has not been reported in adults. Investigation involving adults is still anticipated.

References

1. Kamisawa T, Ando H, Hamada Y, et al. Diagnostic criteria for pancreaticobiliary maljunction 2013. J Hepatobiliary Pancreat Sci. 2014;21:159–61.
2. Kamisawa T, Ando H, Suyama M, et al. Japanese clinical practice guidelines for pancreaticobiliary maljunction. J Gastroenterol. 2012;47:731–59. https://doi.org/10.1007/s00535-012-0611-2.
3. Itoh S, Fukushima H, Takada A, et al. Assessment of anomalous pancreaticobiliary ductal junction with high-resolution multiplanar reformatted images in MDCT. AJR Am J Roentgenol. 2006;187:668–75.
4. Todani T, Watanabe Y, Narusue M, et al. Congenital bile duct cysts: classification operative procedures, and review of thirty-seven cases including cancer arising from choledochal cyst. Am J Surg. 1977;134:263–9.
5. Guo WL, Huang SG, Wang J, et al. Imaging findings in 75 pediatric patients with pancreatobiliary maljunction: a retrospective case study. Pediatr Surg Int. 2012;28:983–8. https://doi.org/10.1007/s00383-012-3159-6.
6. Okada T, Sasaki F, Honda S, et al. Usefulness of axial planes of helical computed tomography for diagnosis of pancreaticobiliary maljunction in early infants with negative findings on magnetic resonance cholangiopancreatography. J Pediatr Surg. 2008;43:579–82.
7. Fumino S, Ono S, Kimura O, et al. Diagnostic impact of computed tomography cholangiography and magnetic resonance cholangiopancreatography on pancreaticobiliary maljunction. J Pediatr Surg. 2011;46:1373–8.
8. Saito T, Terui K, Mitsunaga T, et al. Significance of imaging modalities for preoperative evaluation of the pancreaticobiliary system in surgery for pediatric choledochal cyst. J Hepatobiliary Pancreat Sci. 2016;23:347–52.
9. Fumino S, Tokiwa K, Katoh T, et al. New insight into bile flow dynamics in anomalous arrangement of the pancreaticobiliary duct. Br J Surg. 2002;89:865–9.
10. Lam WW, Lam TP, Saing H, et al. MR cholangiography and CT cholangiography of pediatric patient with choledochal cysts. AJR Am J Roentgenol. 1999;173:401–5.

Chapter 17
Elevation of Pancreatic Enzymes in Bile of PBM

Takaaki Fujimoto, Takao Ohtsuka, and Masafumi Nakamura

Abstract Pancreaticobiliary maljunction (PBM) is a congenital anomaly in which the reciprocal reflux between pancreatic and bile juice occurs because the confluence of the pancreatic and bile ducts lies outside of the area of contractile influence of the sphincter of Oddi. The reflux of pancreatic juice into the bile duct and subsequent elevated pancreatic enzyme level in bile are usually recognized in PBM. Amylase is the most popular pancreatic enzyme for assessment in daily practice, and assessment of amylase level in bile is useful to definitively confirm the presence of PBM, and the mixture of pancreatic and bile juices may produce various physiological and pathological alterations. In PBM, the amylase level in bile in patients with biliary cancers has been reported to be higher than that with benign biliary diseases; however, the relationship between the amylase level in bile and development of biliary diseases has not been well documented. Recently, several studies have demonstrated that some patients with a normal morphological pancreaticobiliary junction have a high amylase level and biliary carcinoma. This suggests the possibility that pancreaticobiliary reflux can occur even in patients without PBM and result in the development of biliary carcinoma in the same manner as in patients with PBM.

Keywords Pancreaticobiliary reflux · Pancreaticobiliary maljunction · Occult pancreaticobiliary reflux · Gallbladder carcinoma · Biliary carcinoma

T. Fujimoto · T. Ohtsuka · M. Nakamura (✉)
Department of Surgery and Oncology, Graduate School of Medical Sciences, Kyushu University, Fukuoka, Japan
e-mail: mnaka@surg1.med.kyushu-u.ac.jp

T. Kamisawa, H. Ando (eds.), *Pancreaticobiliary Maljunction and Congenital Biliary Dilatation*, https://doi.org/10.1007/978-981-10-8654-0_17

17.1 Significance of Elevated Biliary Amylase Level in Pancreaticobiliary Maljunction

In pancreaticobiliary maljunction (PBM), the sphincter of Oddi fails to control the contractile function at the junction of the pancreatic and bile duct, and the pancreatic juice (PJ) usually refluxes into the bile tract because of the higher intraluminal pressure in the pancreatic duct compared with the bile duct. Therefore, determining the elevated pancreatic enzyme level in bile, especially the amylase level, is one of the definitive diagnostic features for PBM according to Japanese clinical practice guidelines [1]. Activated phospholipase A2 in PJ from bile produces strong cytotoxic substances such as lysolecithin, which induces inflammation and regeneration of the bile tract mucosa, and enhanced cell cycle turnover [2]. These mucosal injuries to the biliary system ultimately result in the development of cancer by the genetic mutations at KRAS, p53 [1, 3]. In addition, pancreaticobiliary stones may occur because of stasis of the pancreatic or the bile juices. Taken together, PBM may cause various pancreaticobiliary diseases; however, the mechanism of the development of these pancreaticobiliary diseases has not been fully clarified.

17.1.1 Methods of Collecting Bile Juice

There are various procedures for collecting bile juice (BJ) to assess the amylase levels in bile. Aspiration of the BJ in gallbladder/bile duct under laparotomy or percutaneous transhepatic gallbladder/biliary drainage had been performed in the initial period [4], and collecting bile under endoscopic retrograde cholangiopancreatography (ERCP) [5, 6] has been carried out in the recent most cases. During ERCP, BJ is collected immediately after insertion of the cannula into the bile duct without using contrast media. If contrast media is used during several attempts at cannulation, the initial aspirated fluid in cannula should be discarded and the subsequent aspirated fluid collected and stocked [7]. Method during operation or by percutaneous technique is the most reliable because there is no possibility of contamination of PJ in bile, although it is relatively invasive. However, ERCP may also have an advantage for detailed assessment of pancreaticobiliary junction by cholangiopancreatography, but there is the possibility of contamination of pancreatic enzyme into the bile because it is a retrograde procedure and carries a risk of ERCP-related pancreatitis.

17.1.2 Bile Amylase Level

Although the amylase level in BJ of within the normal upper limit of serum amylase level has been considered as "normal" in the several previous reports [8–10], there is no conclusive evidence of this. Large-scale retrospective studies in Japan

Table 17.1 Gallbladder or bile duct amylase levels in patients with pancreaticobiliary maljunction

	Amylase levels (IU/L)				
	n	Gallbladder	*n*	Bile duct	Authors (year)
Adults (≧20)					
Congenital biliary dilatation	997	98,700[a]	997	78,900[a]	Kamisawa et al. [1]
PBM without biliary dilatation	514	66,000[a]	514	60,000[a]	Kamisawa et al. [1]
Congenital biliary dilatation			47	172,988[b]	Kamisawa et al. [14]
PBM without biliary dilatation			34	93, 898[b]	Kamisawa et al. [14]
PBM			11	102,686[b]	Sai et al. [6]
Congenital biliary dilatation	10	73,148[b]	11	85,345[b]	Jeong et al. [12]
Children (<18)					
Congenital biliary dilatation	950	35,800[a]	950	18,622[a]	Kamisawa et al. [1]
PBM without biliary dilatation	68	17,400[a]	68	10,900[a]	Kamisawa et al. [1]
Congenital biliary dilatation			54	29,400[a]	Jung et al. [13]
Various					
Congenital biliary dilatation			190	65,249[a]	Ragot and Mabrut [11]
PBM			14	28,028[b]	Motosugi et al. [9]
PBM	10	108,000[b]	9	146,000[b]	Sugiyama et al. [4]

PBM pancreaticobiliary maljunction
[a]Median
[b]Mean

and Europe have reported BJ amylase levels in PBM over 50,000 IU/L [1, 11], and others reported values over 10,000 IU/L [4, 6, 9, 12, 13] (Table 17.1). However, some patients with PBM have normal bile amylase levels, possibly because of the disruption of exocrine pancreatic function due to pancreatitis [1, 5]. BJ amylase level in the gallbladder is considered to be higher than that in the bile duct because of the condensing function of the gallbladder [1, 7]. Others have showed that biliary amylase level in the bile duct was higher than that in the gallbladder [4, 12]. Furthermore, according to one nationwide survey in Japan, BJ amylase in PBM without biliary dilatation is significantly higher than that with biliary dilatation [15]. However, in the gallbladder with PBM, the BJ amylase level is significantly higher with biliary dilatation than that without dilatation. Furthermore the BJ amylase level in the common bile duct in PBM with biliary dilatation is the same as that without dilatation [1]. Adult patients with PBM have significantly higher amylase levels in the biliary tract (common bile duct or gallbladder) than children with PBM, irrespective of the presence or absence of biliary dilatation [1].

Further investigation is needed to clarify the relationship between the morphology of PBM (PBM with or without biliary dilatation) and the distribution of amylase concentration in bile, which may affect the location where biliary diseases including carcinoma are more likely to occur.

17.1.3 Relationship Between the Degree of Amylase Level in Bile and Pancreaticobiliary Diseases

It is well known that high BJ amylase levels are related to the 17% incidence of biliary malignancies in patients with PBM [15]. However, even in patients without PBM, the development of various pancreaticobiliary diseases such as cancer and stones seems to be associated with the high amylase level in BJ [7, 10, 16, 17].

Beltrán et al. [16] and Sakamoto et al. [10] reported that among patients with benign pancreaticobiliary diseases without PBM, those with choledocholithiasis have the highest BJ amylase levels (mean, 4578 and 16,360 IU/L, respectively). These reports also demonstrated that patients with acute calculous cholecystitis (mean, 800–2000) had higher amylase levels in BJ than those with asymptomatic cholecystolithiasis or chronic cholecystitis (mean, 400). The BJ amylase level in patients with gallbladder cancer is higher than in those with benign pancreaticobiliary diseases [5, 6, 16, 17]. These reports demonstrated that BJ amylase levels of 10,000 IU/L or higher are observed in patients with gallbladder cancer, irrespective of the presence or absence of PBM. With regard to bile duct cancer (mean, 1952 IU/L), there was no significant difference in BJ amylase levels, compared with other pancreaticobiliary diseases (mean, 4162 IU/L) [17]. It remains unclear whether the risk of developing biliary tract cancer might depend on amylase levels in BJ.

In addition, the relationship between the high amylase in BJ and pancreatic diseases such as pancreatitis, pancreatolithiasis, and pancreatic cancer has not been clarified in patients with PBM. The reflux of bile into the pancreatic duct may occur in PBM in certain patients, which might induce pancreatic damage and result in various pancreatic diseases including cancer. In fact, the mechanism of pancreatic carcinogenesis by PBM has been demonstrated in animal experiments [18], and the incidence of pancreatic cancer in patients with PBM is reported to be higher than that in the overall population in Japan [1]. Therefore, the possibility of pancreatic cancer development in patients with PBM cannot be overlooked.

17.2 Other Pancreatic Enzymes

PJ includes several pancreatic enzymes such as lipase, phospholipase A2, trypsin, and elastase 1, in addition to amylase. Lipase levels in bile have been well documented (Table 17.2). A median BJ lipase level of 172,104 IU/L was noted in 190 patients with congenital biliary dilatation [11]. In addition, 54 patients under

Table 17.2 Gallbladder or bile duct lipase levels in patients with pancreaticobiliary maljunction

	Lipase levels (IU/L)				
	n	Gallbladder	*n*	Bile duct	Author (year)
Adults (≧20)					
Congenital biliary dilatation	8	52,175[a]	8	49,375[a]	Jeong et al. [12]
Children (<18)					
Congenital biliary dilatation			54	81,300[b]	Jung et al. [13]
Various					
Congenital biliary dilatation			190	172,104[b]	Ragot and Mabrut [11]

[a]Mean
[b]Median

18 years old with PBM had BJ lipase levels of 81,300 [13]. In a Japanese nationwide survey, the BJ lipase levels in adults with PBM were higher than those in children, which is consistent with the bile amylase levels as described in the aforementioned studies. However, there are no differences in lipase levels in the common bile duct or gallbladder between patients with PBM with malignancy and those with benign disease [19].

17.3 Occult Pancreaticobiliary Reflux

Occult pancreaticobiliary reflux (OPR), which is characterized by pancreaticobiliary reflux (PBR) in spite of a normal pancreaticobiliary junction (NPJ), has recently been identified [7, 10, 16, 17]. OPR is defined as a high BJ amylase level over the normal upper limit of serum amylase level in the presence of normal pancreaticobiliary anatomy in which the pancreatic duct is not visible on tip contrast imaging of ERCP (Fig. 17.1). PBR in patients with OPR may also cause reciprocal reflux between PJ and BJ, which may induce chronic inflammation and genetic alterations in the pancreaticobiliary epithelium, as is seen in patients with PBM. Although the effect of OPR on the development of biliary or pancreatic neoplasms remains unclear, Horaguchi et al. [17] have recently shown that patients with high amylase levels with NPJ had gallbladder carcinoma (GBC), and thus OPR may also be a risk factor for the development of GBC.

17.3.1 Biliary Amylase Level in Patients with Occult Pancreaticobiliary Reflux

Our group [5] has shown that the amylase level in BJ in patients with PBM ($n = 12$; median, 27,686 IU/L) is higher than that in patients with OPR ($n = 22$; median, 790 IU/L). We have also found that all the patients with NPJ and gallbladder

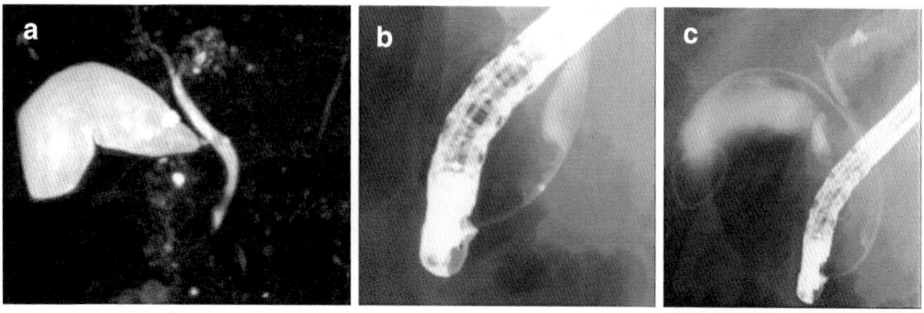

Fig. 17.1 Normal pancreaticobiliary junction with occult pancreaticobiliary reflux. (**a**) Magnetic resonance cholangiopancreatography shows a morphologically normal pancreaticobiliary junction (NPJ). (**b**) Endoscopic retrograde cholangiography demonstrates NPJ anatomy in which the pancreatic duct is not visible on tip contrast imaging. Bile amylase level in common bile duct was 3325 IU/L, indicating the presence of occult pancreaticobiliary reflux. (**c**) Subsequently, an endoscopic nasal gallbladder drainage tube was inserted into the gallbladder. Bile amylase level in the gallbladder was 1288 IU/L

Table 17.3 Relationship between pancreaticobiliary diseases and bile amylase levels in patients with normal pancreaticobiliary junction

	Amylase levels (IU/L)				
Lesion	*n*	Malignant	*n*	Benign	Authors (year)
Gallbladder	9	$1363^{a,*}$	22	$414^{a,*}$	Fujimoto et al. [5]
	32	$19,709^{b,*}$	388	$2,475^{b,*}$	Horaguchi et al. [17]
			196	$4,919^{b}$	Sakamoto et al. [10]
	7	$64,318^{b,*}$	52	$478^{b,*}$	Beltrán et al. [16]
	2	20.5^{b}	39	742.9^{b}	Itokawa et al. [7]
Bile duct	71	1952^{b}	409	4162^{b}	Horaguchi et al. [17]
			17	$1,609^{b}$	Itokawa et al. [7]

PBM pancreaticobiliary maljunction
$^{*}p$-value <0.01
^{a}Median
^{b}Mean

carcinoma (GBC) have high amylase levels in BJ, and the BJ amylase levels in patients with GBC ($n = 9$; median, 1363 IU/L) are significantly higher than in those with benign lesions ($n = 22$; median, 414 IU/L) among the anatomically normal group (Table 17.3). In addition, Horaguchi et al. [17] and Beltrán et al. [16] reported that the amylase level in BJ in patients with GBC was significantly higher than that in patients with benign lesions (Table 17.3). Therefore, the presence of OPR may be a risk factor for the development of GBC. However, OPR patients with choledocholithiasis also had high amylase levels ($n = 17$, mean 4578) [16], and the rate of high amylase level in BJ (≥216 IU/L) in patients with choledocholithiasis (44%) was higher than that in other benign pancreaticobiliary diseases such as acute cholecystitis (6%), adenomyomatosis (13%), and gallbladder polyp (0%) [10]. However, with regard to bile duct diseases, there was no significant difference in amylase level between patients with malignant diseases and those with benign diseases [17].

17.3.2 Occult Pancreaticobiliary Reflux and Carcinogenesis

PBR is also reported to induce injury of the biliary epithelium and may ultimately cause carcinogenesis as described above in PBM session. In fact, patients with OPR are reported to have hyperplasia, dysplasia, or metaplasia of the gallbladder mucosa [7, 10, 20]. In addition, patients with GBC who had OPR were significantly older than those with PBM [5], and it is speculated that the difference in age at carcinogenesis in different types of PBR may be caused by differences in the magnitude of PBR. OPR-induced GBC development may take longer than PBM-induced GBC development because of the smaller amount of PJ reflux in OPR compared with PBM. It is ideal to detect OPR without invasive examinations such as ERCP, or percutaneous transhepatic cholangiography for the assessment of the presence of OPR, although the necessity of prophylactic treatments such as cholecystectomy or biliary diversion remains an unresolved problem in OPR patients.

References

1. Kamisawa T, Ando H, Suyama M, et al. Japanese clinical practice guidelines for pancreaticobiliary maljunction. J Gastroenterol. 2012;47:731–59.
2. Shimada K, Yanagisawa J, Nakayama F. Increased lysophosphatidylcholine and pancreatic enzyme content in bile of patients with anomalous pancreaticobiliary ductal junction. Hepatology. 1991;13:438–44.
3. Tuchida A, Itoi T. Carcinogenesis and chemoprevention of biliary tract cancer in pancreaticobiliary maljunction. World J Gastrointest Oncol. 2010;2:130–5.
4. Sugiyama Y, Kobori H, Hakamada K, et al. Altered bile composition in the gallbladder and common bile duct of patients with anomalous pancreaticobiliary ductal junction. World J Surg. 2000;24:17–21.
5. Fujimoto T, Ohtsuka T, Nakashima Y, et al. Elevated bile amylase level without pancreaticobiliary maljunction is a risk factor for gallbladder carcinoma. J Hepatobiliary Pancreat Sci. 2017;24:103–8.
6. Sai JK, Suyama M, Kubokawa Y, et al. Gallbladder carcinoma associated with pancreatobiliary reflux. World J Gastroenterol. 2006;12:6527–30.
7. Itokawa F, Itoi T, Nakamura K, et al. Assessment of occult pancreatobiliary reflux in patients with pancreaticobiliary disease by ERCP. J Gastroenterol. 2004;39:988–94.
8. Donaldson LA, Joffe SN, Mclntosh W, et al. Amylase activity in human bile. Gut. 1979;20:216–8.
9. Motosugi U, Ichikawa T, Araki T, et al. Secretin-stimulating MRCP in patients with pancreatobiliary maljunction and occult pancreatobiliary reflux: direct demonstration of pancreatobiliary reflux. Eur Radiol. 2007;17:2262–7.
10. Sakamoto H, Mutoh H, Ido K, et al. Intestinal metaplasia in gallbladder correlates with high amylase levels in bile in patients with a morphologically normal pancreaticobiliary duct. Hum Pathol. 2009;40:1762–7.
11. Ragot E, Mabrut JY. Ouaïssi, et al. Pancreaticobiliary Maljunctions in European patients with bile duct cysts: results of the multicenter study of the French Surgical Association (AFC). World J Surg. 2017;41:538–45.
12. Jeong IH, Jung YS, Kim H, et al. Amylase level in extrahepatic bile duct in adult patients with choledochal cyst plus anomalous pancreatico-biliary ductal union. World J Gastroenterol. 2005;11:1965–70.

13. Jung SM, Seo JM, Lee SK. The relationship between biliary amylase and the clinical features of choledochal cysts in pediatric patients. World J Surg. 2012;36:2098–101.
14. Kamisawa T, Suyama M, Fujita N, et al. Pancreatobiliary reflux and the length of a common channel. J Hepatobiliary Pancreat Sci. 2010;17:865–70.
15. Tashiro S, Imaizumi T, Ohkawa H, et al. Pancreaticobiliary maljunction: retrospective and nationwide survey in Japan. J Hepato-Biliary-Pancreat Surg. 2003;10:345–51.
16. Beltrán MA, Vracko J, Cumsille MA, et al. Occult pancreaticobiliary reflux in gallbladder cancer and benign gallbladder diseases. J Surg Oncol. 2007;96:26–31.
17. Horaguchi J, Fujita N, Kamisawa T, et al. Pancreatobiliary reflux in individuals with a normal pancreatobiliary junction: a prospective multicenter study. J Gastroenterol. 2014;49:875–81.
18. Adachi T, Tajima Y, Kuroki T, et al. Bile-reflux into the pancreatic ducts is associated with the development of intraductal papillary carcinoma in hamsters. J Surg Res. 2006;136:106–11.
19. Morine Y, Shimada M, Takamatsu H, et al. Clinical features of pancreaticobiliary maljunction: update analysis of 2nd Japan-nationwide survey. J Hepatobiliary Pancreat Sci. 2013;20:472–80.
20. Itoi T, Tsuchida A, Itokawa F, et al. Histologic and genetic analysis of the gallbladder in patients with occult pancreatobiliary reflux. Int J Mol Med. 2005;15:425–30.

Part V
Pancreaticobiliary Complication

Chapter 18
Pancreaticobiliary Complication Biliary Cancer in Pancreaticobiliary Maljunction and Congenital Biliary Dilatation

Ryota Higuchi, Takehisa Yazawa, and Masakazu Yamamoto

Abstract Pancreaticobiliary maljunction (PBM) and congenital biliary dilatation (CBD) are important risk factors of biliary cancers. According to the nationwide survey in Japan, the biliary cancer incidence of PBM was 21.6% in patients with CBD and 42.4% in patients without CBD. In patients with PBM and CBD, resection and reconstruction of the extrahepatic bile duct (flow-diversion surgery) is a basic surgical procedure for preventing the high occurrence of bile duct and gallbladder cancer. On the contrary, in patients with PBM but without CBD, no consensus has been reached about whether it is better to perform cholecystectomy alone or flow-diversion surgery. After surgery, a reported 0.5–2.0% of patients who undergo cyst excision develop bile duct carcinoma. Although the incidence of cancer after surgery is lower than that before surgery, it is 120–200 times higher than that of the entire population. Therefore, long-term follow-up is needed in patients with PBM and/or CBD.

Keywords Congenital biliary dilatation · Pancreaticobiliary malunion · Choledochal Anomalous · Biliary cancer · Gallbladder cancer · Bile duct cancer · Cholangiocarcinoma

18.1 Introduction

Pancreaticobiliary maljunction (PBM) is a congenital anomaly in which the pancreatic duct and bile duct join anatomically outside the duodenal wall [1]. Congenital biliary dilatation (CBD) is a congenital malformation involving local dilatation of the extrahepatic bile duct, including the common bile duct and PBM [2].

R. Higuchi · T. Yazawa · M. Yamamoto (✉)
Department of Surgery, Institute of Gastroenterology, Tokyo Women's Medical University, Shinjuku-ku, Tokyo, Japan
e-mail: yamamoto.masakazu@twmu.ac.jp

T. Kamisawa, H. Ando (eds.), *Pancreaticobiliary Maljunction and Congenital Biliary Dilatation*, https://doi.org/10.1007/978-981-10-8654-0_18

In PBM, the Oddi sphincter muscles do not influence the confluence of the pancreatic duct and the bile duct, causing various conditions such as flow disturbances of the bile and pancreatic juices, reciprocal reflux between them, and biliary system malignancy [2]. Among them, a major clinical problem is biliary tract cancer, which occurs at a high rate. Therefore, here we describe biliary cancer occurring in patients with PBM and CBD, especially the mechanism, frequency, characteristics, and incidence of biliary cancer after surgery.

18.2 Mechanism of Carcinogenesis in PBM Patients with Biliary Tract Cancer

18.2.1 Mechanism

Sustained inflammation and regeneration of the biliary mucosa results in biliary cancer in PBM patients [1]. Because the papillary Oddi sphincter cannot control the pancreaticobiliary junction, there is regurgitation of pancreatic juice and bile [1]. Therefore, the biliary mucosa is continually damaged by pancreatic enzymes and the induced mutagenic substance in the dilated bile ducts and gallbladder by mixing of refluxed pancreatic juice with the bile [3, 4]. In the dilated bile duct and gallbladder, cell cycle turnover is enhanced by persistent inflammation and regeneration, which has been suggested to induce the development of hyperplasia, dysplasia, and malignancy [1].

It is reported that strong cytotoxic substances (such as lysolecithin) are produced when phospholipase A2 in the pancreatic juice mixes with bile, while chronic inflammation causes repetitive injury–healing cycles in the biliary mucosal epithelium. These changes (predominantly hyperplasia) in the mucosal epithelium, alone or in combination with DNA mutation, are thought to ultimately cause cancer of the tissue [5].

The carcinogenesis of PBM-associated biliary cancer is thought to be due to the hyperplasia–dysplasia–carcinoma pathway induced by chronic inflammation caused by contamination of the bile and pancreatic juice [1]. This mechanism is thought to differ from the adenoma–carcinoma sequence or de novo carcinogenesis related to biliary cancer in a population without PBM [1].

18.2.2 Changes in Biliary Mucosa in Patients with PBM

It has been reported that epithelial hyperplasia is frequently observed in the gallbladders of patients with PBM but not in patients without it [6]. The incidence of epithelial hyperplasia was significantly higher in the gallbladders of patients in whom the major pancreatic duct joined the common bile duct (P-C type) than in patients in whom the common bile duct joined the pancreatic duct (C-P type) [6]. In the early childhood of patients with PBM, early mucosal changes in the gallbladder that may be related to the development of gallbladder cancer also reportedly occur [7]. In this report, there was a significant difference in the Ki-67 labeling index, a nuclear antigen that is present in proliferating cells, in pediatric patients with and without PBM. The Ki-67 labeling index and the incidence of epithelial hyperplasia of the gallbladder were significantly higher in pediatric patients with PBM with the P-C-type than the C-P-type anomaly [7]. Cellular proliferative activity was also increased in children with PBM, especially those with the P-C-type anomaly [7].

In the dilated bile duct wall of CBD patients, an increase in collagen fiber deposition, wall thickening, inflammatory cell infiltration, and pseudopyloric gland metaplasia of the bile ducts' mucous gland are often observed [1]. Dysplasia and/or cancer may develop in such cases [1].

Many oncogenes and tumor suppressor genes have been identified and are reportedly involved in carcinogenesis, especially the K-ras oncogene and the p53 suppressor gene. Several K-ras mutations appear to be nonessential for hyperplasia but have been reported as early events of carcinogenesis. The p53 mutation is suggested to be involved in carcinogenesis of the bile duct epithelium in patients with PBM [8, 9].

18.3 Surgery for PBM with or Without CBD

When PBM is diagnosed, because it is a high-risk factor for the development of biliary tract cancer, there is an indication for preventive surgery regardless of the presence or absence of symptoms. In patients with PBM and CBD, resection and reconstruction of the extrahepatic bile duct (flow-diversion surgery) is a basic surgical procedure. On the contrary, in patients with PBM but without CBD, there are two opinions and, therefore, two different surgical procedures that are followed. One procedure involves only cholecystectomy because most of the complicated cancers are gallbladder cancer, and there are few reports on the occurrence of bile duct cancer after cholecystectomy. The other procedure involves resection and reconstruction of the extrahepatic bile duct because it is considered that there is a potential risk of carcinogenesis in nondilated bile ducts.

18.4 Frequency and Location of Biliary Tract Cancer in Patients with PBM

Patients with PBM have a high rate of biliary tract cancers. Morine et al. reported on the nationwide survey ($n = 2561$) in Japan of patients with PBM performed by the Japanese Study Group and the Committee from 1 January 1990 to 31 December 2007 at 141 institutes [10]. There were 1511 adult patients included: 997 with

Table 18.1 Occurrence rates of the associated cancers [10]

	Adult (n = 1511)	
	With biliary dilatation (n = 997)	Without biliary dilatation (n = 514)
Biliary cancers, n (%)	215 (21.6)	218 (42.4)
Liver cancer, n (%)	5 (0.5)	12 (2.3)
Pancreatic cancer, n (%)	9 (0.9)	5 (1.0)
Others, n (%)	7 (0.7)	14 (2.7)

Reprinted with permission from (Partial modification)
Data are presented as number and percentages

Table 18.2 Location of the associated biliary cancers [10]

	Adult biliary cancer patients (n = 433)	
	With biliary dilatation (n = 215)	Without biliary dilatation (n = 218)
Biliary cancers, n (%)	134 (62.3)	192 (88.1)
Liver cancer, n (%)	69 (32.1)	16 (7.3)
Pancreatic cancer, n (%)	10 (4.7)	9 (4.1)
Others, n (%)	2 (0.9)	1 (0.5)

Reprinted with permission from (Partial modification)
Data are presented as number and percentages

biliary dilatation and 514 without biliary dilatation. The biliary cancer incidence of PBM was 21.6% in patients with CBD and 42.4% in patients without biliary dilatation (Table 18.1). The main malignancies were gallbladder cancer and bile duct cancer, and the rate of each disease in patients with congenital biliary dilatation was 62.3% and 32.1%, respectively, while that of cancers in patients without biliary dilatation was 88.1% and 7.3%, respectively (Table 18.2). Gallbladder cancer was the most frequent cancer in this series [10], and its incidence increased recently [10].

Sastry et al. reported in a review of 5780 reported choledochal cyst patients, of whom nearly 85% were from Asia, 8.6% were from the United States, and 5.8% were from Europe [11]. In this review, 434 patients had cancer, and the incidence of malignancy in adults was 11.4%. In this review, bile duct (70.4%, 255 patients) and gallbladder cancer (23.5%, 85 patients) were also the most common malignancies [11].

18.5 Characteristics of Biliary Tract Cancer Occurring in Patients with PBM

18.5.1 Age at the Time Cancer Was Discovered

According to the Japanese nationwide survey, the mean age of PBM patients who are reported to develop biliary cancer and gallbladder carcinoma is 60.1 ± 10.4 years, bile duct cancer is 52.0 ± 15.0 years old in patients with CBD, and that of gallbladder cancer is 58.6 ± 9.6 years and that of bile duct cancer is 63.3 ± 6.8 years in

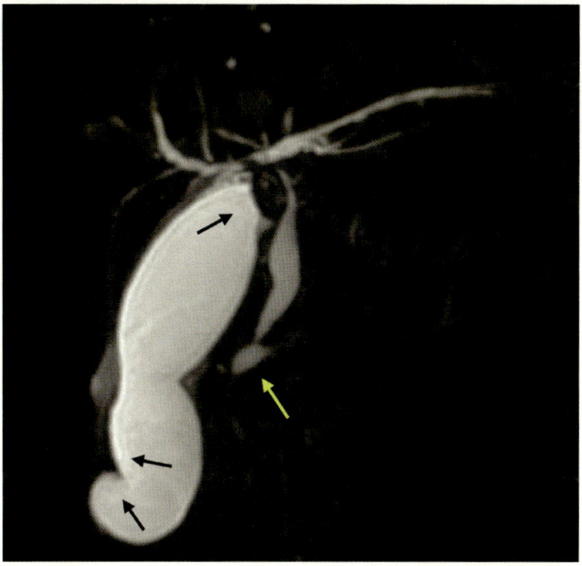

Fig. 18.1 A 49-year-old woman with gallbladder cancer of the neck and fundus (*black arrows*) and pancreaticobiliary maljunction (*yellow arrow*) without biliary dilatation underwent extended cholecystectomy with resection and reconstruction of the bile duct and postoperative chemotherapy and immunotherapy. The pathological diagnosis was adenosquamous cell carcinoma T3a N1 M1 (no. 16 lymph node metastasis). She died of multiple lymph node metastasis 36 months postoperatively

patients with PBM but without biliary dilation [10]. The age of patients with PBM accompanied by biliary tract cancer is significantly higher than those with PBM but no biliary tract cancer [10, 12]. In another review, the median age for the diagnosis of cancer associated with CBD was reportedly 42 years [11]. Biliary cancer associated with PBM may occur more than 10–20 years earlier than in cases without PBM (Fig. 18.1) [1, 13, 14].

18.5.2 Risk Factors

It is currently unknown whether the risk factors for biliary tract cancer are related to the amylase level in the gallbladder or bile duct [1]. In one report, age ≥45 years, P-C type, and a biliary lipase level ≥45,000 IU/L are significantly associated with PBM-related biliary tract cancer [15].

18.5.3 Survival

In patients with gallbladder cancer who underwent curative resection, the presence or absence of PBM is not an independent prognostic factor, so it has been reported that there was no difference in survival rate in gallbladder cancer patients with or without PBM [13, 16]. In patients with bile duct cancer arising from a choledochal cyst, the reported survival rate was generally equivalent to that of patients with bile duct cancer [17].

18.5.4 Occurrence of Synchronous Multiple or Double Cancers

Synchronous multiple or double cancers occur more frequently in patients with PBM than in those without PBM. Of the 37 patients with simultaneous and/or metachronous double biliary cancers, 19 (51.4%) were associated with PBM [1]. Metachronous double cancers are also frequently reported in PBM patients [1, 13, 17].

18.5.5 Rate of Gallstones in Gallbladder Cancer

Gallbladder cancer in patients with PBM reportedly has a significantly lower rate of gallstones (about 10%) compared to gallbladder cancer in patients without PBM [1, 13].

18.6 Incidence of Biliary Cancer After Flow-Diversion Surgery

In recent years, the occurrence of cancer in the residual hepatic duct, intrahepatic bile duct, or residual intrapancreatic bile duct after cyst excision is a serious problem [2]. Bile duct carcinoma occurs in an estimated 0.5–2.0% [2, 17–20] of patients who undergo cyst excision, an incidence that is 120–200 times higher than that of the entire population [2]. Carcinogenesis is frequently observed in cases of repeated cholangitis, intrahepatic calculus, and residual extended bile duct due to insufficient biliary tract resection [2].

18.6.1 Biliary Cancer After Dilated Bile Duct Resection in Patients with PBM and CBD

Ando recently reported the aggregated results of 107 Japanese patients with PBM and CBD (conference record included) with biliary cancer after dilated bile duct resection [20] as follows: (1) The age at first surgery was 5–72 years (mean, 34.8 years); 16 patients underwent the initial surgery at 1–15 years of age, and even if the patient underwent surgery during childhood, the cancer occurred. (2) The age at the time of cancer discovery was 18–83 years (mean, 47.2 years old), while the male/female ratio was 28:65 (unclear in 14). (3) The time from the initial surgery to cancer discovery was 8–38 years (mean, 12 years). He also reported the aggregated results of 75 cases of biliary cancer after dilated bile duct resection in patients with PBM and CBD that occurred more than 5 years after the initial surgery [20]. (4) As the age at surgery increased, the period until carcinogenesis tended to be shorter.

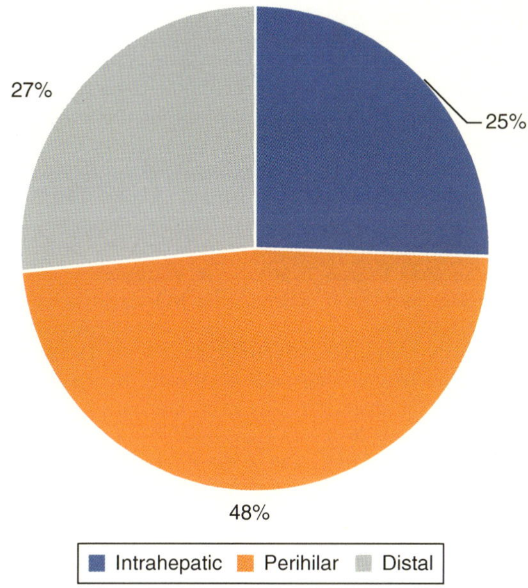

Fig. 18.2 Site of biliary tract cancer development after resection of the dilated bile duct ($n = 98$) [20]. Reprinted with permission from (Partial modification)

(5) Among the 92 patients whose type was clear, 28 (30.4%) were type I and 64 (69.6%) were type IVA. (6) The 98 cases in which the details were clear involved cancer in 25 intrahepatic bile ducts, 47 hepatic or bile ducts, and 26 intrapancreatic ducts (Fig. 18.2). (7) Cancer was found in 47 patients among the resected 2354 cases at 24 facilities in a paper in which the total number of resections was mentioned, and the carcinogenic rate was 2.0%. Cholangitis and intrahepatic calculi coexisted in 38 of 80 cases of symptomatic cancer.

18.6.2 Carcinogenesis of the Bile Duct After Cholecystectomy in Patients Without CBD

In general, in cases of PBM without gallbladder dilation, cholecystectomy only is performed and bile ducts are preserved; therefore, postoperative bile duct cancer is the main concern. However, few reports on the occurrence of such carcinoma are available [1].

18.7 Conclusion

PBM is an important risk factor of biliary cancers, and prophylactic surgery will be indicated when it is diagnosed. After surgery for PBM and CBD, long-term follow-up is needed in patients with PBM or CBD because the incidence of cancer after surgery is rather high.

References

1. Kamisawa T, Ando H, Suyama M, Shimada M, Morine Y, Shimada H, Working Committee of Clinical Practice Guidelines for Pancreaticobiliary Maljunction. Japanese clinical practice guidelines for pancreaticobiliary maljunction. J Gastroenterol. 2012;47:731–59.
2. Ishibashi H, Shimada M, Kamisawa T, Fujii H, Hamada Y, Kubota M, Urushihara N, Endo I, Nio M, Taguchi T, Ando H, Japanese Study Group on Congenital Biliary Dilatation (JSCBD). Japanese clinical practice guidelines for congenital biliary dilatation. J Hepatobiliary Pancreat Sci. 2017;24:1–16.
3. Matsubara T, Tsuji T, Miyama A, Yamaguchi H, Funabiki T. Mutagenicity of bile and pancreatic juice from patients with pancreatico-biliary maljunction. Hepatogastroenterology. 1995;42:113–6.
4. Kato T, Matsuda K, Kayaba H, Enomoto S, Hebiguchi T, Koyama K, Hachiya N, Takizawa Y. Pathology of anomalous junction of the pancreaticobiliary ductal system: mutagenicity of the contents of the biliary tract and nuclear atypia of the biliary epithelium. Keio J Med. 1989;38:167–76.
5. Shimada K, Yanagisawa J, Nakayama F. Increased lysophosphatidylcholine and pancreatic enzyme content in bile of patients with anomalous pancreaticobiliary ductal junction. Hepatology. 1991;13:438–44.
6. Tokiwa K, Iwai N. Early mucosal changes of the gallbladder in patients with anomalous arrangement of the pancreaticobiliary duct. Gastroenterology. 1996;110:1614–8.
7. Ono S, Tokiwa K, Iwai N. Cellular activity in the gallbladder of children with anomalous arrangement of the pancreaticobiliary duct. J Pediatr Surg. 1999;34:962–6.
8. Matsumoto Y, Fujii H, Itakura J, Matsuda M, Yang Y, Nobukawa B, Suda K. Pancreaticobiliary maljunction: pathophysiological and clinical aspects and the impact on biliary carcinogenesis. Langenbecks Arch Surg. 2003;388:122–31.
9. Hanada K, Itoh M, Fujii K, Tsuchida A, Ooishi H, Kajiyama G. K-ras and p53 mutations in stage I gallbladder carcinoma with an anomalous junction of the pancreaticobiliary duct. Cancer. 1996;77:452–8.
10. Morine Y, Shimada M, Takamatsu H, Araida T, Endo I, Kubota M, Toki A, Noda T, Matsumura T, Miyakawa S, Ishibashi H, Kamisawa T, Shimada H. Clinical features of pancreaticobiliary maljunction: update analysis of 2nd Japan-nationwide survey. J Hepatobiliary Pancreat Sci. 2013;20:472–80.
11. Sastry AV, Abbadessa B, Wayne MG, Steele JG, Cooperman AM. What is the incidence of biliary carcinoma in choledochal cysts, when do they develop, and how should it affect management? World J Surg. 2015;39:487–92.
12. Cho MJ, Hwang S, Lee YJ, Kim KH, Ahn CS, Moon DB, Lee SK, Kim MH, Lee SS, Park DH, Lee SG. Surgical experience of 204 cases of adult choledochal cyst disease over 14 years. World J Surg. 2011;35:1094–102.
13. Chang J, Jang JY, Kang MJ, Jung W, Shin YC, Kim SW. Clinicopathologic differences in patients with gallbladder cancer according to the presence of anomalous biliopancreatic junction. World J Surg. 2016;40:1211–7.
14. Hasumi A, Matsui H, Sugioka A, Uyama I, Komori Y, Fujita J, Aoki H. Precancerous conditions of biliary tract cancer in patients with pancreaticobiliary maljunction: reappraisal of nationwide survey in Japan. J Hepatobiliary Pancreat Surg. 2000;7:551–5.
15. Park JS, Song TJ, Park TY, Oh D, Lee HK, Park do H, Lee SS, Seo DW, Lee SK, Kim MH. Predictive factors of biliary tract cancer in anomalous union of the pancreaticobiliary duct. Medicine (Baltimore). 2016;95:e3526.
16. Lim H, Seo DW, Park DH, Lee SS, Lee SK, Kim MH, Hwang S. Prognostic factors in patients with gallbladder cancer after surgical resection: analysis of 279 operated patients. J Clin Gastroenterol. 2013;47:443–8.

17. Lee SE, Jang JY, Lee YJ, Choi DW, Lee WJ, Cho BH, Kim SW, Korean Pancreas Surgery Club. Choledochal cyst and associated malignant tumors in adults: a multicenter survey in South Korea. Arch Surg. 2011;146:1178–84.
18. Takeshita N, Ota T, Yamamoto M. Forty-year experience with flow-diversion surgery for patients with congenital choledochal cysts with pancreaticobiliary maljunction at a single institution. Ann Surg. 2011;254:1050–3.
19. Watanabe Y, Toki A, Todani T. Bile duct cancer developed after cyst excision for choledochal cyst. J Hepatobiliary Pancreat Surg. 1999;6:207–12.
20. Ando H. Problems of the surgical treatment for the congenital biliary dilatation taken into consideration from postoperative carcinogenesis. Tan Sui Biliary Tract Pancreas. 2017;38:381–5. (in Japanese)

Chapter 19
Biliary Cancer in Children with Pancreaticobiliary Maljunction and Congenital Biliary Dilatation

Masayuki Kubota

Abstract In order to clarify the clinical characteristics of children with cancer of the extrahepatic biliary tract (EHBT) associated with congenital biliary dilatation (CBD) and/or pancreaticobiliary maljunction (PBM), a comprehensive literature search for this subject was carried out in the English and Japanese literatures. The upper age limit of the children was set at 20 years of age in this study. As a result of the literature search, 17 patients (8 males and 9 females) were identified, specifically 15 patients with CBD with or without PBM and 2 patients with PBM without CBD. The median age of these 17 patients was 15 years (95% confidence interval, 11.7–16.6 years). A questionnaire was then sent to the authors of the reports of these 17 patients to determine the type of CBD and PBM, stage of cancer, and its prognosis. Taking together all data from the literature and the replies to the questionnaire, the site of cancer was the common bile duct in 14 CBD patients, while 2 patients with PBM without CBD and 1 with CBD showed cancer in the gallbladder. The stage of EHBT cancer and prognosis were identified in eight CBD patients with cancer in the common bile duct. The stages of the three survivors were IA in two and IIB in one, while those of the five dead patients were IIA in one, IIB in one, and IV in three. Survivors were found only in Stage IA and IIB patients, indicating the importance of complete resection of the tumor, even in children.

Keywords Congenital biliary dilatation · Pancreaticobiliary maljunction · Cancer Extrahepatic biliary tract · Children

M. Kubota
Department of Pediatric Surgery, Niigata University Graduate School of Medical and Dental Sciences, Niigata City, Niigata, Japan
e-mail: kubotama@med.niigata-u.ac.jp

T. Kamisawa, H. Ando (eds.), *Pancreaticobiliary Maljunction and Congenital Biliary Dilatation*, https://doi.org/10.1007/978-981-10-8654-0_19

19.1 Introduction

Pancreaticobiliary maljunction (PBM) and/or congenital biliary dilatation (CBD) are well-known risk factors for cancer of the extrahepatic biliary tract (EHBT). According to the registration data in the Japanese Study Group of PBM, EHBT cancer was found at the time of radical operation in 2.3% and 5.7% of PBM patients in their 20s and 30s, respectively. However, in patients in their 40s, the cancer association rate increased to 22.5% [1]. In contrast, in people without PBM, the incidence of EHBT cancer first exceeds 10% when they pass 65 years of age [2]. Therefore, the age of developing EHBT cancer is 20–30 years younger in PBM patients than in non-PBM patients. However, the incidence and prognosis of EHBT cancer in children with PBM and CBD are still unknown.

Therefore, a literature review of EHBT cancer in children was conducted to examine the clinical characteristics of EHBT cancer in this population. The upper age limit of children was set at 20 years of age to examine as many patients as possible.

19.2 Patients and Methods

A literature search for EHBT cancer patients ≤20 years of age was performed using PubMed and Ichushi for the English and Japanese literature, respectively. The key words used in the literature search were choledochal cyst, congenital biliary dilatation, congenital dilatation of bile duct, pancreaticobiliary maljunction, cancer, bile duct, and extrahepatic biliary tract for the PubMed search, and the corresponding Japanese words were used for the Ichushi search.

The Japanese literature search included abstracts of meetings. The proceedings of the annual meeting of the Japanese Study Group of pancreaticobiliary maljunction were also surveyed up to 2015.

The present study included patients whose EHBT cancer was found at the time of radical surgery for PBM or CBD. The patients who developed metachronous cancer after radical surgery or after an internal drainage operation of CBD were excluded. A questionnaire was then sent to the authors of the identified papers to determine the type of CBD based on Todani classification [3], the type of PBM based on Komi classification [4], and the stage of EHBT cancer based on the Japanese classification of the biliary tract cancers, 6th Japanese edition published in 2013 [5].

This study protocol was approved by the Ethics Committee of Niigata University for medical and health research involving human subjects (No. 2544).

19.3 Results

A total of 17 patients (8 males and 9 females) ≤20 years of age with EHBT cancer found at the radical operation for CBD and/or PBM were identified in the present literature search (Table 19.1) [6–21]. The median age at operation was 15.0 years of age (95% confidence interval, 11.7–16.6 years). All patients were Japanese, and all

Table 19.1 List of 17 children with cancer of the extrahepatic biliary tract

Case no	Author	Institute	Journal	Year	Age	Sex	Classification
1	Tsuchiya [6]	Second Department of Surgery, Nagasaki University School of Medicine	Ann Surg	1977	5	F	CBD
2	Tobita[a] [7]	Division of Surgery, Miyazaki Prefectural Nobeoka Hospital	J Jpn Surg Assoc[a]	1980	16	M	CBD
3	Nakasako[a] [8]	Institute of Gastroenterology, TWMU	Jpn J Gastroenterol	1982	14	M	CBD
4	Niimoto[a] [9]	Department of Gastroenterological Surgery, University of Fukui Hospital	Proc (JSG on PBM)	1983	18	F	CBD, PBM
5	Takanashi[a] [10]	First Department of Internal Medicine, Hiraka General Hospital	Jpn J Gastroenterol	1984	18	M	CBD
6	Ohyama[a] [11]	Division of Surgery, Miyazaki Prefectural Nobeoka Hospital	J Jpn Soc Pediatr Surg	1985	10	F	CBD
7	Shiraishi[a] [12]	First Department of Surgery, Faculty of Medicine, Fukuoka University	Jpn J Gastroenterol	1986	18	M	CBD, PBM
8	Haraoka[a] [13]	Department of Surgery, Faculty of Medicine, Saga University	Proc (JSG on PBM)	1988	19	M	CBD
9	Fujiwara[a] [14]	First Department of Surgery, School of Medicine, Dokkyo University	Proc (JSG on PBM)	1989	18	M	CBD
10	Iwai [15]	Division of Surgery, Children's Research Hospital, Kyoto Prefectural University of Medicine	J Pediatr Surg	1990	12	F	CBD
11	Kuriyama[a] [16]	Division of Pediatric Surgery, Matsudo City Hospital	J Jpn Soc Pediatr Surg	1997	15	F	CBD
12	Yamashita[a] [17]	Department of Surgery, Tokyo Medical University Hospital	J Jpn Soc Pediatr Surg	1998	15	F	PBM
13	Yamashita[a] [17]	Department of Surgery, Tokyo Medical University Hospital	J Jpn Soc Pediatr Surg	1998	20	F	PBM
14	Ueda[a] [18]	Division of Surgery, Maizuru Kyosai Hospital	Journal of Biliary Tract & Pancreas	2000	13	F	CBD, PBM
15	Tanaka [19]	Department of Pediatric Surgery, Niigata University	J Pediatr Surg	2006	11	M	CBD
16	Nakamura [20]	Division of Hepato-Biliary Pancreatic Surgery, Department of Surgery, Tohoku University Graduate School of Medicine	J Hepatobiliary Pacreatic Surg	2008	15	F	CBD, PBM
17	Saikusa [21]	Department of Pediatric Surgery, Niigata City General Hospital	J Pediatr Surg	2009	3	M	CBD

F female, *M* male, *CBD* congenital biliary dilatation, *PBM* pancreaticobiliary maljunction
[a]Indicate the papers written in Japanese

papers were reported from Japan. The year of publication ranged from 1977 to 2009, giving an annual incidence of EHBT cancer in patients ≤20 years of age associated with CBD and/or PBM of 0.53. Five patients were reported in the English literatures, while the remaining 12 were reported in Japanese papers. Sixteen papers were reports of a single case, while one paper described two cases (case Nos. 12 and 13). Case No. 15 was our own case. A questionnaire was sent to 15 institutes, and responses were obtained from 12. However, in 4 of the 12 institutes, the hospital no longer had the medical records related to the reported case. Taking together all available data from the publications and the newly obtained data from the questionnaire, 15 patients were diagnosed as CBD with or without PBM (Table 19.2), and 2 patients were diagnosed as PBM not associated with CBD (Table 19.3).

Table 19.2 List of 15 CBD children with cancer of the extrahepatic biliary tract

Case no	Site of cancer	Pathology	Todani	PBM	Komi	Stage	Prognosis	Follow-up period
1	Common bile duct	Botryoid sarcoma	Ic	–	–	–	Alive	
2	Common bile duct	Adenocarcinoma	IV-A	–	–	–	Dead	8 months
3	Common bile duct	Papillary adenocarcinoma	IV-A	–	–	IV	Dead	
4	Common bile duct	Well-differentiated adenocarcinoma	Ia	–	–	–	–	
5	Common bile duct	Adenocarcinoma	–	–	–		–	
6	Gallbladder	Adenocarcinoma	IV-A	–	–	IV	Dead	
7	Common bile duct	Adenosquamous carcinoma	Ia	C-P type	–	–	–	
8	Common bile duct	Adenocarcinoma	–	–	–	–	–	
9	Common bile duct	Tubular adenocarcinoma	IV-A	C-P type	Ib	IA	–	
10	Common bile duct	Adenocarcinoma	Ia	C-P type	–	IIA	Dead	1 year
11	Common bile duct	Well-differentiated tubular adenocarcinoma	Ia	–	–	IIB	Dead	21 months
14	Common bile duct	Carcinoma in situ	Ia	–	IIIa	IA	Alive	4 years and 5 months
15	Common bile duct	Adenocarcinoma	IV-A	C-P type	Ia	IIB	Alive	12 years and 4 months
16	Common bile duct	Differentiated tubular adenocarcinoma	Ia	C-P type	IIIc2	IV	Dead	14 months
17	Common bile duct	Adenocarcinoma	Ia	C-P type	–	IA	Alive	8 years

Todani Todani classification of congenital biliary dilatation, *PBM* pancreaticobiliary maljunction, *Komi* Komi classification of PBM
"–" indicates data not obtained

Table 19.3 List of two PBM patients with cancer of the extrahepatic biliary tract not associated with CBD

No	Site of Cancer	Pathology	PBM	Komi	Stage	Prognosis	Follow-up period
12	Gallbladder	Well-differentiated papillary adenocarcinoma	P-C type	–	–	Alive	16 years
13	Gallbladder	Well-differentiated papillary adenocarcinoma	P-C type	–	–	Alive	13 years

PBM pancreaticobiliary maljunction, *Komi* Komi classification of PBM
"–" indicates data not obtained

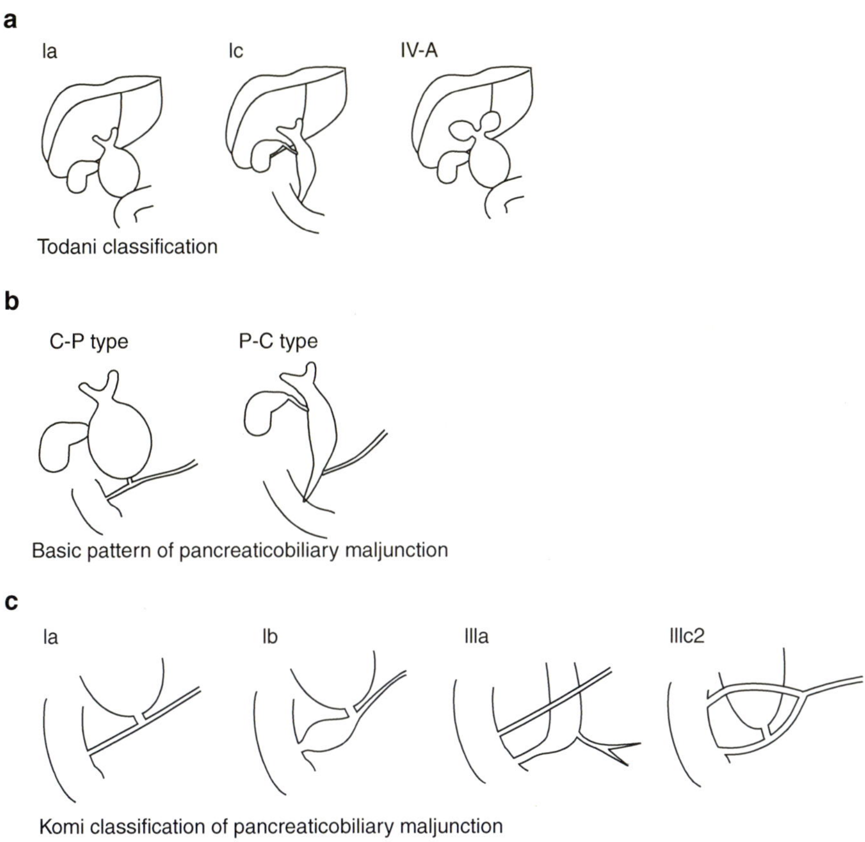

Fig. 19.1 A schematic illustration of Todani classification of CBD, basic pattern of PBM, and Komi classification of PBM introduced in the text. In type A or C-P type, the common bile duct joins the pancreatic duct at a right angle, while in type B or P-C type, the pancreatic duct joins the common bile duct at a right angle. *Ia* A type PBM, *Ib* Ia with dilatation of the common channel, *IIIa* pancreas divisum, *IIIc2* Ia with visualization of the accessory pancreatic duct. (**a**) Todani classification. (**b**) Basic pattern of pancreaticobiliary maljunction. (**c**) Komi classification of pancreaticobiliary maljunction

The 15 CBD patients with EHBT cancer are described in Table 19.2. Cancer was found in the common bile duct in 14 patients, while the remaining patient had gallbladder cancer. Pathological studies have shown that the type of EHBT cancer was adenocarcinoma in 14 cases and botryoid rhabdomyosarcoma in the remaining patient. According to the Todani classification, the number of patients with types Ia, Ic, and IV-A were 7, 1, and 5, respectively (Fig. 19.1a). The type of Todani classification was not defined in two patients due to a lack of information. Seven patients were reported to have PBM. The type of PBM was clarified in six patients and was commonly P-C type in these patients, with the common bile duct seeming to join the pancreatic duct at a right angle (Fig. 19.1b). Further detailed classification of PBM using Komi classification was only possible in four patients (one each with Ia, Ib, IIIa, and IIIc2) (Fig. 19.1c). The stage of EHBT cancer and prognosis were defined in nine and ten patients, respectively. Both the stage and prognosis were defined in eight patients. The survivors were two Stage IA patients and one Stage IIB patient, while one Stage IIA patient, one Stage IIB patient, and three Stage IV patients died.

In two PBM patients without CBD, papillary adenocarcinoma was found in the gallbladder. The type of PBM was C-P type, with the pancreatic duct connecting to the common bile duct at a right angle (Fig. 19.1a). Even though the stage was not clarified, a long-term survival was reported.

19.4 Discussion

In the present study, in order to clarify the characteristics of EHBT cancer in children associated with CBD and/or PBM, a literature search was carried out. To include as many patients as possible, the upper age limit was set at 20. In addition, in the Japanese literature search, the abstracts of meetings or proceedings of the annual meeting of the Japanese Study Group of pancreaticobiliary maljunction were included. Despite conducting such an intensive literature search, only 17 patients could be found among the published papers, clearly indicating a paucity of EHBT cancer in children associated with CBD and/or PBM.

Of the 17 EHBT cancer children, 15 were CBD patients with or without PBM, and 2 were PBM patients without CBD. According to the Todani classification [3], 12 of the 13 CBD patients whose Todani classification was identified were either type Ia or IV-A, suggesting cystic dilatation of the common bile duct, except for 1 case of type Ic with fusiform dilatation of the common bile duct. Types Ia, Ic, and IV-A were reported to be associated with PBM [3]. Therefore, we suspect that these 15 CBD children might be associated with PBM.

In adult PBM patients without CBD, cancer occurs in the gallbladder in 90% of cases [22]. In the present study, two of three patients with gallbladder cancer were not associated with CBD. PBM is considered to be a causative factor for carcinogenesis in the sense that the activated pancreatic enzymes are stocked and concentrated in the gallbladder, which induces a cascade of hyperplasia-dysplasia-carcinoma sequence [23]. In adult patients associated with both PBM and CBD, the ratio of gallbladder cancer drops to 60%, and the ratio of common bile duct cancer increases to 30% [22].

In the present 15 CBD patients, cancer was found in the common bile duct in 14 cases and in the gallbladder in 1 case. In adult PBM patients, the association rate of CBD was 66%, while this ratio increased to 93.3% in children <15 years of age [22]. The basic patterns of PBM were classified into two types: type A (C-P type) and type B (P-C type), as shown in Fig. 19.1a. The basic pattern of PBM was found in 6 of 15 CBD patients. They were all type A cases. In adult PBM patients, the ratios of types A and B were 57.3% and 32.7%, respectively, when associated with CBD. The corresponding ratios of types A and B in children <15 years of age were 57.5% and 31.1%, respectively. However, this ratio reversed when not associated with CBD. The ratios of types A and B in PBM patients without CBD were 31.5% and 58.6%, respectively, and the corresponding values in children were 25.0% and 55.9%, respectively. Therefore, in the CBD children with EHBT cancer, the type of PBM is more likely to be type A than B, and cancer occurrence is mainly found in the common bile duct.

The pathological diagnosis was adenocarcinoma of EHBT in 16 patients, while 1 patient was diagnosed with botryoid rhabdomyosarcoma. Reportedly, 1% of rhabdomyosarcoma occurs in EHBT, which constitutes the highest incidence of EHBT tumor in children [24]. Only fetal-type rhabdomyosarcoma occurs in EHBT with a botryoid appearance [25].

A major limitation associated with the present study is the relatively low number of cases identified. Seventeen patients are not large enough to draw any definitive conclusion. The year of publication ranged from 1977 to 2009. This long study period may be the reason for the missing data in some institutes. It was also difficult to evaluate the collected data on the same clinical basis because the method of the diagnosis and treatment protocols vary considerably across such a long study period. While we wanted to investigate the prognosis of EHBT cancer children with CBD and/or PBM, combined data on the stage and prognosis could be obtained in only eight patients. The most advanced stage among the surviving cases was Stage IIB, while another Stage IIB patient died. This discrepancy in outcomes suggests that we lacked sufficient data concerning the prognosis of the EHBT cancer children with CBD and/or PBM for a comparison with adult EHBT cancer patients. Therefore, the surgical strategy for EHBT cancer in children should be as strict as that for adult EHBT cancer patients. Early detection and complete resection of the tumor might be necessary for a favorable outcome.

References

1. Watanabe Y, Toki A, Todani T. Bile duct cancer developed after cyst excision for choledochal cyst. J Hepatobiliary Pancreat Surg. 1999;6(3):207–12.
2. Utada M, Ohno Y, Tamaki T, Sobue T, Endo G. Long-term trends in incidence and mortality of intrahepatic and extrahepatic bile duct cancer in Japan. J Epidemiol. 2014;24(3):193–9.
3. Todani T, Watanabe Y, Toki A, Morotomi Y. Classification of congenital biliary cystic disease: special reference to type Ic and IVA cysts with primary ductal stricture. J Hepatobiliary Pancreat Surg. 2003;10(5):340–4.
4. Komi N. Analysis of 50 cases with pancreaticobiliary maljunction associated with congenital biliary dilatation-supplement of Komi classification. Suizo (Japanese). 1991;6(3):234–44.

5. Classification of the biliary tract cancers established by Japanese Society Hepato-Biliary-Pancreatic Surgery. 6th English edition. J Hepatobiliary Pancreat Sci. 2017, Kanehara, Tokyo.
6. Tsuchiya R, Harada N, Ito T, Furukawa M, Yoshihiro I. Malignant tumors in choledochal cysts. Ann Surg. 1977;186(1):22–8.
7. Tobita K, Matsueda K, Kawaguchi T, Narita F, Komorita Y, Hirota S. A case of congenital biliary dilatation associated with biliary cancer. J Jpn Surg Assoc (Japanese). 1980;41(5):87.
8. Nakasako T, Takada T, Sato Y, Uchiyama K, Ohashi M, Suzuki E, et al. The youngest case of biliary tract cancer with congenital biliary dilatation. Jpn J Gastroenterol (Japanese). 1982;79(3):926–7.
9. Niimot S, Shimada H, Kinoshita M, Kojima Y, Miwa K, Nakagawara Y, et al. Pathology of pancreaticobiliary maljunction. Proc (JSG on PBM)(Japanese). 1983;6:80.
10. Takahashi M, Ohkubo T, Nakajima K, Mizuno K, Miyazaki Y, Murakami T, et al. A case of congenital biliary dilatation associated with biliary tract cancer. Jpn J Gastroenterol (Japanese). 1984;81(1):145.
11. Ohyama T, Fukuda S, Kondo C, Kojima A, Maeda M, Kawachi J. Five cases with congenital biliary dilatation, especially about 5-year-old case associated with cancer. J Jpn Soc Pediatr Surg (Japanese). 1985;18(2):534.
12. Shiraishi M, Watanabe D, Ikeda S, Shimura K, Sakaguchi S, Ymamoto T, et al. A case of congenital biliary dilatation associated with early cancer of biliary tract (adenosquamous carcinoma). Jpn J Gastroenterol (Japanese). 1986;83(2):299.
13. Haraoka S, Satoh Y, Hidaka K, Harada S, Hisatsugu T. A case of juvenile congenital biliary dilatation associated with unresectable biliary cancer when clinical symptom appeared. Proc (JSG on PBM)(Japanese). 1988;11:84.
14. Fujiwara T, Kobayashi K, Ikeda S, Nobuta S, Miyano T, Saotome I. A case of pancreaticobiliary maljunction associated with bile duct cancer. Proc (JSG on PBM)(Japanese). 1989;12:32–3.
15. Iwai N, Deguchi E, Yanagihara J, Iwai M, Matsuo H, Todo S, et al. Cancer arising in a choledochal cyst in a 12-year-old girl. J Pediatr Surg. 1990;25(12):1261–3.
16. Kuriyama Y, Kawamura K, Enomoto H, Asanuma K. A case of 15-year-old girl with congenital biliary dilatation with bile duct cancer. J Jpn Soc Pediatr Surg (Japanese). 1997;33(2):314–8.
17. Yamashita Y, Kajimura K, Kajiyana T, Tamada N, Nishio A, Yamamoto T, et al. A case of juvenile gallbladder cancer with pancreaticobiliary maljunction followed for one year. Jpn J Gastroenterol (Japanese). 1986;83(4):915.
18. Ueda M, Neduka H, Yamamot S, Yoshimitsu Y, Isobe Y, Yamaguchi N, et al. A case of 13-year-old girl of congenital biliary dilatation and pancreaticobiliary maljunction associated with early stage bile duct cancer. Tan to Sui (Japanese). 2000;21(7):593–7.
19. Tanaka S, Kubota M, Yagi M, Okuyama N, Ohtaki M, Yamazaki S, et al. An 11-year-old male patient demonstrating cholangiocarcinoma associated with congenital biliary dilatation. J Pediatr Surg. 2006;41(1):e15–9.
20. Nakamura H, Katayose Y, Rikiyama T, Onogawa T, Yamamoto K, Yoshida H, et al. Advanced bile duct carcinoma in a 15-year-old patient with pancreaticobiliary maljunction and congenital biliary cystic disease. J Hepatobiliary Pancreat Surg. 2008;15(5):554–9.
21. Saikusa N, Naito S, Iinuma Y, Ohtani T, Yokoyama N, Nitta K. Invasive cholangiocarcinoma identified in congenital biliary dilatation in a 3-year-old boy. J Pediatr Surg. 2009;44(11):2202–5.
22. Morine Y, Shimada M, Takamatsu H, Araida T, Endo I, Kubota M, al s. Clinical features of pancreaticobiliary maljunction: update analysis of 2nd Japan-nationwide survey. J Hepatobiliary Pancreat Sci. 2013;20(5):472–80.
23. Tsuchida A, Itoi T. Carcinogenesis and chemoprevention of biliary tract cancer in pancreaticobiliary maljunction. World J Gastrointest Oncol. 2010;2(3):130–5.
24. Zampieri N, Camoglio F, Corroppolo M, Cecchetto M, Ornis S, Ottolenghi A. Botryoid rhabdomyosarcoma of the biliary tract in children: a unique case report. Eur J Cancer Care (Engl). 2006;15(5):463–6.
25. Levy AD. Malignant liver tumors. Clin Liver Dis. 2002;6(1):147–64.

Chapter 20
Carcinogenesis of the Biliary Tract in PBM

Yuichi Nagakawa, Yatsuka Sahara, Chie Takishita, and Akihiko Tsuchida

Abstract Pancreaticobiliary maljunction (PBM) complicates biliary tract cancer at a high rate because of continuous biliary reflux of pancreatic juice. Pathological findings suggest a hyperplasia-dysplasia-carcinoma sequence in carcinogenesis of PBM. This appears to be a different mechanism from that of usual gallbladder cancer without PBM, which develops by an adenoma-carcinoma sequence or by de novo carcinogenesis. Molecular biological analysis revealed a high incidence of cellular proliferation-activating factors, such as COX-2, in the hyperplasia stage. In addition, cellular proliferative activity including Ki-67 was significantly higher in normal gallbladder mucosa without PBM. Furthermore, a high incidence of K-ras gene mutation was seen in hyperplasia (13–63%), and microsatellite instability was observed in 60% of cases with dysplasia. In cancerous lesions, a high rate of cyclin D1 and p53 overexpression and p53 gene mutation have been recognized. These results suggest that a multistep carcinogenetic process contributes to the carcinogenesis of PBM. Overexpression of COX-2 is observed in PBM. Therefore, COX-2 inhibitors, such as NSAIDs, may play an important role in preventing carcinogenesis.

Keywords Pancreaticobiliary maljunction · Congenital biliary dilatation · Carcinogenesis · K-ras · p53 · Cyclooxygenase-2

20.1 Introduction

As pancreaticobiliary maljunction (PBM) causes continuous biliary reflux of pancreatic juice, it complicates biliary tract cancer at a high rate. Congenital bile duct dilatation (CBD) co-occurs with PBM, but some PBM patients do not have dilatation of the bile duct [1]. PBM patients with CBD show an extremely high incidence

Y. Nagakawa · Y. Sahara · C. Takishita · A. Tsuchida (✉)
Department of Gastrointestinal and Pediatric Surgery, Tokyo Medical University, Shinjuku-ku, Tokyo, Japan
e-mail: akihikot@tokyo-med.ac.jp

T. Kamisawa, H. Ando (eds.), *Pancreaticobiliary Maljunction and Congenital Biliary Dilatation*, https://doi.org/10.1007/978-981-10-8654-0_20

of biliary tract cancer, and the incidence is 5–35 times higher than that of cases with biliary tract cancer [2]. It is also reported that the age of cancer development in patients with PBM is more than 10 years earlier than that of common biliary tract cancer in patients without PBM. Given these facts, the carcinogenic process in PBM patients is different at a pathological and molecular level from that in common biliary tract cancer patients without PBM. In addition, various studies using carcinogenic models have revealed certain genetic defects involved in the carcinogenesis. We review the carcinogenic mechanism in PBM based on previously reported histopathological and molecular biological studies.

20.2 Mechanism of Biliary Epithelial Damage in PBM

In PBM, as the main pancreatic duct and the common bile duct join one another outside the duodenal wall, the joint lies outside the sphincter of Oddi, possibly leading to reciprocal reflux of pancreatic juice and bile. If bacterial infection and increased intrapressure in the pancreatic or bile duct occur simultaneously, pancreatic enzymes can be easily activated. Among these enzymes, amylase and lipase have little damaging effect on the biliary mucosa, but trypsin together with Ca^{2+} activates phospholipase A2. This pancreatic enzyme has a stronger destructive effect on the pancreatic duct and biliary mucosa than do others and changes biliary lecithin to lysolecithin or free fatty acids that have a strong damaging effect on cellular membranes [3]. Furthermore, bile acids also have a damaging effect on these tissues, and secondary bile acids have a particularly damaging effect and appear to enhance the activity of phospholipase A2 [4]. These effects cause long-term damage to the biliary mucosa and enhance the cell cycle, resulting in various epithelial changes such as hyperplasia or dysplasia. If carcinogenesis-promoting factors are involved in this process, it is sufficiently conceivable that malignant transformation could be facilitated. Thus, the biliary mucosa, in PBM cases, is constantly exposed to damaging substances and is considered to be in a precancerous state.

20.3 Morphological Change in the Biliary Mucosa in PBM

In pathological findings of the gallbladder in PBM, hyperplastic changes are observed in many epitheliums. The causes of hyperplasia have been reported as reactive changes due to increased intrapressure in the gallbladder associated with pancreatic juice reflux or constant pancreatic juice exposure that enhances the cell cycle of the gallbladder mucosal cells, resulting in changes to the mammillary forms [5]. Since gallbladder cancer patients with PBM have dysplasia twice as frequently as those without PBM, dysplasia seems to be a common tumoral change in PBM.

Given the continuous reciprocal reflux of pancreatic juice and bile, age is an important factor in evaluating histopathological findings in PBM. We classified patients with PBM into the following three groups according to their ages: group A (0–3 years), group B (4–39 years), and group C (over 40 years). Hyperplastic changes were noted in groups A, B, and C at high rates, though the rates were lower in groups B and C than in A. Meanwhile, dysplasia was only found in groups B and C. Additionally, most dysplasia was noted in the mucosae around gallbladder cancer [6]. Therefore, hyperplastic epithelium is present at early childhood or at birth, and dysplasia appears with age. Although it is still unclear whether hyperplastic epithelium is a precancerous state, the presence of the hyperplasia-dysplasia-carcinoma sequence is strongly suggested in the cancerization process of PBM. This appears to be a different mechanism from that of usual gallbladder cancer without PBM, which develops by an adenoma-carcinoma sequence or by de novo carcinogenesis [7] (Fig. 20.1).

20.4 Cellular Proliferative Activity

Many reports have described that the cell proliferation of gallbladder mucosa in PBM patients in evaluation using proliferating cell nuclear antigen or Ki-67 immunohistological staining was higher in PBM patients than that in non-PBM patients

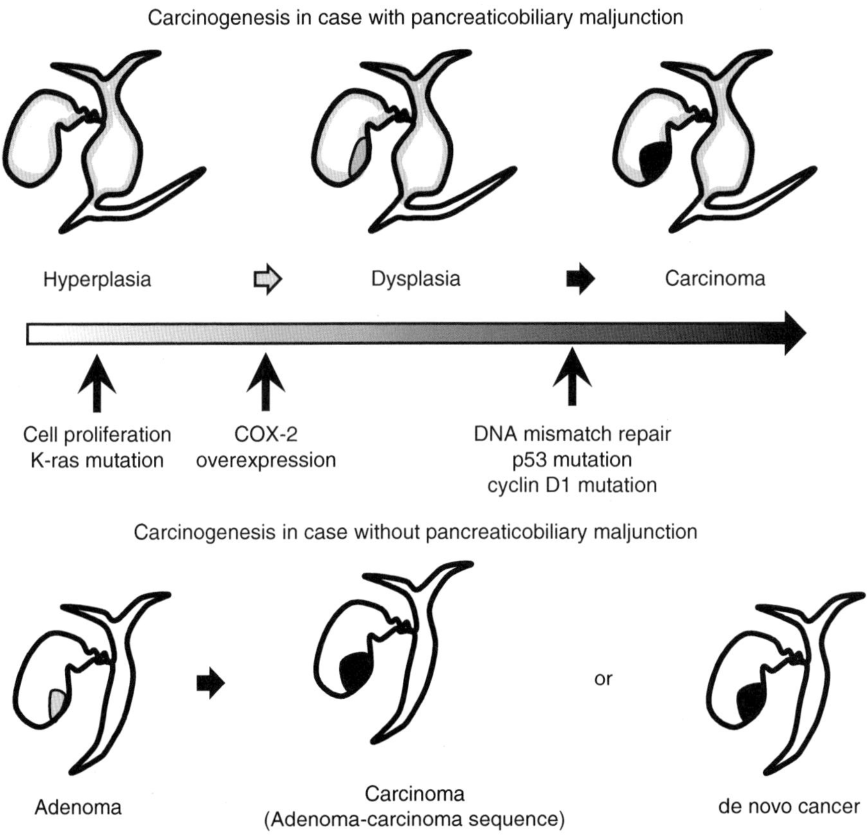

Fig. 20.1 Differences in carcinogenesis of the biliary tract in cases with and without PBM

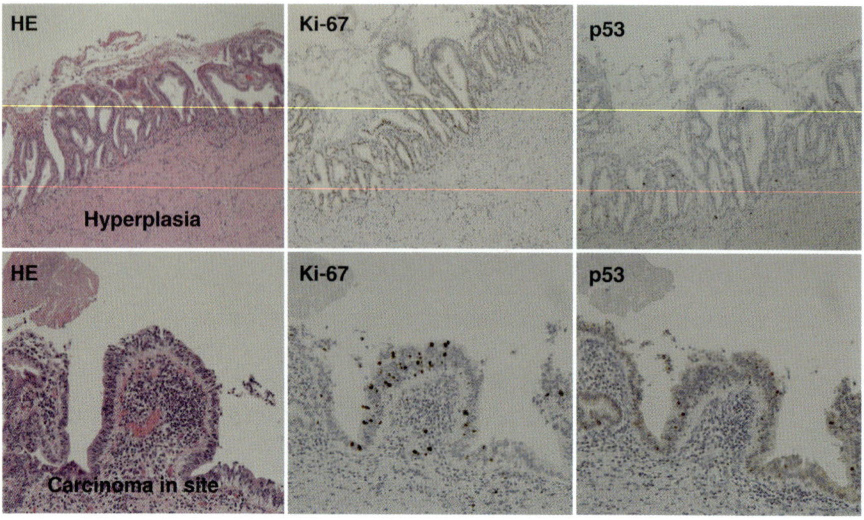

Fig. 20.2 Pathological findings in gallbladder mucosa and p53 and Ki-67 staining in patient with PBM. In the hyperplastic epithelium, many epithelial cells are stained with Ki-67. Thus, it is confirmed that the cell proliferation was promoted at the stage of hyperplasia. However, overexpression of p53 is not observed (figure above). In carcinoma in situ, not only Ki-67 staining is observed in many cells, but overexpression of p53 is also observed in some cells

[5, 8, 9]. In addition, Hanada et al. [8] reported that the cell proliferation of gallbladder mucosa was significantly more enhanced with a thicker mucosa in PBM patients than in non-PBM cases (Fig. 20.2). Furthermore, Tokiwa et al. [5] reported that hyperplastic changes in the mucosa already exist during childhood at a high incidence, with almost the same activity as the cell proliferation of adult gallbladder mucosa. As the gallbladder mucosa is constantly destroyed and repaired as a result of continuous reciprocal reflux of bile and pancreatic juice in PBM patients, the cell cycle seems to be enhanced. However, it is unknown whether this enhancement of the cell cycle is directly related to carcinogenesis.

20.5 Various Gene Mutations

20.5.1 K-ras

Gallbladder cancer patients with PBM show an incidence of K-ras mutation of 33–83%, which is higher than that in gallbladder cancer patients without PBM [8, 10]. Additionally, K-ras mutation is also found at a high rate in even normal mucosa in PBM patients. Iwase et al. [11] reported that 36% of hyperplastic epithelium had K-ras mutation in evaluation using polymerase chain reaction-single-strand conformation polymorphism (PCR-SSCP) method. Matsubara et al. [10] reported that K-ras mutation was found in 31.6% of inflammatory epithelia and 47.6% of hyperplastic and metaplastic epithelium in the PCR-SSCP method. Our previous study [5] also showed mutations in 64% of hyperplastic and 17% of dysplastic epithelia according to a polymerase chain reaction-enzyme-linked mini-sequence assay. As described above, as K-ras mutation was noted in non-tumor mucosa such as the normal and hyperplastic mucosa, they are thought to exist in genetically precancerous conditions and are considered to be in the early stages of multistep carcinogenesis.

Tomishige et al. [12] reported that a 1-month-old patient with PBM had K-ras mutation, suggesting that genetic alteration occurs early in life. Furthermore, they suggested that the incidence of K-ras mutation has no correlation with age. Our previous study also revealed no significant difference between child group and adult group in the frequencies of K-ras mutation of non-tumor gallbladder mucosa [5]. If the damages to the gallbladder mucosa accumulate with age, and the incidence of genetic mutation increases accordingly, the frequency of occurrence of K-ras mutation should increase with the increase in the patient's age. However, according to previously reported results, the frequency of K-ras mutation shows almost no change with age; thus, this mutation alone does not seem to be a direct promotor of carcinogenesis. Therefore, additional genetic alterations, such as p53 mutation, are required for cancer development.

20.5.2 p53

Hanada et al. [13] reported that 50% of patients with stage I gallbladder cancer and PBM had mutation in exons 7 and 8 in analysis of exons 5–8 using PCR-SSCP. They also observed that p53 overexpression was noted in 67% of patients with stage I gallbladder cancer. Our results showed that p53 gene mutation was noted in 34.8% of inflammatory epithelia, 47.6% of hyperplasia and metaplasia, and 60% of cancers and that it was mainly found in exons 5, 6, and 8 [5]. Additionally, p53 overexpression was found in 8.3% of inflammatory epithelium, 33.3% of hyperplasia and metaplasia, and 80% of cancers (Fig. 20.2). The higher positive rates in their reports than in others are considered attributable to their immunostaining criteria, which determined a positive result even when only small portions were stained. These results demonstrated that the benign epithelium in PBM patients had almost no p53 overexpression but was associated with gene mutation at a high frequency. Based on the result, p53 overexpression is considered to occur as a late event in the cancerization process of PBM patients.

20.5.3 Cyclin D1

DNA integrity is usually checked during the G1 or G2 phases, which serve as checkpoints for repair of damaged DNA. Regulators in the G1 phase referred to as G1 cyclins are particularly important, because their overexpression or genetic alteration is noted in various cancers. G1 cyclins combine with cyclin-dependent kinases to form complexes, playing important roles not only in the progress of the G1 phase and transition to the S phase in the cell cycle but also in malignant transformation. Cyclin D1, one of the G1 cyclins, shows abnormality in a variety of cancers. According to a report by Hui et al. [14] and our report [15], cyclin D1 mutation is a critical event in malignant transformation of usual gallbladder cancer, and this factor defines the prognosis and the degree of progression. Overexpression of cyclin D1 was found in gallbladder cancer cases complicated by PBM at a high frequency, but was not seen in nonmalignant epithelium regardless of the presence of cancer or PBM complication. This could be explained by activated ras causing overexpression of cyclin D1 predominantly in the epithelial cells extracted from a normal rat intestine or murine mammary glands in in vitro experiments [16]. This suggests that the high frequency of K-ras mutation in PBM might lead to overexpression of cyclin D1 in gallbladder cancer.

20.5.4 COX-2

A lower prevalence of various malignant tumors has been reported among habitual users of nonsteroidal anti-inflammatory drugs (NSAIDs), which inhibit cyclooxygenase (COX). Furthermore, overexpression of COX-2 is noted in various types of tumors, including colorectal tumors, which indicates a strong relationship between COX-2 expression and tumor growth and invasive potential. Several examinations of the direct effect of COX-2 activity on tumor cell growth have been performed in vitro or in animal experiments; however, many aspects of the effect of COX-2 remain unclear, as the reactivity varies depending on the types or conditions of cells. COX-2 expression in stromal cells has been suggested to enhance production of angiogenic or growth factors, including VEGF, b-FGF, and PDGF, thereby potentially participating indirectly in the growth or invasion of epithelial cells. We previously performed immunohistochemical staining of COX-2 and VEGF in the gallbladder epithelia of 65 patients with PBM to examine the relationship between the two factors [17]. Positive expression of COX-2 was found in 11.1% of hyperplasia without atypia, 86.4% of hyperplasia with mild atypia, 75% of dysplasia, and 75% of cancerous lesions. In addition, VEGF was highly expressed in 27.8% of hyperplasia without atypia, 86.4% of hyperplasia with mild atypia, 66.7% of dysplasia, and 75% of cancerous lesions. The rates of both COX-2 and VEFG overexpression were significantly higher in hyperplasia with atypia, dysplasia, and cancerous lesions than in hyperplasia without atypia. Furthermore, there was a statistically significant correlation between COX-2 and VEGF overexpression in six of eight patients of all histological types, in whom both COX-2 and VEGF were stained in almost exactly the same locations. These results demonstrate a strong relationship between COX-2 and VEGF overexpression in PBM. Therefore, chemoprevention via the suppression of angiogenesis with a COX-2 inhibitor may be effective in PBM [18].

20.5.5 Microsatellite Instability

Molecular biological studies of hereditary nonpolyposis colorectal cancer have revealed that there are some cancers in which mismatch repair gene abnormalities can be recognized. When a mismatch repair gene becomes altered, replication errors in DNA may be passed on to daughter cells through cell division, and this change sequentially causes alterations in oncogenes and/or cancer suppressor genes, resulting in carcinogenesis. In human DNA, there are 104–105 repeated sequences of single base units, such as (A)n or (CA)n, and multiple base units, which are designated microsatellites. Mismatch repair gene abnormalities can readily lead to the misreading of repeated sequences, which induces changes to the length of the microsatellite (microsatellite instability, MSI). Nagai et al. [19] showed that MSI played an important role in carcinogenesis of the gallbladder mucosa in patients with PBM. MSI was detected by 13 microsatellite markers in 16 (69.6%) of all 23 samples. Mutations in the transforming growth factor type II receptor (TGF-β RII) were detected in 8 samples (50%), mutations in the insulin-like growth factor type II receptor gene were detected in 2 samples (12.5%), and loss of heterozygosity was detected in 4 samples (25%), 2 (12.5%) at the hMSH2 locus and 2 (12.5%) at the hMLH1 locus. No TGF-β RII mutations or loss of heterozygosity in hMSH2 or hMLH1 were detected in MSI-negative samples. Nagai et al. also reported that MSI was detected in 0% of hyperplasia, 57.1% of dysplasia, and 52% of cancerous lesions. These results suggested that MSI may contribute to the late phase of carcinogenesis in the gallbladder mucosa of PBM patients.

20.6 Conclusion

Reflux of pancreatic juice into the bile duct leads to production of mutagenic compounds, causing continuous inflammation in the bile duct mucosa. Subsequently, the abnormalities in oncogenic-related genes, such as K-ras, and abnormal expression of a specific protein, COX-2, accumulate, which result in mucosal hyperplasia. During the change from hyperplasia to dysplasia, p53 abnormality seems to partly contribute to the subsequent carcinogenesis. In addition, given that analysis of MSI and telomerase is advancing, new molecular abnormalities that elucidate the pathology of PBM are expected to be observed in the future.

References

1. Aoki T, Tsuchida A, Kasuya K, Endo M, Kitamura K, Koyanagi Y. Is preventive resection of the extrahepatic duct necessary in cases of pancreaticobiliary maljunction without dilatation of the bile duct? Jpn J Clin Oncol. 2001;31:107–11.
2. Reveille RM, VanStiegmann G, Everson GT. Increased secondary bile acids in choledochal cyst; possible role in biliary metaplasia and carcinoma. Gastroenterology. 1990;99:525–7.

3. Narita H, Hashimoto T, Suzuki T, Kamiya Y, Murata Y, Hayashi S, Tsuruga N, Yura J. Clinical and experimental studies on the activation mechanism of pancreatic enzymes refluxing into the biliary tract with an anomoalous pancreatico-biliary ductal junction (in Japanese). J Jpn Soc Pediatr Surg. 1990;26:609–15.
4. Narisawa T. Bile acids and colon cancer (in Japanese). Igaku no Ayumi. 1988;147:395–8.
5. Tokiwa K, Iwai N. Early mucosal changes of the pancreaticobiliary duct. Gastroenterology. 1996;110:1614–8.
6. Masuhara S, Kasuya K, Aoki T, Yoshimatsu A, Tsuchida A, Koyanagi Y. Relation between K-ras codon mutation and p53 protein overexpression in gallbladder cancer and biliary ductal epithelia in patients with pancreaticobiliary maljunction. J Hepato-Biliary-Pancreat Surg. 2000;7:198–205.
7. Kamisawa T, Kuruma S, Chiba K, Tabata T, Koizumi S, Kikuyama MJ. Biliary carcinogenesis in pancreaticobiliary maljunction. Gastroenterology. 2017;52:158–63.
8. Hanada K, Itoh M, Fujii K, Tsuchida A, Hirata M, Ishimaru S, Iwao T, Eguchi N, Kajiyama G. Pathology and cellular kinetics of gallbladder with an anomalous junction of the pancreaticobiliary duct. Am J Gastroenterol. 1996;91:1007–11.
9. Itoi T, Itokawa F, Takei K, Kasuya K, Watanabe H, Nakamura K, Sofuni A, Tsuchida A, Aoki T. Clinicopathological aspects of carcinogenesis of pancreaticobiliary maljunction. In: Koyanagi Y, Aoki T, editors. Pancreaticobiliary maljunction. Tokyo: Igaku Tosho; 2002. p. 261–8.
10. Matsubara T, Sakurai Y, Sasayama Y, et al. K-ras point mutations in cancerous and noncancerous biliary epithelium in patients with pancreaticobiliary maljunction. Cancer. 1996;77:1752–7.
11. Iwase T, Nakazawa S, Yamao K, Yoshino J, Inui K, Yamachika H, Kanemaki N, Fujimoto M, Okushima K, Miyoshi H, Taki N, Nakamura Y, Mizutani S, Horibe Y, Masui T, Tatematsu M. Ras gene point mutations in gallbladder lesions associated with anomalous connection of pancreaticobiliary ducts. Hepato-gastroenterol. 1997;44:1457–62.
12. Tomishige H, Kishikawa T, Hara F, Nishikawa O, Nishida Y, Kongo M, Li SF. Point mutations of K-ras gene in children with congenital biliary dilatation. J Jpn Soc Pediatr Surg. 1999;35:215–20.
13. Hanada K, Itoh M, Fujii K, Tsuchida A, Ooishi H, Kajiyama G. K-*ras* and p53 mutations in stage I gallbladder carcinoma with an anomalous junction of the pancreaticobiliary duct. Cancer. 1996;77:452–8.
14. Hui AM, Li X, Shi YZ, Takayama T, Torzilli G, Makuuchi M. Cyclin D1 overexpression in a critical event in gallbladder carcinogenesis and independently predicts decreased survival for patients with gallbladder carcinoma. Clin Cancer Res. 2000;6:4272–7.
15. Itoi T, Shinohara Y, Takeda K, Nakamura K, Takei K, Sanada J, Horibe T, Saito T, Kasuya K, Ebihara Y. Nuclear cyclin D1 overexpression is a critical event associated with cell proliferation and invasive growth in gallbladder carcinogenesis. J Gastroenterol. 2000;35:142–9.
16. Filmus J, Robles AI, Shi W, Wong MJ, Colombo LL, Conti CJ. Induction of cyclin D1 overexpression by activated ras. Oncogene. 1994;9:3627–33.
17. Tsuchida A, Nagakawa Y, Kasuya K, Itoi T, Endo M, Ozawa T, Aoki T, Koyanagi Y. Immunohistochemical analysis of cyclooxygenase-2 and vascular endothelial growth factor in pancreaticobiliary maljunction. Oncol Rep. 2003;10:339–42.
18. Tsuchida A, Itoi T. Carcinogenesis and chemoprevention of biliary tract cancer in pancreaticobiliary maljunction. World J Gastrointest Oncol. 2010;2:130–5.
19. Nagai M, Kawarada Y, Watanabe M, Iwase T, Muneyuki T, Yamao K, Fukutome K, Yatani R. Analysis of microsatellite instability, TGF-beta type II receptor gene mutations and hMSH2 and hMSH1 allele losses in pancreaticobiliary maljunction-associated biliary tract tumors. Anticancer Res. 1999;19:1765–8.

Chapter 21
Carcinogenesis of Biliary Tract in Pancreaticobiliary Maljunction

Keigo Yada, Hiroki Mori, Hiroki Ishibashi, and Mitsuo Shimada

Abstract Pancreaticobiliary maljunction (PBM) is a high-risk factor for biliary tract cancer. Because of the excessive length of the common channel in PBM, sphincter action does not directly affect the pancreaticobiliary junction, which allows pancreatic juice to reflux into the biliary tract. The refluxed pancreatic juice injures the epithelium of the biliary tract and promotes the development of the cancer. Indeed, a nationwide survey in Japan revealed that biliary cancers were detected in 21.6 and 42.4% of PBM patients with and without biliary dilatation, respectively. The mechanism of carcinogenesis in PBM is considered to be the "hyperplasia-dysplasia-carcinoma sequence" which differs from the usual biliary carcinogenesis (the "adenoma-carcinoma sequence" or "de novo carcinogenesis") in the population without PBM. Hyperplastic changes of the biliary epithelium were observed even in children with PBM, and the Ki-67 labeling index was higher. Several gene mutations were reported to be related in biliary carcinogenesis of PBM.

Keywords Congenital biliary dilatation · Biliary cancer · Hyperplasia · Dysplasia

21.1 Introduction

The sphincter of Oddi is normally located at the distal end of the pancreatic and bile ducts and regulates the flow of their output. Pancreaticobiliary maljunction (PBM) is a congenital anomaly defined as a junction of the pancreatic and bile ducts located outside the duodenal wall, usually forming a markedly long common channel. This in turn causes histological changes such as hyperplastic

K. Yada (✉) · H. Mori · H. Ishibashi · M. Shimada
Department of Surgery, The University of Tokushima, Tokushima City, Tokushima, Japan
e-mail: k-yada@tokushima-u.ac.jp

T. Kamisawa, H. Ando (eds.), *Pancreaticobiliary Maljunction and Congenital Biliary Dilatation*, https://doi.org/10.1007/978-981-10-8654-0_21

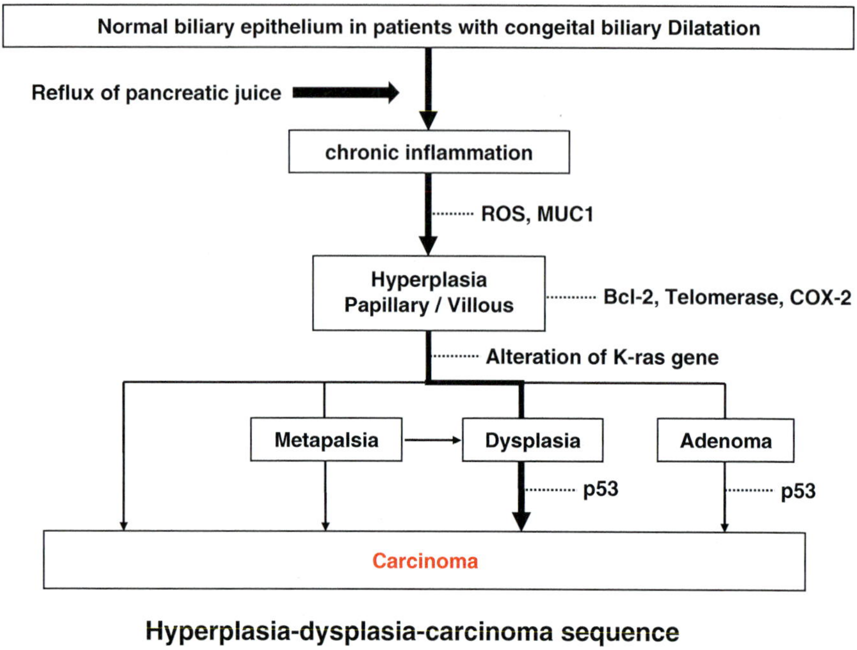

Fig. 21.1 Hyperplasia-dysplasia-carcinoma sequence in PBM carcinogenesis

epithelium (hyperplasia), metaplastic epithelium (metaplasia), and dysplastic epithelium (dysplasia), ultimately resulting in biliary carcinogenesis. These changes are called the "hyperplasia-dysplasia-carcinoma sequence" (Fig. 21.1). In PBM, the long common channel allows regurgitation of pancreatic and bile juices in the biliopancreatic tract causing PBM to be a high-risk factor for biliary tract cancer [1].

PBM is classified as either PBM with biliary dilatation (congenital biliary dilatation) or PBM without biliary dilatation. A nationwide survey reported that the prevalence of bile duct and gallbladder cancers was 6.9% and 13.4% of adult patients with congenital biliary dilatation and 3.1% and 37.4% of those with PBM without biliary dilatation, respectively [1]. In general, patients with PBM develop biliary cancer 15–20 years earlier than patients without PBM.

To assess the biliary dilatation, the maximum diameter of the bile duct is measured using nonpressure imaging modalities such as US or MRCP. Accordingly, when PBM is diagnosed, the standard treatment consists of cholecystectomy and resection of the dilated extrahepatic bile duct to prevent carcinogenesis. However, for PBM without dilatation of the extrahepatic bile duct, cholecystectomy alone is often performed since the incidence of bile duct cancer is low in such cases. The treatment for PBM without biliary tract dilatation, that is, a cholecystectomy alone or total excision of the extrahepatic biliary tract with biliary reconstruction, is still controversial. Thus, it is important to elucidate the carcinogenesis pathway to prevent biliary cancer in patients with PBM.

21.2 The Carcinogenesis of Biliary Cancer in Patients with PBM

The pathophysiology of carcinogenesis in PBM is considered to be the persistent reflux of pancreatic juice into the biliary tract. Because of the increased pressure in the biliary tract or bacterial infection, activation of pancreatic enzymes occurs. It is suggested that phospholipase A2 in refluxed pancreatic juice produces lysophosphatidylcholine, which is known to have a cytotoxic effect, and an increased concentration of lysophosphatidylcholine gives rise to cell damage causing mucosal hyperplasia and metaplasia [2] (e.g., "hyperplasia-dysplasia-carcinoma sequence," Fig. 21.1). As well, in the bile of patients with PBM, there is an increase of deoxycholic acid (DCA), lithocholic acid (LCA), and unconjugated bile acid fractions which are known to have a cancer-promoting effect [3].

On the other hand, the usual biliary carcinogenesis in the population without PBM is considered to be the "adenoma-carcinoma sequence" or "de novo carcinogenesis" [4, 5]. It is well known that gallstones are associated with gallbladder carcinoma; however, the pathologic mechanism of how gallstone contributes to carcinoma is yet to be clarified [6].

21.3 Pathological Changes of the Biliary Epithelium in PBM

Owing to the persistent reflux of pancreatic juice to the bile duct, various histopathological changes such as inflammation, hyperplasia, metaplasia, and dysplasia have been observed in the biliary epithelium in PBM. Hyperplasia and dysplasia, especially, have been frequently observed with a corresponding increase in cellular kinetics [7]. Hyperplasia of the gallbladder epithelium was observed in 38.5– 91% of patients with PBM [8, 9]. Hyperplastic changes in the biliary epithelium were observed even in children with PBM [10], and the mucosal cell kinetic markers, Ki-67 labeling index, bromodeoxyuridine labeling index, and PCNA scoring were significantly higher [10].

21.4 Gene Mutation

The mechanism of carcinogenesis in PBM is considered to be the "hyperplasia-dysplasia-carcinoma sequence" (Fig. 21.1) which differs from the usual biliary carcinogenesis ("adenoma-carcinoma sequence" or "de novo carcinogenesis") in the population without PBM. As part of the carcinogenesis pathway in PBM, several gene mutations or expressions were reported to be related in the biliary carcinogenesis of PBM.

K-ras point mutations are the most evident changes in the biliary epithelium of PBM. In fact, mutation of the K-ras gene is more frequently observed in early-stage gallbladder cancer tissue of patients with PBM than in patients without PBM [11]. Furthermore, K-ras mutations are observed in the non-cancerous biliary epithelium of PBM patients [12]. Therefore, K-ras mutations are estimated to occur in the early stage of carcinogenesis in PBM [13] (Fig. 21.1).

The mutation of tumor-suppressor gene p53 is known to be related to biliary carcinoma. Inactivity of p53 induces dysfunction of the cell cycle, DNA repair, and apoptosis control thereby facilitating the proliferation of abnormal cells to occur. It is reported that p53 mutation was detected in 39% of the non-cancerous biliary epithelium of the patients with PBM [14], while another report related that the mutation of p53 gene was not detected in the non-cancerous biliary epithelium of the patients without PBM [15]. Compared with the K-ras mutation, p53 mutation is relatively lower in the non-cancerous biliary epithelium of PBM. Therefore, it is unclear whether p53 mutation occurs in non-cancerous biliary epithelium in PBM or not, although p53 mutation is estimated to occur in the late stage of carcinogenesis in PBM [16].

Mucin core protein (MUC1), which is overexpressed in various cancers, is a glycoprotein on the apical surface of epithelial cells. MUC1 is frequently expressed in the non-cancerous/cancerous areas of the gallbladder epithelium of patients, even children, with PBM [17].

Cyclooxygenase (COX)-2 is an enzyme that is responsible for the formation of prostanoids. COX-2 is highly expressed in the non-cancerous biliary epithelium, for example, hyperplasia with mild atypia or dysplasia, of patients with PBM [18]. Furthermore, in an animal model using Syrian hamsters, COX-2 prevented the occurrence of carcinoma in situ of the biliary epithelium [19].

Recently, telomerase activity, which adds telomeric sequences to chromosome ends, has been known to be a marker of precancerous lesions. Also, Bcl-2, which is located in the mitochondria membrane, is reported to enhance telomerase activity. In the cases of non-PBM gallbladder cancer, Bcl-2 expression and telomerase activity are increased only in cancerous lesions, whereas both non-cancerous and cancerous areas have this increased activity in the cases of PBM gallbladder cancer [20]. These facts suggest that Bcl-2 expression and telomerase activation might be the relatively early events in the carcinogenesis of PBM (Fig. 21.1).

Nagai et al. reported that microsatellite instability (MSI) was detected in 0% of hyperplasia, 86% of dysplasia, and 80% of cancerous lesions of the biliary epithelium of patients with PBM [15].

21.5 Epigenetic Regulation

Histone deacetylase (HDAC) is strongly associated with epigenetic regulation and carcinogenesis. Histone acetylation, one of the epigenetic regulations, is a post-translational modification of nucleosomal histones that affects chromatin structure and modulates gene expression. The acetylation status of histones is modulated by histone acetyltransferases and HDACs. HDACs comprise an ancient family of enzymes that play crucial roles in numerous biological processes. The dynamic interplay of acetylation and deacetylation serves as a key regulatory mechanism governing the control of gene expression, differentiation, and development. HDACs contribute to cancer initiation and progression through their epigenetic regulatory activities on cell cycle progression, epithelial differentiation, angiogenesis, metastasis, and apoptosis and have been found to be overexpressed in many types of tumors.

We have been already reported that patients with both dilated and non-dilated types of PBM have a possibility of carcinogenic potential for biliary tract cancer through the expression of HDAC, even in the pediatric patients. These findings suggest that patients with PBM have a possibility of carcinogenic potential for biliary tract cancer through epigenetic regulation (Fig. 21.2).

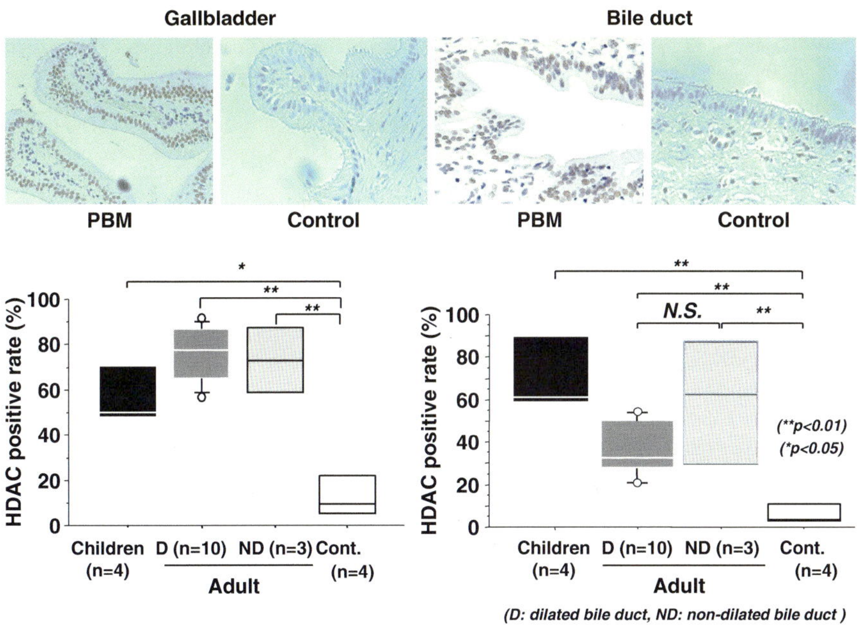

Fig. 21.2 The expression of HDAC in gallbladder/bile duct epithelium. The expression of HDAC in the dilated/non-dilated/children groups significantly increased compared to that in control group, and the level of the expression of HDAC was almost equal between the dilated group and the non-dilated group. Values are expressed as median

21.6 Conclusions

The biliary-carcinogenesis pathway in PBM is multifactorial. The harmful substrate in the bile duct is followed by the mutation/overexpression of various genes, for example, both tumor suppressor and oncogenic and cell cycle acceleration. Furthermore, epigenetic regulation through HDAC might play a role in this pathway. This carcinogenesis pathway can be phrased as the "hyperplasia-dysplasia-carcinoma sequence." To elucidate the precise and detailed pathway, further investigations will be needed.

References

1. Morine Y, Shimada M, Takamatsu H, Araida T, Endo I, Kubota M, et al. Clinical features of pancreaticobiliary maljunction: update analysis of 2nd Japan-nationwide survey. J Hepatobiliary Pancreat Sci. 2013;20(5):472–80.
2. Shimada K, Yanagisawa J, Nakayama F. Increased lysophosphatidylcholine and pancreatic enzyme content in bile of patients with anomalous pancreaticobiliary ductal junction. Hepatology. 1991;13(3):438–44.
3. Funabiki T, Sugiue K, Matsubara T, Amano H, Ochiai M. Bile acids and biliary carcinoma in pancreaticobiliary maljunction. Keio J Med. 1991;40(3):118–22.
4. Kozuka S, Tsubone N, Yasui A, Hachisuka K. Relation of adenoma to carcinoma in the gallbladder. Cancer. 1982;50(10):2226–34.
5. Watanabe H, Date K, Itoi T, Matsubayashi H, Yokoyama N, Yamano M, et al. Histological and genetic changes in malignant transformation of gallbladder adenoma. Ann Oncol. 1999;10(Suppl 4):136–9.
6. Tazuma S, Kajiyama G. Carcinogenesis of malignant lesions of the gall bladder. The impact of chronic inflammation and gallstones. Langenbecks Arch Surg/Deutsche Gesellschaft fur Chirurgie. 2001;386(3):224–9.
7. Hanada K, Itoh M, Fujii K, Tsuchida A, Hirata M, Ishimaru S, et al. Pathology and cellular kinetics of gallbladder with an anomalous junction of the pancreaticobiliary duct. Am J Gastroenterol. 1996;91(5):1007–11.
8. Yamamoto M, Nakajo S, Tahara E, Ito M, Taniyama K, Shimamoto F, et al. Mucosal changes of the gallbladder in anomalous union with the pancreatico-biliary duct system. Pathol Res Pract. 1991;187(2–3):241–6.
9. Tanno S, Obara T, Fujii T, Mizukami Y, Shudo R, Nishino N, et al. Proliferative potential and K-ras mutation in epithelial hyperplasia of the gallbladder in patients with anomalous pancreaticobiliary ductal union. Cancer. 1998;83(2):267–75.
10. Tokiwa K, Ono S, Iwai N. Mucosal cell proliferation activity of the gallbladder in children with anomalous arrangement of the pancreaticobiliary duct. J Hepato-Biliary-Pancreat Surg. 1999;6(3):213–7.
11. Hanada K, Itoh M, Fujii K, Tsuchida A, Ooishi H, Kajiyama G. K-ras and p53 mutations in stage I gallbladder carcinoma with an anomalous junction of the pancreaticobiliary duct. Cancer. 1996;77(3):452–8.
12. Matsubara T, Sakurai Y, Zhi LZ, Miura H, Ochiai M, Funabiki T. K-ras and p53 gene mutations in noncancerous biliary lesions of patients with pancreaticobiliary maljunction. J Hepato-Biliary-Pancreat Surg. 2002;9(3):312–21.
13. Funabiki T, Matsubara T, Miyakawa S, Ishihara S. Pancreaticobiliary maljunction and carcinogenesis to biliary and pancreatic malignancy. Langenbecks Arch surg/Deutsche Gesellschaft fur. Chirurgie. 2009;394(1):159–69.

14. Matsubara T, Funabiki T, Jinno O, Sakurai Y, Hasegawa S, Imazu H, et al. p53 gene mutations and overexpression of p53 product in cancerous and noncancerous biliary epithelium in patients with pancreaticobiliary maljunction. J Hepato-Biliary-Pancreat Surg. 1999;6(3):286–93.
15. Nagai M, Watanabe M, Iwase T, Yamao K, Isaji S. Clinical and genetic analysis of noncancerous and cancerous biliary epithelium in patients with pancreaticobiliary maljunction. World J Surg. 2002;26(1):91–8.
16. Kamisawa T, Kuruma S, Chiba K, Tabata T, Koizumi S, Kikuyama M. Biliary carcinogenesis in pancreaticobiliary maljunction. J Gastroenterol. 2017;52(2):158–63.
17. Yamato T, Kurumaya H, Ohama K, Yamamichi N, Watanabe Y, Harada K, et al. Frequent expression of mucin core protein MUC1 in non-neoplastic gallbladder mucosa from patients with pancreaticobiliary maljunction. Liver. 1999;19(4):281–7.
18. Tsuchida A, Nagakawa Y, Kasuya K, Itoi T, Endo M, Ozawa T, et al. Immunohistochemical analysis of cyclooxygenase-2 and vascular endothelial growth factor in pancreaticobiliary maljunction. Oncol Rep. 2003;10(2):339–43.
19. Tsuchida A, Itoi T, Kasuya K, Endo M, Katsumata K, Aoki T, et al. Inhibitory effect of meloxicam, a cyclooxygenase-2 inhibitor, on N-nitrosobis (2-oxopropyl) amine induced biliary carcinogenesis in Syrian hamsters. Carcinogenesis. 2005;26(11):1922–8.
20. Ichikawa Y, Kamiyama M, Sekido H, Ishikawa T, Miura Y, Kamiya N, et al. Telomerase activity and Bcl-2 expression in gallbladders of pancreaticobiliary maljunction patients: a preliminary study. J Hepato-Biliary-Pancreat Surg. 2004;11(1):34–9.

Chapter 22
Pancreatitis and Biliary Stone in PBM

Kenitiro Kaneko

Abstract In patients with pancreaticobiliary maljunction (PBM), acute pancreatitis occurs more frequently in children (30%) than adults (9%). Pancreatitis in these cases is typically mild. Most cases reveal no evidence of pancreatitis on imaging or at surgery. This is referred to as fictitious pancreatitis or pseudopancreatitis. Increased biliary pressure caused by protein plug obstruction causes cholangiovenous reflux, by which regurgitated amylase in bile passes into the bloodstream. Biliopancreatic reflux can cause true pancreatitis, but rarely. Another factor seems necessary for the severity to advance. Chronic pancreatitis complicates PBM in 3% of patients but differs from alcoholic chronic pancreatitis in clinical and imaging points.

Gallstones have been reported to complicate PBM (adults, 25%, children, 9%). However, many reported gallstones in children must have included protein plugs stained with bile. Though rare, PBM can produce fatty acid calcium stones. Activated pancreatic enzymes in bile may release fatty acids from lecithin. Free fatty acids combine with calcium ions in bile and turn into stones. Gallstones in adults may be only coincident or form unrelated to pancreaticobiliary reflux but related to bile stasis and/or sphincter insufficiency as a result of aging. Brown pigment stones often occur after excision of the bile duct because of bile stasis and β-glucuronidase from enteric bacteria.

Keywords Pancreaticobiliary maljunction · Acute pancreatitis · Chronic pancreatitis · Gallstones · Fatty acid calcium stones

22.1 Pancreatitis

Pancreatitis has been frequently reported to complicate pancreaticobiliary maljunction (PBM). A Japanese nationwide study (n = 2529) demonstrated that acute pancreatitis occurs in 30% of children with PBM and 9% of adults with PBM and thus

K. Kaneko
Division of Pediatric Surgery, Department of Surgery, Aichi Medical University, Nagakute, Aichi, Japan
e-mail: kkaneko@aichi-med-u.ac.jp

T. Kamisawa, H. Ando (eds.), *Pancreaticobiliary Maljunction and Congenital Biliary Dilatation*, https://doi.org/10.1007/978-981-10-8654-0_22

is more frequent in children [1]. Elevated levels of serum amylase are seen in 40% of children with PBM, usually accompanied by abdominal pain and diagnosed as acute pancreatitis [2]. Acute pancreatitis complicating PBM is mild in most patients. Imaging such as computed tomography rarely shows pancreatic enlargement or other abnormal findings indicating pancreatitis. Surgery soon after the symptoms subside fails to reveal fat necrosis or changes in the pancreatic tissue. This state of hyperamylasemia without pancreatic lesions has been called fictitious pancreatitis or pseudopancreatitis [3, 4]. Increased biliary pressure by protein plug obstruction causes abdominal pain as well as cholangiovenous reflux, by which regurgitated amylase in the bile passes into the bloodstream at the liver (see Chap. 8). The mechanism of this has been confirmed by experimental studies using animals [5, 6].

Biliopancreatic reflux causes true pancreatitis in a few patients. In my experience of 225 pediatric patients with PBM, more than 30% presented with an elevated level of serum amylase, but only 2% showed pancreatic enlargement with fluid collection on computed tomography (Fig. 22.1). However, there were no cases of severe acute pancreatitis. Necrotizing pancreatitis is also extremely rare in adult patients. In addition to re-reflux of activated pancreatic enzymes regurgitated in bile into the pancreatic duct, another factor seems necessary for advancing the severity of pancreatitis [7]. Small gallstones occurring unrelated to PBM are one of the candidates as an aggravating factor, as described in Opie's paper from 1901 [8].

According to the aforementioned nationwide study, chronic pancreatitis complicates PBM in 3% of children and 3% of adults and in 3% of patients with congenital

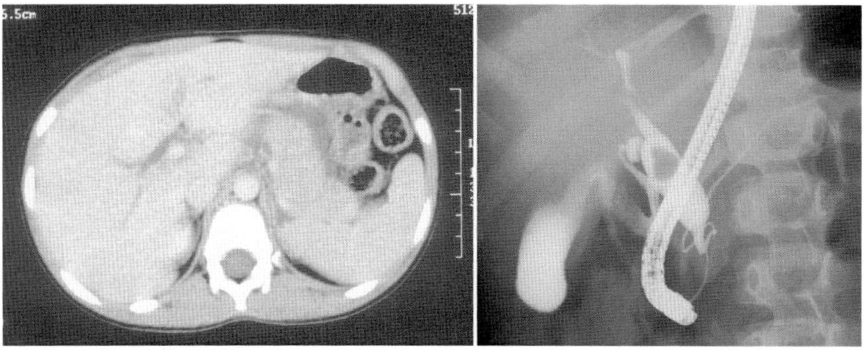

Fig. 22.1 A rare case of true pancreatitis. A 6-year-old girl had acute abdominal pain and vomited several times. Serum levels of transaminase, amylase, and lipase were elevated. Computed tomography showed pancreatic enlargement and adjacent fluid collection (*left*). Six weeks later when symptoms subsided, endoscopic retrograde cholangiopancreatography showed a dilated common bile duct with pancreaticobiliary maljunction and a large filling defect in the dilated bile duct (*right*). After 2 weeks, the patient underwent surgery. Operative cholangiography showed the filing defect had disappeared, but many white fragments of protein plugs were found in the bile. Protein plugs are generally fragile. The plugs blocking the common channel usually flow out spontaneously before causing true pancreatitis, but in this case, plugs must have been more stubborn than usual

biliary dilatation (CBD) but in 0.7% of patients without CBD [1]. The reason for the rarity in non-dilated PBM is unknown. It is also unknown whether repeating acute pancreatitis progresses into chronic pancreatitis. More fundamentally, it is uncertain whether PBM truly causes chronic pancreatitis. Unlike alcoholic chronic pancreatitis, in which pancreatic stones are radiopaque and distributed diffusely, in chronic pancreatitis under PBM, pancreatic stones (i.e., protein plugs) are mostly radiolucent and detected only in the dilated common channel or in the main pancreatic duct near the common channel [9]. Patients with chronic pancreatitis complicating PBM infrequently show pancreatic insufficiency. The details on chronic pancreatitis complicating PBM remain largely unknown.

22.2 Gallstones

Gallstones have long been reported to complicate PBM. In 1980, Yamaguchi reported that 111 (8%) of 1433 patients with choledochal cyst had gallstones [10]. According to the nationwide survey on PBM in 2013, 9% of children and 25% of adults with PBM had gallstones [1]. In children, pancreaticobiliary reflux frequently produces protein plugs made of lithostathine in the biliary tract (see Chap. 8). These protein plugs are stained with bile pigment and resemble gallstones (Fig. 22.2). Many stained plugs must have been mistaken for gallstones in children. In my experience of pediatric PBM, except for protein plugs and fatty acid calcium stones discussed below, gallstones were found only in patients who had undergone biliary

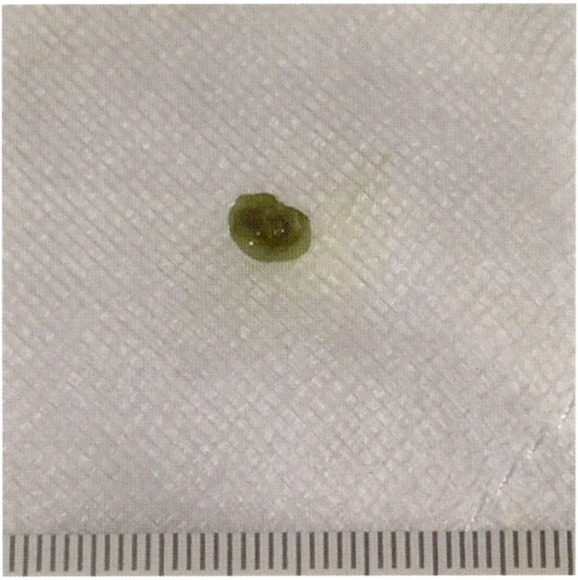

Fig. 22.2 A bile-stained protein plug similar to a gallstone. Protein plugs themselves are white but are stained yellow or green with bile

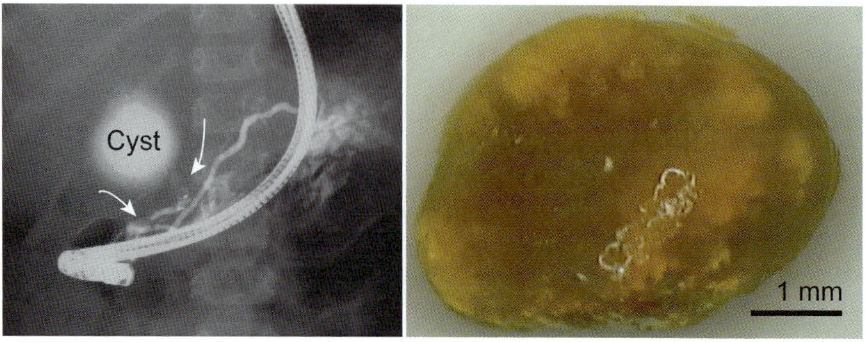

Fig. 22.3 A fatty acid calcium stone as another cause of obstruction besides protein plugs. A 4-year-old boy underwent endoscopic retrograde cholangiopancreatography because of persistent abdominal pain and elevated levels of transaminase and amylase (*left*). A filling defect was found in the narrow segment and another was present in the common channel (*arrows*). Endoscopic insertion of a biliary stent tube relieved his symptoms immediately, but 18 days later, his symptoms recurred. Surgery disclosed a choked tube and many stones harder than protein plugs. Infrared absorption spectrometry showed the stone was composed of fatty acid calcium (*right*). Gas chromatography showed that 54% of fatty acids were palmitic acid

surgery including cyst-enterostomy and bile duct excision with biliary reconstructions. These postoperative gallstones are brown pigment stones, which are created by bile stasis and β-glucuronidase from enteric bacteria [11] (see Chap. 29). Oddi's sphincter keeps enteric bacteria from entering the biliary tract, even though PBM and CBD exist in children, and prevents brown pigment stones from forming in spite of bile stagnation [11].

In children, pancreaticobiliary reflux also produces fatty acid calcium stones though very rarely (Fig. 22.3). In my experience of PBM in children, only two patients (0.9%) had fatty acid calcium stones. The main fatty acid of the stones was palmitic acid [12]. Fatty acid calcium stones are rare gallstones and are usually seen in the elderly without PBM. These stones are created by a combination of free fatty acids and calcium ions [13]. The main fatty acid is palmitic acid. Calcium palmitate has also been found as a major component of brown pigment stones [14]. In both stone formations, free fatty acids are caused by bacterial phospholipase, which releases fatty acids from phosphatidylcholine (lecithin), a major phospholipid in bile [14]. In PBM cases, stones are mainly composed of calcium palmitate, but bacteria may be unrelated, because bile in patients with PBM is sterile [11]. Pancreatic enzymes including phospholipases and bile salt-activated lipase are regurgitated and activated in the biliary tract. These activated pancreatic enzymes most likely release free fatty acids from lecithin, which combine with calcium ions in bile and turn into stones.

Most stones reported to complicate PBM in adults were located in the gallbladder or a dilated bile duct [15]. More than half of the stones (65%) are pigmented and followed by cholesterol stones (31%) [15]. Gallstones in adults appear to form independent of pancreaticobiliary reflux but are related to bile stasis and/or sphincter insufficiency resulting from aging or are only coincident with PBM. Gallstones cause obstructive symptoms such as protein plugs in children and are important as they provide an opportunity to diagnose PBM in adults.

References

1. Morine Y, Shimada M, Takamatsu H, et al. Clinical features of pancreaticobiliary maljunction: update analysis of 2nd Japan-nationwide survey. J Hepatobiliary Pancreat Sci. 2013;20:472–80.
2. Kaneko K, Ando H, Ito T, Watanabe Y, Seo T, Harada T, Ito F. Protein plugs cause symptoms in patients with choledochal cysts. Am J Gastroenterol. 1997;92:1018–21.
3. Stringel G, Filler RM. Fictitious pancreatitis in choledochal cyst. J Pediatr Surg. 1982;17:359–61.
4. Todani T, Urushihara N, Watanabe Y, Toki A, Uemura S, Sato Y, Morotomi Y. Pseudopancreatitis in choledochal cyst in children: intraoperative study of amylase levels in the serum. J Pediatr Surg. 1990;25:303–6.
5. Ohkawa H, Sawaguchi S, Khalil B, Ishikawa A, Yamazaki Y. Cholangio-venous reflux as a cause of recurrent hyperamylasemia in choledochal dilatation with anomalous pancreaticobiliary ductal union: an experimental study. J Pediatr Surg. 1985;20:53–7.
6. Urushihara N, Todani T, Watanabe Y, Uemura S, Morotomi Y, Wang ZQ. Does hyperamylasemia in choledochal cyst indicate true pancreatitis? An experimental study. Eur J Pediatr Surg. 1995;5:139–42.
7. Kamisawa T, Egawa N, Tsuruta K, Okamoto A. Gallbladder carcinoma associated with pancreaticobiliary maljunction presenting as severe acute pancreatitis. J Gastroenterol. 2005;40:659–60.
8. Opie EL. The etiology of acute hemorrhagic pancreatitis. Johns Hopkins Hosp Bull. 1901;12:182–8.
9. Kamisawa T, Matsukawa M, Amemiya K, Tu Y, Egawa N, Okamoto A, Aizawa S. Pancreatitis associated with pancreaticobiliary maljunction. Hepatogastroenterology. 2003;50:1665–8.
10. Yamaguchi M. Congenital choledochal cyst. Analysis of 1,433 patients in the Japanese literature. Am J Surg. 1980;140:653–7.
11. Kaneko K, Ando H, Seo T, Ono Y, Ochiai K, Ogura Y. Bile infection contributes to intrahepatic calculi formation after excision of choledochal cysts. Pediatr Surg Int. 2005;21:8–11.
12. Kaneko K, Ono Y, Tainaka T, Sumida W, Ando H. Fatty acid calcium stones in patients with pancreaticobiliary maljunction/choledochal cyst as another cause of obstructive symptoms besides protein plugs. J Pediatr Surg. 2008;43:564–7.
13. Cowie AGA, Sutor DJ, Wooley SE, Clark CG. The calcium palmitate gallstone. Br J Surg. 1973;60:16–8.
14. Nakano T, Yanagisawa J, Nakayama F. Phospholipase activity in human bile. Hepatology. 1988;8:1560–4.
15. Funabiki T, editor. Pancreaticobiliary maljunction. Its consensus and controversy. Tokyo: Igakutoshoshuppan; 1997.

Part VI
Treatment

Chapter 23
Standard Surgical Procedure for CBD

Tsugumichi Koshinaga

Abstract Total cyst excision (extrahepatic bile duct resection including cholecystectomy) with biliary tract reconstruction is regarded as the standard surgical procedure for congenital choledochal cyst. Most congenital choledochal cysts accompany with pancreato-biliary maljunction (PBM), which causes varied pathologies such as biliary tract cancer, cholangitis, and pancreatitis. Carcinoma arises also from the intrahepatic bile duct and the pancreatic duct even after total cyst excision.

When relative stenosis occurs in the hepatic duct near the hepatic hilum, it is necessary to extend incision to the wall of the left and right at the hepatic duct branch level, creating a large anastomotic opening. There is no consensus regarding whether or not hepatectomy should be considered at the primary surgery for congenital choledochal cysts, particularly in children. The risks have been also noted on cancer arising from the residual bile duct in the pancreas, pancreatitis, and pancreatic stone. It is necessary to resect the distal end of the common bile duct near the junction with the pancreatic duct so as not to remain the intrapancreatic bile duct.

Keywords Congenital choledochal cysts · Total cyst excision · Extrahepatic bile duct resection · Intrapancreatic bile duct · Hepatic hilum · Relative stenosis Biliary tract cancer

23.1 Introduction

Total cyst excision (extrahepatic bile duct resection including cholecystectomy) with biliary tract reconstruction is regarded as the standard surgical procedure for congenital choledochal cyst [1, 2]. Cyst-intestine anastomosis (internal fistula production) is rather contraindicated at present because of an increase in the risk of cholangitis and biliary cancer [2, 3]. Most congenital choledochal cysts accompany

T. Koshinaga
Department of Pediatric Surgery, Nihon University School of Medicine, Tokyo, Japan
e-mail: koshinaga.tsugumichi@nihon-u.ac.jp

T. Kamisawa, H. Ando (eds.), *Pancreaticobiliary Maljunction and Congenital Biliary Dilatation*, https://doi.org/10.1007/978-981-10-8654-0_23

with pancreato-biliary maljunction (PBM), which causes varied pathologies such as biliary tract cancer, cholangitis, and pancreatitis. Biliary tract cancer is noted to arise in the cyst and gall bladder at a high rate [4]. According to the Japanese national registry of PBM [5], the incidence of biliary tract carcinoma yielded 10.6% arising in patients with PBM and 21.6% especially in adult patients with PBM. The distribution of the cancer varied from 32.1% in the bile ducts and 62.3% in the gallbladder. Carcinoma arises also from the intrahepatic bile duct and the endocrine pancreatic duct even after total cyst excision [6, 7]. Bilioenteric anastomosis itself is a risk factor for cholangiocarcinoma reportedly [8]. A long-term follow-up is mandatory after total cyst excision.

The risks have been also noted on cancer arising from the residual bile duct in the pancreas, pancreatitis, and pancreatic stone [9, 10]. In the operative technique, it is necessary to resect the distal end of the common bile duct near the junction with the pancreatic duct so as not to remain the intrapancreatic bile duct [11]. In cases of cystic type of biliary dilation, the distal portion of the bile duct in the pancreas is usually narrow, making it relatively easy to resect the bile duct near the pancreatic duct confluence. However, in the spindle-shaped or cylindrical type, the narrow portion is shortened and thin, sometimes unclear. This increases a risk of pancreatic duct injury when dissecting the bile duct, leading to postoperative pancreatic fistula, pancreatitis, or pancreatic duct stenosis. Several methods have been described to avoid these complications, including intraoperative cholangiography using a metal clip [11], and choledochoscopy (using cystoscopy) for confirming the biliary distal end point [12].

When relative stenosis occurs in the hepatic duct near the hepatic hilum, it is necessary to extend incision to the wall of the left and right at the hepatic duct branch level, creating a large anastomotic opening. Recently, hepatectomy has been increasingly reported as the primary surgery in cases when the biliary dilation extends to the intrahepatic bile duct [13–16]. According to a comparative study of the patients with only total cyst resection versus concomitant hepatectomy as the primary surgeries for congenital choledochal cysts with dilation of the intrahepatic bile duct, the need of reoperation for intrahepatic stones and stenosis was significantly lower in adults than in children in primary hepatectomy [15]. Other report [16] suggested an additional hepatectomy should be considered in adults because of a potential risk of intrahepatic bile duct carcinoma arising. There is no consensus regarding whether or not hepatectomy should be considered at the primary surgery for congenital choledochal cysts, particularly in children.

23.2 Surgical Techniques and Key Points

23.2.1 Skin Incision

With the patient in the supine position, laparotomy is performed via a transverse incision in the right upper abdomen.

23.2.2 *Mobilization of the Gallbladder from the Liver Bed*

The appearance of the extrahepatic biliary tree and the liver and pancreas should be noted, if there is no anatomical anomaly. A large biliary cyst is readily evident, with further gained by displacing the hepatic flexure of the colon and the duodenum. The gallbladder is mobilized from the liver bed; the cystic artery is identified and ligated. Then the cystic duct is identified extending from the biliary cyst and ligated at the proximal side of the infundibulum at this point. We usually remove the gallbladder so as not to interfere with the view of the surgical field.

23.2.3 *Exposure of the Total Biliary Cyst*

The hepatoduodenal ligament is incised after a Kocher maneuver. The exposed cyst often extends behind the proximal duodenum. In a case of fusiform type of cyst with no adhesion between the cyst and the surrounding tissue, the cyst is easily mobilized. Once encircled, taping of the cyst allowed better exposure and further dissection of the surrounding tissues. However, the cyst dissection is difficult in a case of cystic type with dense adhesion and venous engorgement of the anterior cyst wall after inflammation. A great care is necessary for the cyst excision. The "opencut method," cutting open the anterior wall of the cyst transversely prior to dissection of the posterior wall of the cyst, is a good choice of the procedure for a case of large cyst (Fig. 23.1).

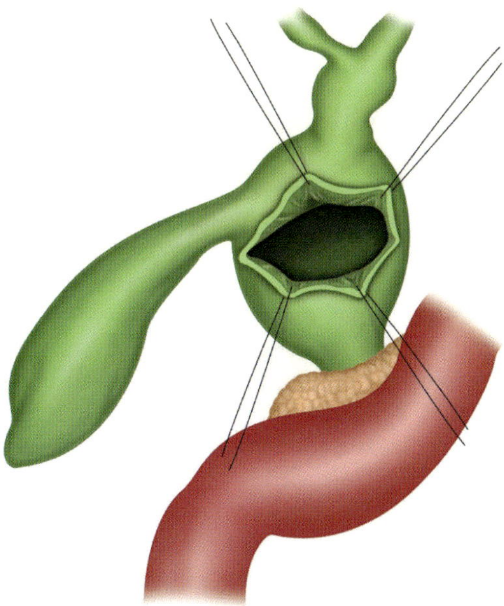

Fig. 23.1 The "opencut method." The anterior wall of the cyst is cut open transversely prior to dissection of the posterior wall of the cyst

23.2.4 Incision and Transection of the Common Bile Duct

Near the junction of the cystic duct and biliary cyst, where the diameter of the common bile duct is the largest, the anterior wall of the cyst is transversely incised ("opencut method"). One can see directly the posterior wall of the cyst from the inside. Dissection of the lateral and posterior wall of the cyst is much easier. The opencut method can also prevent the damage of the portal vein and pancreas. This technique is very similar to transection of a hernia sac in pediatric inguinal hernias, as most pediatric surgeons experience. Due to the presence of a collateral circulation of the portal vein at the posterior wall of the cyst, careful ligation of small veins is also important. Dissection should always be performed precisely close to the posterior wall; the trick is to dissect the plane right outer to the posterior wall of the cyst. If the cyst is extremely inflamed and adhesions dense, mucosectomy should be performed.

23.2.5 Dissection and Excision of the Cyst in the Pancreas

It is important to excise the distal end of the biliary duct up close to the pancreatic duct confluence buried in the pancreatic parenchyma. Protein plugs and debris associated with PBM must be removed, if there is evident during the intraoperative exploration as well as preoperative imaging. Since protein plugs are generally fragile, they tend to disappear spontaneously before surgery in half the cases. In cases when a protein plug is visible by cholangiopancreatography or endoscopy during surgery, it is removed by flushing into the duodenum by irrigation with saline through the narrow segment beneath the cyst with a Fogarty catheter or removed through the narrow segment using a blunt spoon [17, 18]. When the plugs are too large or too hard to be removed through the narrow segment, an incision in the main pancreatic duct is required. The narrow segment is used as a flap to prevent ductal stricture after primary repair of the pancreatic duct [17]. There is also a report using a small diameter endoscope to remove protein plugs in the common duct. However, despite the consensus regarding the need for elimination of protein plugs during flow-diversion surgery, there are no studies on probabilities of sequelae such as pancreatitis occur, if residual plugs remain postoperatively. No protein plug reforms after complete excision of the intrapancreatic bile duct [11]. Conversely, protein plug reforms even if there is an intrapancreatic biliary remnant after flow-diversion surgery.

By cholangiopancreatography or endoscopy via the opened bile duct, the resection line of the distal end of the common bile duct is to be determined. If there is a possible protein plug, the ductal lumen should be checked visually and flushing using an endoscope. Cholangiopancreatography or endoscopy should be repeated if

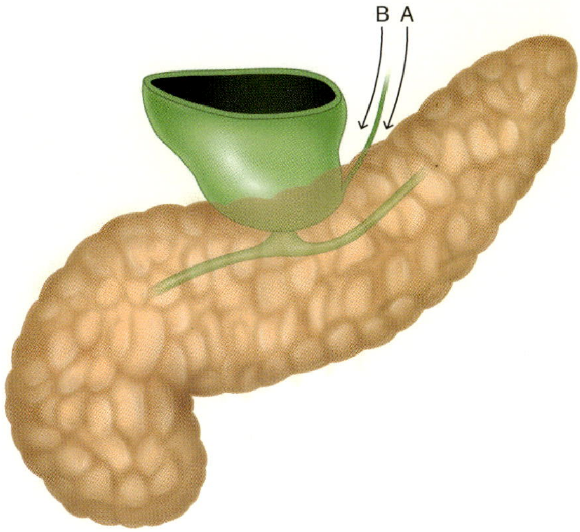

Fig. 23.2 Dissection of the cyst buried in the pancreas. Dissection of the intrapancreatic bile duct should always be performed precisely outer the wall of the bile duct (Line **a**); however, mucosectomy should be performed if dense adhesion due to inflammation (Line **b**)

necessary to determine the resection line accurately. While proceeding the dissection of the intrapancreatic bile duct, thin blood vessels, running on the outer surface of the bile duct, should be properly treated just on the bile duct wall. While proceeding closer to the junction with the pancreatic duct, a field of view should be tried to secure for dissection of the bile duct in the pancreas. Care must be taken to ensure that the dissection plane never made away from the wall of the bile duct. Dissection of the intrapancreatic bile duct should always be performed precisely outer the wall of the bile duct; however, mucosectomy should be performed if dense adhesion due to inflammation (Fig. 23.2). When dissection reaches near the junction with the pancreatic duct, the resection line is finally determined by direct viewing or contrast imaging of the junction. For resection, the distal end of the bile duct is ligated with nonabsorbable suture (silk, etc.) as close as possible to directly above its confluence with the pancreatic duct. An absorbable suture (4–0 proline, etc.) is added as transfixing at the stump.

23.2.6 Dissection of the Bile Duct on the Side of the Liver and Creation of an Anastomosis

Cholangitis and intrahepatic stones after total cyst excision are caused by anastomotic strictures and intrahepatic biliary dilatation with stenosis [19]. Bile duct stenosis is found in 80% of congenital choledochal cysts at the hepatic hilum to the liver [20]. Bile duct stenosis includes membrane-like stenosis and funicular

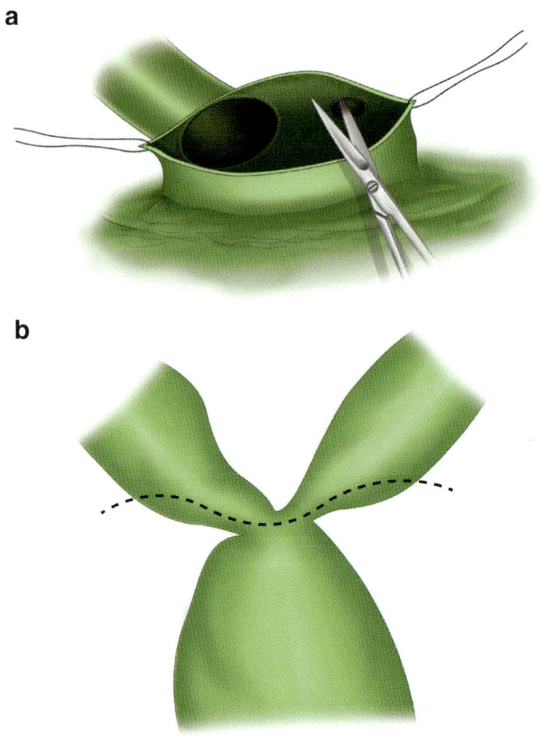

Fig. 23.3 The treatment of the stenosis of the bile duct at the hepatic hilum. A membrane-like stenosis of the bile duct is resected (**a**). Incision (dotted line) should be intended to extend along the lateral wall of both the hepatic ducts for a wide anastomosis (**b**)

stenosis, often found near the hilar region of the liver. Ando et al. [20] has recommended resection of the stenosis of the bile duct or biliary reconstruct at the initial surgery because of cholangitis and intrahepatic stones following extrahepatic bile duct resection. The treatment the stenosis includes resection of a strand or a membrane-like stenosis from the inside of the opened common hepatic duct [21], and incision extending along the lateral wall of both the hepatic ducts to permit a wide anastomotic stoma of choledochojejunostomy [2, 22] (Fig. 23.3a, b). As the procedure of choice for type IV-A cysts presenting with relative stenosis in hepatic hilum, partial resection of the wall of the intrahepatic cyst combined with excision of the intrahepatic cyst is recommended [23]. There is consensus that treating with stenosis of the bile duct is necessary if it is; however, there are few evidence that choledochojejunostomy must be create always at the hepatic hilum in all case of choledochal cyst. The posterior wall of the cyst is dissected toward the hepatic hilum by control of thin blood vessels. It is important to have the direct view of the lumen of the cyst. A care must be taken for possible accessory hepatic ducts to confirm if there are aberrant bile ducts while proceeding dissection of the posterior wall of the cyst. An endoscopic examination is performed if necessary. A large anastomotic opening should be created by extending incision along with the wall of the hilar bile duct (Fig. 23.4).

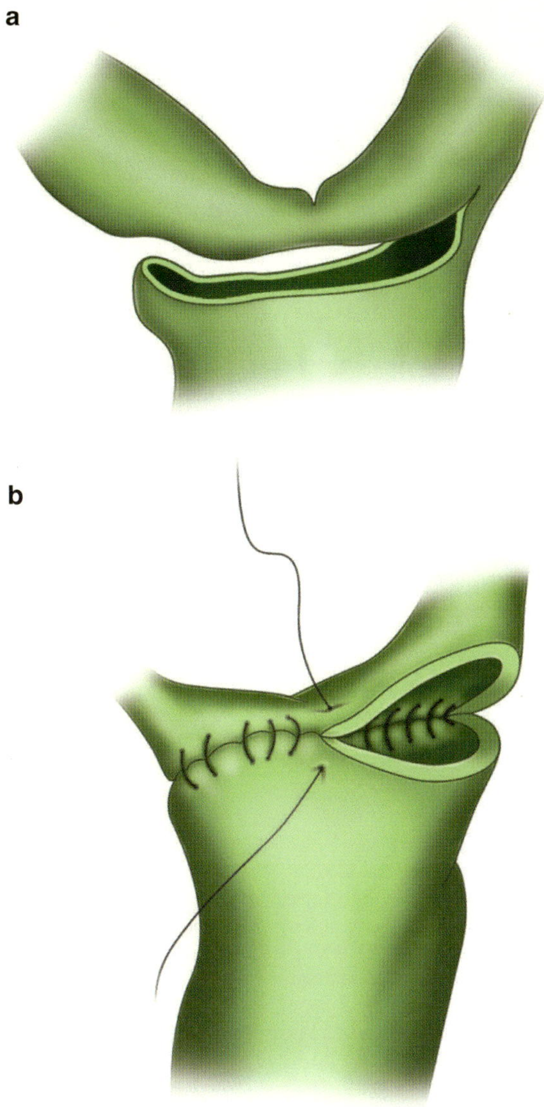

Fig. 23.4 Biliary reconstruction. A large anastomotic opening should be created (**a**). End-to-end hepaticojejunostomy is performed by using full-thickness, single-layer, and monofilament absorbable sutures (**b**)

23.2.7 Biliary Reconstruction

The intestine used for biliary reconstruction is the duodenum or jejunum. However, hepaticojejunostomy is the standard procedure for reconstruction in Japan. The anastomotic technique used is end-to-side or end-to-end hepaticojejunostomy. We use a 40-cm length of jejunum for Roux-en-Y conduit. The conduit is brought through a retrocolica window. The hepaticojejunostomy is performed by using full-thickness, single-layer, and monofilament absorbable sutures.

References

1. Todani T, Watanabe Y, Narusue M, Tabuchi K, Okajima K. Congenital bile duct cysts: classification, operative procedures, and review of thirty-seven cases including cancer arising from choledochal cyst. Am J Surg. 1977;134(2):263–9.
2. Lilly JR. Total excision of choledochal cyst. Surg Gynecol Obstet. 1978;146(2):254–6.
3. Todani T, Watanabe Y, Toki A, Urushihara N. Carcinoma related to choledochal cysts with internal drainage operations. Surg Gynecol Obstet. 1987;164(1):61–4.
4. Todani T, Tabuchi K, Watanabe Y, Kobayashi T. Carcinoma arising in the wall of congenital bile duct cysts. Cancer. 1979;44(3):1134–41.
5. Morine Y, Shimada M, Takamatsu H, et al. Clinical features of pancreaticobiliary maljunction: update analysis of 2nd Japan-nationwide survey. J Hepatobiliary Pancreat Sci. 2013;20(5):472–80.
6. Kobayashi S, Asano T, Yamasaki M, Kenmochi T, Nakagohri T, Ochiai T. Risk of bile duct carcinogenesis after excision of extrahepatic bile ducts in pancreaticobiliary maljunction. Surgery. 1999;126(5):939–44.
7. Watanabe Y, Toki A, Todani T. Bile duct cancer developed after cyst excision for choledochal cyst. J Hepato-Biliary-Pancreat Surg. 1999;6(3):207–12.
8. Strong RW. Late bile duct cancer complicating biliary-enteric anastomosis for benign disease. Am J Surg. 1999;177(6):472–4.
9. Yoshikawa K, Yoshida K, Shirai Y, et al. A case of carcinoma arising in the intrapancreatic terminal choledochus 12 years after primary excision of a giant choledochal cyst. Am J Gastroenterol. 1986;81(5):378–84.
10. Urushihara N, Fukumoto K, Fukuzawa H, et al. Long-term outcomes after excision of choledochal cysts in a single institution: operative procedures and late complications. J Pediatr Surg. 2012;47(12):2169–74.
11. Ando H, Kaneko K, Ito T, et al. Complete excision of the intrapancreatic portion of choledochal cysts. J Am Coll Surg. 1996;183(4):317–21.
12. Miyano T, Yamataka A, Kato Y, Kohno S, Fujiwara T. Choledochal cysts: special emphasis on the usefulness of intraoperative endoscopy. J Pediatr Surg. 1995;30(3):482–4.
13. Pal K, Singh VP, Mitra DK. Partial hepatectomy and total cyst excision is curative for localized type IV-a biliary duct cysts – report of four cases and review of management. Eur J Pediatr Surg. 2009;19(3):148–52.
14. Kawarada Y, Das BC, Tabata M, Isaji S. Surgical treatment of type IV choledochal cysts. J Hepato-Biliary-Pancreat Surg. 2009;16(5):684–7.
15. Zheng X, Gu W, Xia H, et al. Surgical treatment of type IV-A choledochal cyst in a single institution: children vs. adults. J Pediatr Surg. 2013;48(10):2061–6.
16. He XD, Wang L, Liu W, et al. The risk of carcinogenesis in congenital choledochal cyst patients: an analysis of 214 cases. Ann Hepatol. 2014;13(6):819–26.
17. Ando H, Kaneko K, Ito F, et al. Surgical removal of protein plugs complicating choledochal cysts: primary repair after adequate opening of the pancreatic duct. J Pediatr Surg. 1998;33(8):1265–7.
18. Diao M, Li L, Zhang JS, Cheng W. Laparoscopic-assisted clearance of protein plugs in the common channel in children with choledochal cysts. J Pediatr Surg. 2010;45(10):2099–102.
19. Todani T, Watanabe Y, Urushihara N, Noda T, Morotomi Y. Biliary complications after excisional procedure for choledochal cyst. J Pediatr Surg. 1995;30(3):478–81.
20. Ando H, Ito T, Kaneko K, Seo T. Congenital stenosis of the intrahepatic bile duct associated with choledochal cysts. J Am Coll Surg. 1995;181(5):426–30.
21. Ando H, Kaneko K, Ito F, Seo T, Ito T. Operative treatment of congenital stenoses of the intrahepatic bile ducts in patients with choledochal cysts. Am J Surg. 1997;173(6):491–4.
22. Todani T, Watanabe Y, Mizuguchi T, Fujii T, Toki A. Hepaticoduodenostomy at the hepatic hilum after excision of choledochal cyst. Am J Surg. 1981;142(5):584–7.
23. Todani T, Narusue M, Watanabe Y, Tabuchi K, Okajima K. Management of congenital choledochal cyst with intrahepatic involvement. Ann Surg. 1978;187(3):272–80.

Chapter 24
Laparoscopic Surgery for Congenital Biliary Dilatation in Children

Hiroyuki Koga and Atsuyuki Yamataka

Abstract The treatment of choice for congenital biliary dilatation is complete excision with Roux-en-Y hepaticojejunostomy, a procedure that is now being performed laparoscopically. We describe our technique (laparoscopic dilated bile duct dissection, distal common bile duct ligation, intrahepatic bile duct and common channel protein plug clearance, and customizing the length of the Roux-en-Y loop) and discuss attendant issues from our wealth of experience of treating this condition using both open and minimally invasive surgery.

In summary, laparoscopic excision of the bile duct and Roux-en-Y hepaticojejunostomy is feasible and safe, associated with lower postoperative morbidity and less blood loss, in the hands of experts. With continued advancement in technology and improvement in surgical skills with experience, it is only a matter of time before minimally invasive surgery becomes the mode of choice for treating congenital biliary dilatation.

Keywords Congenital biliary dilatation · Hepaticojejunostomy · Laparoscopy · Children

24.1 Introduction

Minimally invasive surgery has gained acceptance for treating pediatric congenital biliary dilatation because of comparative advantages over more conventional open surgery, such as, better cosmesis, less requirement for analgesia, a more rapid return to baseline functional status, quicker rehabilitation, and less likelihood of complications secondary to postoperative adhesions. Surgical intervention for congenital biliary dilatation necessitates an exhaustive understanding of anatomic variations centered on the porta hepatis and mastery of skills appropriate for dealing them.

H. Koga · A. Yamataka (✉)
Department of Pediatric General and Urogenital Surgery, Juntendo University School of Medicine, Tokyo, Japan
e-mail: yama@juntendo.ac.jp

T. Kamisawa, H. Ando (eds.), *Pancreaticobiliary Maljunction and Congenital Biliary Dilatation*, https://doi.org/10.1007/978-981-10-8654-0_24

In 1995, Ferallo et al. first described laparoscopic resection and Roux-en-Y hepaticojejunostomy in a 6-year-old case with congenital biliary dilatation [1]. Although their technique has been modified by the advent of finer instruments and the adoption of novel maneuvers, it is the standard viable option for treating congenital biliary dilatation using minimally invasive surgery [2, 3].

The authors will introduce their laparoscopic technique for dilated bile duct excision. A distinguishing feature of their technique is intraoperative endoscopy of the common channel and intrahepatic bile ducts that is performed routinely to examine for biliary debris/stones and protein plugs that are cleared by irrigation with normal saline to prevent mid- to long-term postoperative cholangitis, pancreatitis, and stone formation [4–6].

24.2 Surgical Technique

24.2.1 Laparoscopic Excision

24.2.1.1 Patient/Port Positioning and Initial Preparation

Under general anesthesia, the patient is placed in the reverse Trendelenburg position. A GelPOINT® mini advanced access platform. (Applied Medical, Rancho Santa Margarita, USA) inserted in a 2 cm umbilical incision is used to introduce a 30° 5 or 10 mm laparoscope into the abdomen. Pneumoperitoneum is established with CO_2 insufflated at a flow rate of 0.5–1.0 L/min at a pressure of 8 mmHg, increasing to 12 mmHg if required. Two additional 5 mm trocars are inserted in the right upper quadrant and left upper quadrant, respectively (Fig. 24.1). A percutaneous stay suture is introduced just below the xiphoid process to snare the falciform ligament and retract/elevate the liver to improve exposure. A pair of Babcock forceps is inserted through the left subcostal port in the anterior axillary line to grasp and elevate the gallbladder to expose the porta hepatis and allow the dilated bile duct to be dissected free from surrounding structures, such as the portal vein and hepatic artery. Usually, there are more adhesions between a cystic bile duct and the portal vein and hepatic artery than with a fusiform bile duct, especially in older children.

In adolescents and adults, adhesions can be very dense and complicate dissection. When adhesions are extremely dense, an additional trocar inserted in the lateral right subcostal area can be used for an assistant to grasp the bile duct and facilitate safe dissection (Fig. 24.2). If the adhesion bile duct is inflamed and there are dense adhesions, the anterior wall of the bile duct can be incised at any time during bile duct dissection to allow the posterior wall of the bile duct to be dissected safely under direct vision.

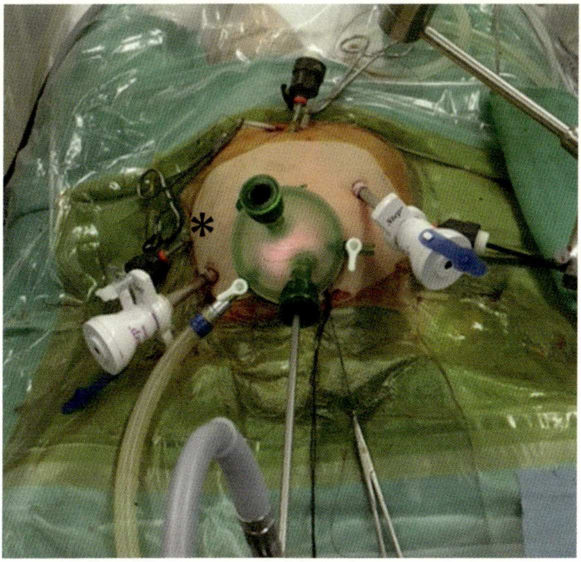

Fig. 24.1 Trocar positions. A 30° 5 or 10 mm laparoscope is introduced through a GelPOINT® mini advanced access platform. (Applied Medical, Rancho Santa Margarita, USA) inserted in a 2 cm umbilical incision. Two additional 5 mm trocars are inserted in the right upper quadrant and left upper quadrant, respectively, as working trocars. The left upper quadrant trocar (left subcostal trocar in the anterior axillary line) is inserted to expose the porta hepatis. An additional 3.9 mm trocar is placed in the left epigastrium for intraoperative endoscopy. Another additional 3.9 mm trocar (*asterisk*) may be placed in the lateral right subcostal area for an assistant to grasp the bile duct to facilitate safe dissection of the bile duct by the surgeon

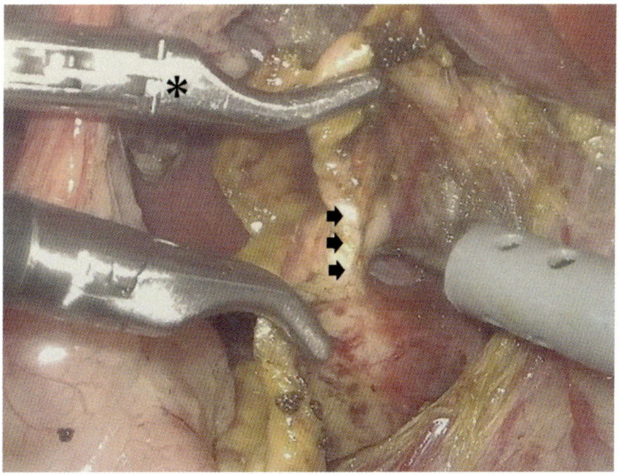

Fig. 24.2 Severely dense adhesions. If the adhesion is inflamed and there are dense adhesions, the anterior wall of the bile duct may be incised at any time during dissection to allow the posterior wall (*arrows*) of the bile duct to be dissected safely under direct vision. An additional trocar (*asterisk*) in the lateral right subcostal area may be placed for an assistant to grasp the bile duct during dissection

24.2.2 Intraoperative Cholangiography

Intraoperative cholangiography is performed if preoperative magnetic resonance cholangiopancreatography is not available or fails to delineate the anatomy of the hepatopancreaticobiliary ducts, especially the anatomy of the pancreaticobiliary junction, and the presence of debris or protein plugs in the intrahepatic bile ducts and common channel. Preoperative magnetic resonance cholangiopancreatography is the investigation of choice and is accurate in the majority of cases.

24.2.3 Intraoperative Endoscopy

For intraoperative endoscopy, an additional 3.9 mm trocar is inserted in the left epigastrium for the introduction of a fine pediatric ureteroscope [7]. We use a pediatric ureteroscope specifically because it allows normal saline to flow continuously through a dedicated side channel, allowing constant visualization and irrigation. While some surgeons suggest that laparoscopic examination is sufficient, we find that a constant flow of saline dilates the lumen to allow safe examination and assists in clearing debris and protein plugs. Without a constant flow of saline, the lumen collapses, greatly compromising both examination and clearing, and side channels on flexible scopes are essentially designed only for flushing and are inadequate for inspection and irrigation.

Intraoperative endoscopy is particularly valuable during excision of fusiform type congenital biliary dilatation to ensure that any wide intrapancreatic choledochus is excised adequately as any remnant may contribute to stone formation that may cause postoperative pancreatitis in the long-term. It is less important in cystic type congenital biliary dilatation, since the intrapancreatic choledochus is short and narrow and the patient does not often present with pancreatitis, probably because there are no debris in the common channel. Intraoperative endoscopy is performed routinely in all congenital biliary dilatation patients unless the ureteroscope cannot be inserted into the intrapancreatic choledochus and common channel from the distal part of the bile duct because they are too narrow.

24.2.4 Complete Excision

The cystic artery is identified and divided. Dissection of the dilated bile duct is initiated by removing the adjacent peritoneum using monopolar electrocautery and a Maryland dissector to establish a plane of dissection, beginning on the anterior/lateral wall and continuing to the distal sides and then to the posterior portion.

The exact level of transection of the distal common bile duct is determined by intraoperative endoscopy when the orifice of the pancreatic duct can be identified with the ureteroscope [8] and with intraoperative cholangiography if the orifice of the pancreatic duct cannot be identified.

During intraoperative endoscopy, the part of the ureteroscope emerging externally from the trocar is held with mosquito forceps and pulled very gently from the pancreatic duct to the level where the distal dissection was ceased under laparoscopic view (Fig. 24.3). Because there is a light source at the tip of the ureteroscope, the laparoscopic surgeon can measure the actual length of the intrapancreatic part of the dilated bile duct from the pancreatic duct orifice to the point where dissection was ceased. If the intrapancreatic part is longer than 5 mm, the distal end of the bile duct is dissected further caudally toward the intrapancreatic duct orifice. This procedure is repeated until the intrapancreatic part is 5 mm or less in length. To prevent erroneous measurement, an exteriorized silk suture is fixed by clamping with a pair of mosquito forceps to ensure constant tension is maintained on the bile duct. Thus, the laparoscopic surgeon can continue to dissect toward the common channel to excise the intrapancreatic part of the bile duct, confident there is no risk for injuring the pancreatic duct because the exact length of the intrapancreatic part of the bile duct is known. Once 5 mm or less in length, the intrapancreatic part is ligated and excised. Once the bile duct has been freed, the distal part is divided as close as pos-

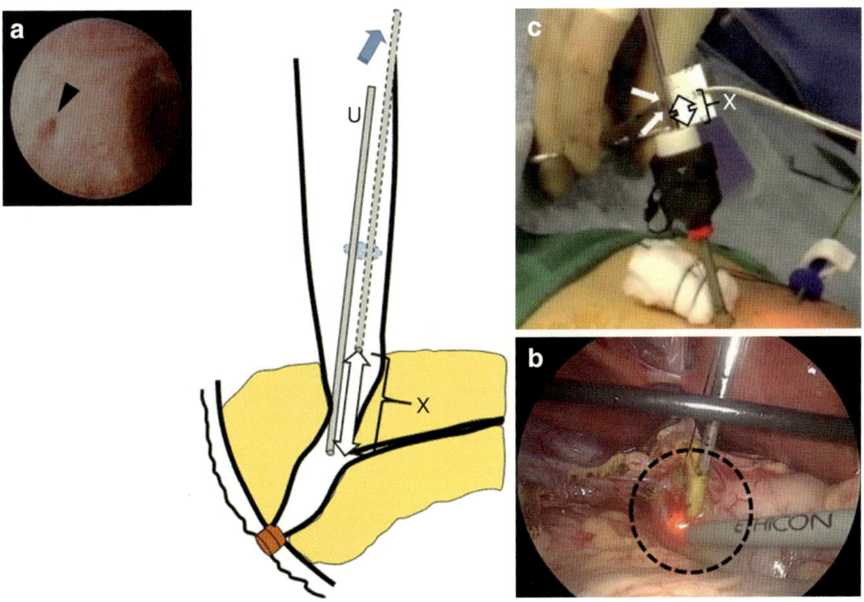

Fig. 24.3 Measuring the intrapancreatic part of the bile duct during laparoscopic excision. After opening the dilated bile duct distally, an ureteroscope (Diagram: U) is inserted to identify the orifice of the pancreatic duct (**a**: *arrowhead*). The part of the ureteroscope emerging externally from the trocar is held with mosquito forceps (**c**: *white arrows*) and pulled very gently (Diagram: *Blue arrow*) from the pancreatic duct to the level where distal dissection was ceased under laparoscopic view (**b**). The laparoscopic surgeon can measure the length X (Diagram and **c**: *double-headed white arrow*) which will be the length of the intrapancreatic part of the congenital biliary dilatation

sible to the pancreaticobiliary junction, and the stump is ligated with an endoloop. When the pancreatic duct orifice cannot be identified, intraoperative cholangiography may be performed by placing an endoscopic metal clip at the distal end of the dissected bile duct to indicate the extent of dissection required further distally, because the clip and the confluence between the common channel, intrapancreatic choledochus, and pancreatic duct can be visualized. If dissection is inadequate, the bile duct can be dissected further distally and intraoperative cholangiography repeated as above until bile duct dissection is considered adequate.

The proximal bile duct is excised leaving 10 mm of common hepatic bile duct for the hepaticojejunostomy. Should the anatomy be more complicated than expected, for example, if there is membranous stenosis in the common hepatic duct, conversion to mini laparotomy for open hepaticojejunostomy should be considered without hesitation.

24.2.5 Extracorporeal Transumbilical Jejunal Roux-en-Y

The ligament of Treitz is identified, and jejunum 15 cm distal to the ligament is exteriorized through the umbilical port site to create the Roux-en-Y jejunal loop extracorporeally. Pneumoperitoneum is interrupted, and the jejunum is divided, and the length of the Roux limb is customized by bringing it up to 1 cm above the xiphoid process on the anterior abdominal wall. Customizing ensures that a Roux limb will grow with the patient and not become tortuous as predetermined lengths of Roux limb (30, 40, or 50 cm) have a tendency to do, leading to stasis and risk for cholangitis. A jejunojejunostomy is performed extracorporeally. The customized Roux limb is approximated to the native jejunum for 8 cm cranially to prevent the contents of the native jejunum from refluxing into the Roux limb. The jejunojejunostomy should fit naturally into the splenic flexure after anastomosis [9]. Finally, an antimesenteric enterotomy is made near the closed end of the Roux limb, and the jejunum returned to the abdominal cavity; the pneumoperitoneum is reestablished; and the jejunal limb is passed through a retrocolic window to lie without tension at the porta hepatis. A scalpel should be used for the enterotomy in the jejunum to prevent thermal injury to the jejunal wall; we never use diathermy with coagulation mode for the enterotomy, since thermal injury can cause scarring [5, 6]. If the enterotomy is made slightly on the anterior side of the jejunum rather than the antimesenteric side, the hepaticojejunostomy is easier, because the mucosa of the posterior wall of the jejunum can be easily identified while performing the anastomosis.

24.2.6 Hepaticojejunostomy

From experience, an additional two ports (3.9/5 mm) are required for hepaticojejunostomy, one lateral right subcostal port and one between the right subcostal and right upper quadrant ports in order to prevent the quality of the anastomosis from deteriorating, especially when the diameter is less than 9 mm. End-to-side hepaticojejunostomy is performed using interrupted 5/0 or 6/0 absorbable sutures with the right upper quadrant port as the needle holder in the right hand, the 5 mm port for the scope, and the 3 mm subcostal port as the needle receiver in the left hand (Fig. 24.4a, b). Both the right and left edge sutures are exteriorized and used as traction sutures during anastomosis of the anterior wall to facilitate accuracy, especially when the hepaticojejunostomy anastomosis diameter is less than 9 mm.

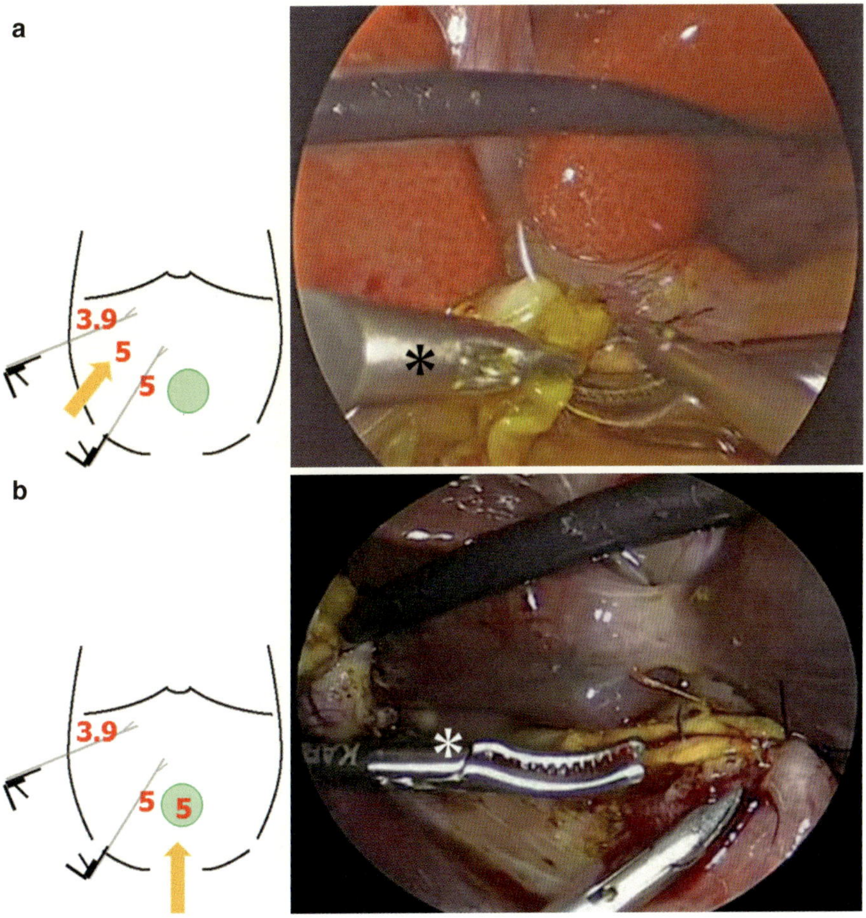

Fig. 24.4 End-to-side hepaticojejunostomy. (**a**) Coaxial ergonomics: hepaticojejunostomy is performed using interrupted 5/0 or 6/0 absorbable sutures with the right upper quadrant port as a needle holder in the right hand, the 5 mm port for the scope (Diagram: *orange arrow*) and the 3.9 mm subcostal port (*asterisk*) as a needle receiver in the left hand. The green circle is the GelPOINT® mini advanced access platform. (**b**) Paraaxial ergonomics: hepaticojejunostomy is performed with the right upper quadrant port as a needle holder in the right hand and the 3.9 mm subcostal port (*asterisk*) as a needle receiver in the left hand. The scope (Diagram: *orange arrow*) has been moved to the GelPOINT® mini advanced access platform.

A tube drain is inserted in the foramen of Winslow. The resected bile duct and gallbladder are extracted through the umbilical port site. The trocars are removed and the wounds closed.

24.2.7 Single-Incision Laparoscopic Excision

First reported in 2012, single-incision laparoscopic surgery for congenital biliary dilatation involves placing all trocars at a single site with a single skin incision instead of multiple skin incisions at separate sites as in conventional laparoscopic surgery [10]. In general, it is more difficult than conventional laparoscopic surgery due to problems related to triangulation and instrument manipulation. To facilitate single-incision laparoscopic surgery, specialized multichannel ports and/or specialized laparoscopic instruments with curved bent tips or rotating mechanisms are used. To date, some 260 cases of successful single-incision laparoscopic surgery for congenital biliary dilatation have been reported [11–13]. Compared with conventional laparoscopic surgery, single-incision laparoscopic surgery would appear to be more efficient based on operative time and postoperative recovery and have better cosmesis [14], although longer follow-up is still needed. Single-incision requires mastery of both laparoscopic and hepaticobiliary surgery to manage potential complications. Such expertise is proportional to experience obtained from performing a large number of conventional laparoscopic hepaticojejunostomies as a team to foster technical proficiency and establish rapport between surgeons and assistants.

24.2.8 Robotic-Assisted Excision

Robotic surgery has been in use for the treatment of congenital biliary dilatation since 2006 [15]. Its advantages include superb visualization and instrument control. The camera provides high magnification with three-dimensional visualization through a stereo endoscope, and the surgeon is assisted by features such as direct control of the visual field, improved dexterity, tremor reduction, motion scaling, and higher degrees of freedom compared with standard laparoscopic instruments. These advantages make dissecting, suturing, and knot-tying easier, and the hepaticojejunostomy anastomosis is facilitated greatly by robotic assistance. For example, the authors recently treated a pediatric case of pancreaticobiliary malunion without dilatation of the common hepatic duct successfully using da Vinci robotic assistance for the hepaticojejunostomy anastomosis with a common hepatic duct only 4 mm in diameter. Such a procedure would have been quite difficult using conventional laparoscopy.

The potential promise of robotic-assisted surgery is that it can encourage surgeons to be more ambitious when planning and performing complex minimally invasive procedures. To date, some 45 pediatric congenital biliary dilatation cases treated by robotic-assisted hepaticojejunostomy have been reported [15–19]. The mean operative time of these cases ranged from 180 to 520 min, significantly longer than for conventional laparoscopic procedures; bile leak was reported in one case. At present, the size of robotic hardware prevents it from being used more generally in pediatric surgery. The hardware is also expensive and maintenance costs are high. With ongoing technical improvements, robotic assistance will enable surgeons to approach the optimal goal of minimally invasive surgery, i.e., atraumatic, scarless treatment.

24.2.9 Laparoscopic Hepaticojejunostomy Versus Laparoscopic Hepaticoduodenostomy

Although hepaticoduodenostomy is an easier, quicker procedure and allows bile to enter the duodenum directly, which is more physiological [20–22], postoperative cholangitis and bile gastritis are known complications with risk for mucosal damage and possible malignant change. Todani et al. [20] reported a patient who underwent bile duct excision and hepaticoduodenostomy at 13 months old and developed hilar bile duct carcinoma 18 years later. Inflammation of the bile duct mucosa was thought to be related to the reflux of duodenal contents (including activated pancreatic enzymes) into the intrahepatic bile ducts though the anastomosis which prompted them to abandoned hepaticoduodenostomy in favor of hepaticojejunostomy. The authors also reported bilious gastritis due to marked duodenogastric bile reflux on upper gastrointestinal endoscopy, and histology of biopsied gastric mucosa showed gastritis [23].

Overall, hepaticojejunostomy is recommended for biliary reconstruction in children requiring congenital biliary dilatation excision, because hepaticoduodenostomy is associated with some degree of duodenal contents reflux into the biliary tree, especially when intrahepatic bile duct dilatation is present. A long-term prospective randomized controlled study is warranted to compare the outcomes of laparoscopic hepaticoduodenostomy and hepaticojejunostomy.

24.2.10 Surgical Outcome

In mid- to long-term follow-up studies published recently [24, 25], experienced laparoscopic surgeons were reported to be able to achieve results similar to open surgery. In a report comparing laparoscopic bile duct excision with open surgery in children [22, 25], the operative time was found to be longer and overall costs higher, but there was significantly less blood loss and duration of hospitalization was shorter. There were no significant differences in the incidences of bile leaks or wound infections. This would appear to suggest that in the hands of skilled laparoscopic surgeons, laparoscopic bile duct excision and Roux-en-Y reconstruction are safe and effective.

24.3 The Authors' Experience

The authors performed 43 laparoscopic congenital biliary dilatation excisions between 2009 and 2017. Cases requiring conversion to open laparotomy ($n = 1$) and minilaparotomy ($n = 2$) were excluded, leaving 40 cases, 32 females and 8 males. Congenital biliary dilatations were fusiform in 21 cases and cystic in 19 cases. Mean age (range) at surgery was 4.8 (0.3–14.1) years, and mean weight at surgery was 17.0 (5.5–47.0) kg. Five patients had intrahepatic bile duct dilatation. There were no intraoperative complications. Estimated mean blood loss was minimal at 15 mL. Hepaticojejunostomy diameters were 6–9 mm in 13/21 fusiform cases and 12/19 cystic cases, more than 10 mm in 8/21 fusiform cases and 7/19 cystic cases.

Intraoperative endoscopy of both the common channel and intrahepatic bile ducts was performed in 25 cases (21 fusiform; 4 cystic); the remaining 15 had intraoperative endoscopy of intrahepatic ducts alone because the ureteroscope could not be inserted into the intrapancreatic choledochus and common channel. Protein plugs were present in the common channel in all 21 fusiform cases (massive in 6, moderate in 12, minimal in 3), successfully cleared by irrigation with normal saline from the side channel of the ureteroscope. Debris were present in all 15 cases who had intraoperative endoscopy of the intrahepatic bile ducts alone (moderate in 6, minimal in 9). There were no debris in the intrahepatic bile ducts of the 25 who had intraoperative endoscopy of both the common channel and intrahepatic bile ducts.

Although all patients are well after a mean follow-up of 4.5 years (range: 6 months to 8.5 years) with cosmetically esthetic wounds, there were three cases of postoperative complications. The first was pancreatitis that developed 8 months postoperatively in a case with massive protein plugs on intraoperative endoscopy, even though all plugs were cleared thoroughly by irrigation. The pancreatitis was treated by conservative medical management, and there have been no further episodes. The cause was attributed to new 3 × 3 mm debris. The second was duodenal obstruction in a cystic case. At exploratory laparoscopy, the third part of the duodenum was found to be compressed by the Roux-en-Y limb that had been inadequately fixed to the colonic mesentery. Once the sutures between the Roux-en-Y limb and colonic mesentery were released laparoscopically, the postoperative recovery was uneventful. The third was anastomotic leak treated by minilaparotomy.

24.4 Conclusion

The authors were the first to report the value of customizing the length of the short Roux loop, performing the hepaticojejunostomy very close to the closed end of the Roux loop blind end, and creating the enterotomy on the anterior side of the Roux loop as part of their routine laparoscopic bile duct excision procedure. Despite extra trocars and longer operative time, postoperative pain is minimized, allowing patients to be discharged earlier. Intraoperative endoscopy is invaluable for reducing mid- to long-term postoperative complications.

References

1. Farello GA, Cerofolini A, Rebonato M, et al. Congenital choledochal cyst: video-guided laparoscopic treatment. Surg Laparosc Endosc. 1995;5:354–8.
2. Liem NT. Laparoscopic surgery for choledochal cysts. J Hepatobiliary Pancreat Sci. 2013;20:487–91.
3. Li L, Feng W, Jing-Bo F, et al. Laparoscopic-assisted total cyst excision of choledochal cyst and Roux-en-Y hepatoenterostomy. J Pediatr Surg. 2004;39:1663–6.
4. Takahashi T, Shimotakahara A, Okazaki T, et al. Intraoperative endoscopy during choledochal cyst excision: extended long-term follow-up compared with recent cases. J Pediatr Surg. 2010;45:379–82.
5. Yamataka A, Lane GJ, Cazares J. Laparoscopic surgery for biliary atresia and choledochal cyst. Semin Pediatr Surg. 2012;21:201–10.
6. Yamataka A, Lane GJ, Koga H, et al. Role of laparoscopy during surgery at the porta hepatis. S Afr Med J. 2014;104:820–4.
7. Miyano G, Koga H, Shimotakahara A, et al. Intralaparoscopic endoscopy: its value during laparoscopic repair of choledochal cyst. Pediatr Surg Int. 2011;27:463–6.
8. Koga H, Okawada M, Doi T, et al. Refining the intraoperative measurement of the distal intrapancreatic part of a choledochal cyst during laparoscopic repair allows near total excision. Pediatr Surg Int. 2015;31:991–4.
9. Yamataka A, Kobayashi H, Shimotakahara A, et al. Recommendations for preventing complications related to Roux-en-Y hepatico-jejunostomy performed during excision of choledochal cyst in children. J Pediatr Surg. 2003;38:1830–2.
10. Diao M, Li L, Dong N, et al. Single-incision laparoscopic Roux-en-Y hepaticojejunostomy using conventional instruments for children with choledochal cysts. Surg Endosc. 2012;26:1784–90.
11. Tang Y, Li F, He G. Comparison of single-incision and conventional laparoscopic cyst excision and Roux-en-Y hepaticojejunostomy for children with choledochal cysts. Indian J Surg. 2016;78:259–64.
12. Diao M, Li L, Li Q, et al. Single-incision versus conventional laparoscopic cyst excision and Roux-Y hepaticojejunostomy for children with choledochal cysts: a case-control study. World J Surg. 2013;37:1707–13.
13. Lin XK, Wu DZ, Cai JL, et al. Transumbilical single-incision laparoscopic surgery in children with conventional instruments: our early experience. J Laparoendosc Adv Surg Tech A. 2016;26:938–41.
14. Son TN, Liem NT, Hoan VX. Transumbilical laparoendoscopic single-site surgery with conventional instruments for choledochal cyst in children: early results of 86 cases. J Laparoendosc Adv Surg Tech A. 2014;24:907–10.

15. Woo R, Le D, Albanese CT, et al. Robot-assisted laparoscopic resection of a type I choledochal cyst in a child. J Laparoendosc Adv Surg Tech A. 2006;16:179–83.
16. Kim NY, Chang EY, Hong YJ, et al. Retrospective assessment of the validity of robotic surgery in comparison to open surgery for pediatric choledochal cyst. Yonsei Med J. 2015;56:737–43.
17. Akaraviputh T, Trakarnsanga A, Suksamanapun N. Robot-assisted complete excision of choledochal cyst type I, hepaticojejunostomy and extracorporeal Roux-en-y anastomosis: a case report and review literature. World J Surg Oncol. 2010;8:87.
18. Alizai NK, Dawrant MJ, Najmaldin AS. Robot-assisted resection of choledochal cysts and hepaticojejunostomy in children. Pediatr Surg Int. 2014;30:291–4.
19. Meehan JJ, Elliott S, Sandler A. The robotic approach to complex hepatobiliary anomalies in children: preliminary report. J Pediatr Surg. 2007;42:2110–4.
20. Todani T, Wantanabe Y, Toki A, Hara H. Hilar duct carcinoma developed aft er cyst excision followed by hepaticoduodenostomy. In: Koyanagi Y, Aoki T, editors. Pancreaticobiliary maljunction. Tokyo: Igaku tosho Shuppan; 2002. p. 17–21.
21. Liem NT, Pham HD, Dung le A, et al. Early and intermediate outcomes of laparoscopic surgery for choledochal cysts with 400 patients. J Laparoendosc Adv Surg Tech A. 2012;22:599–603.
22. Santore MT, Deans KJ, Behar BJ, et al. Laparoscopic hepaticoduodenostomy versus open hepaticoduodenostomy for reconstruction after resection of choledochal cyst. J Laparoendosc Adv Surg Tech A. 2011;21:375–8.
23. Shimotakahara A, Yamataka A, Yanai T, et al. Roux-en-Y hepaticojejunostomy or hepaticoduodenostomy for biliary reconstruction during the surgical treatment of choledochal cyst: which is better? Pediatr Surg Int. 2005;21:5–7.
24. Qiao G, Li L, Li S, et al. Laparoscopic cyst excision and Roux-Y hepaticojejunostomy for children with choledochal cysts in China: a multicenter study. Surg Endosc. 2015;29:140–4.
25. Zhen C, Xia Z, Long L, et al. Laparoscopic excision versus open excision for the treatment of choledochal cysts: a systematic review and meta-analysis. Int Surg. 2015;100:115–22.

Chapter 25
Laparoscopic Surgery of Congenital Biliary Dilatation

Nguyen Thanh Liem

Abstract Laparoscopic surgery has become a common procedure for congenital biliary dilatation. The dilated choledochus should be removed completely just above the confluence of the common biliopancreatic channel at the distal end and approximately 5 mm from the confluence of the right and left hepatic ducts at the proximal end to avoid complications of the its remnant. The operation is feasible and safe. The rate of conversion to open surgery is low. The rate of complication of laparoscopic surgery performed by skilled surgeons is also low, even lower than that of open surgery. There is no difference between hepaticoduodenostomy and hepaticojejunostomy concerning the rate of cholangitis. Gastritis due to bilious reflux occurred with a low rate in hepaticoduodenostomy. Both techniques could be used for congenital biliary dilatation; however, hepaticoduodenostomy should be applied for congenital biliary dilatation without intrahepatic dilatation of biliary tract.

Keywords Congenital biliary dilatation · Laparoscopic surgery · Hepaticoduodenostomy · Hepaticojejunostomy

The first laparoscopic operation to remove the congenital choledochal dilatation (CCD) and hepaticojejunostomy was performed by Farello in 1995, and then the first laparoscopic hepaticoduodenostomy was carried out by Tan in 2003 [1, 2]. Since then many other studies with different modifications have been published [3–19].

N. T. Liem
Vinmec International Hospital, Hanoi, Vietnam

Vinmec Research Institute of Stem Cell and Gene Technology, Hanoi, Vietnam
e-mail: v.liemnt@vinmec.com

T. Kamisawa, H. Ando (eds.), *Pancreaticobiliary Maljunction and Congenital Biliary Dilatation*, https://doi.org/10.1007/978-981-10-8654-0_25

25.1 Indication and Contraindication

25.1.1 Prenatal Detected Congenital Biliary Dilation

- The surgery should be performed around 3 months old if there are no manifestations of biliary obstruction.
- On the contrary, the surgery should be carried out earlier if there are manifestations of biliary obstruction or the choledochal dilatation could not be distinguished from type I of biliary atresia.

25.1.2 Postnatal Detected Congenital Biliary Dilatation

- The surgery can be performed after shortly given good preparation.
- For common biliopancreatic malunion without choledochal dilatation, the surgery is indicated if there is repeated abdominal pain, pancreatitis, or cholangitis.

25.1.3 Contraindication

- Severe hepatic dysfunction
- Perforated choledochal dilatation
- Active cholangitis

25.2 Preoperative Preparation

25.2.1 Confirmation of Diagnosis

- Routine preoperative blood tests and biochemical liver function tests must be conducted.
- The accurate diagnosis should be obtained by abdominal ultrasound and magnetic resonance cholangiopancreatography. However, endoscopic retrograde cholangiopancreatography or the intraoperative cholangiography should be performed if the common biliopancreatic channel is still not identified with abovementioned investigations.

25.2.2 Preparation

- A prolonged prothrombin time secondary to cholestasis should be corrected with intravenous vitamin K.
- Biliary infection has to be well managed.
- Ascaris elimination medicaments should be given if the parasite is present.

25.3 General Operative Principles

- Complete removal of the choledocal dilation and hilar hepaticoenterostomy is the standard treatment for CCD.
- The distal removal should be close to the orifice of common biliopancreatic channel.

25.4 Anesthesia

General anesthesia with endotracheal intubation is standard. Broad-spectrum intravenous antibiotics are best given at induction of anesthesia and continued for 2–5 days postoperatively.

25.5 Operative Techniques

25.5.1 Laparoscopic Complete Removal of Dilated Choledochus and Hepaticojejunostomy

- A nasogastric tube, rectal tube, and Foley urinary catheter are inserted to decompress the stomach, the colon, and the bladder, respectively. The patient is placed in a 30° head-up supine position. The surgeon stands at the lower end of the operating table between the patient's legs. The monitor is positioned at patient's head side.
- A 10-mm trocar is inserted through the umbilicus for the telescope. Three additional 5- or 3-mm trocars are placed for instruments: one at the right flank, one at the left flank, and the final one in the left hypochondrium (Fig. 25.1)
- A carbon dioxide pneumoperitoneum is maintained at a pressure of 8–12 mmHg depending on patient's age. Inspection of the choledochus, gallbladder, and liver is carried out.

25.5.2 Jejunojejunostomy

The ligament of Treitz is identified by laparoscopy. A 5/0 silk stay suture is placed 30 cm distal to the ligament of Treitz. A second 5/0 PDS suture is placed 2.0 cm below the first suture to mark the jejunal limb, which will be anastomosed to the hepatic duct. The jejunal segment with two sutures is grasped with an intestinal grasper. The transumbilical vertical incision is extended 1.0 cm above the umbilicus. The jejunum is exteriorized, and the jejunojejunostomy is carried out extracorporeally. The jejunum is then reintroduced into the abdominal cavity. The extended incision is closed. The laparoscopic instruments are repositioned.

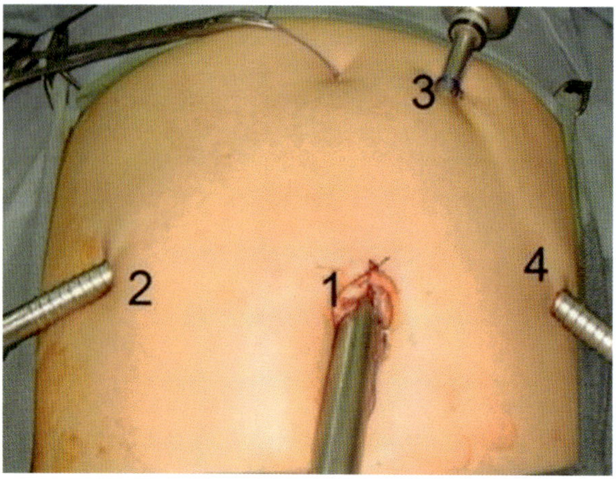

Fig. 25.1 Trocars arrangement

25.5.3 *Complete Removal of Dilated Choledochus*

The liver is secured to the abdominal wall by stay suture placed at the round ligament (Fig. 25.2). The cystic artery and cystic duct are identified, clipped, and divided, respectively. A second traction suture is placed at the distal cystic duct and gallbladder fundus to elevate the liver and splay out the liver hilum.

The duodenum is retracted downward using a dissector through the fourth trocar site. The midportion of the dilated choledochus is dissected circumferentially. Separation of the dilated choledochus from the portal vein is carried out meticulously until a dissector can be passed through the space between the posterior wall of the dilated choledochus and portal vein proceeding from left to right (Fig. 25.3).

The dilated choledochus is then divided at this site. The lower part of the dilated choledochus is detached from the surrounding and pancreatic tissue down to the common biliopancreatic duct using a 3-mm dissector for cautery and dissection. Protein plugs or calculi within the distal dilated choledochus and common channel are washed out and removed. The distal part of the dilated choledochus is opened longitudinally. The interior of the dilated choledochus is inspected to identify the orifice of the common biliopancreatic channel. A small catheter is inserted into the common channel. Irrigation with normal saline via this catheter is performed to eliminate any protein plugs until the catheter can be passed down to the duodenum.

The inspection and irrigation may be performed through a pediatric cystoscope if the common channel is wide enough. The distal dilated choledochus is clipped and divided at the level of the orifice of the common channel.

- The upper part of the dilated choledochus is now dissected up to the common hepatic duct and divided. The dilated choledochus is initially divided below the cystic duct level, and after identifying the orifice of the right and left hepatic ducts by inspecting internally, the definitive division is performed.

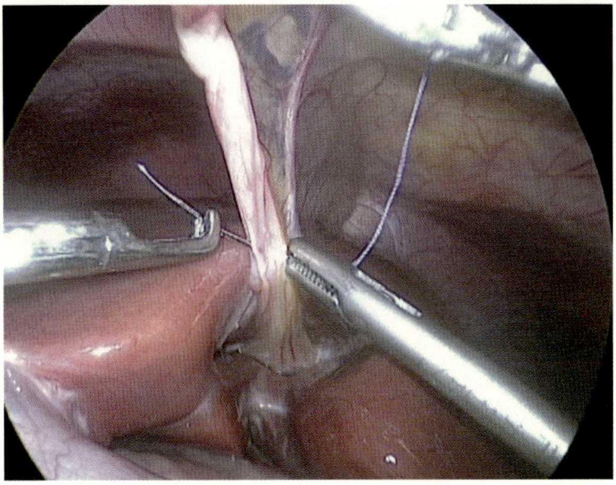

Fig. 25.2 The liver is secured to the abdominal wall by stay suture placed at the round ligament

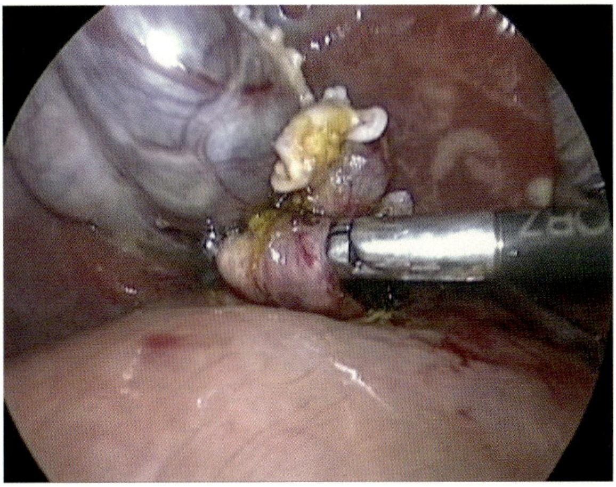

Fig. 25.3 Separation of the dilated choledochus from the portal vein

- Irrigation with normal saline through a small catheter inserted into the right and then into the left hepatic duct is performed to wash out the protein plugs or calculi until the fluid from those ducts is clear.
- With a large dilated choledochus, the dissection starts from the middle portion, proceeding distally. The distal portion of the dilated choledochus is separated from the portal vein. The distal common bile duct is divided above the biliary-pancreatic duct. The distal dilated choledochus is inspected from inside to identify the orifice of the common biliopancreatic duct. A small catheter was inserted through one trocar to the distal end of the cholechocus. Irrigation with normal saline through this catheter is carried out to wash out debris and calculi (Fig. 25.4). The distal common bile duct is then clipped and transected at the level of the common channel orifice.

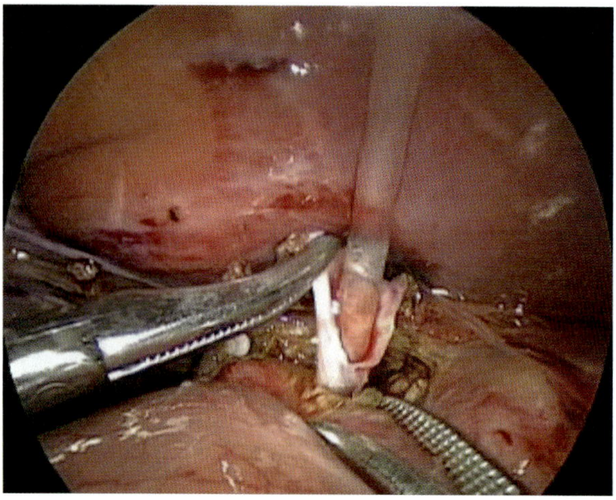

Fig. 25.4 A small catheter was inserted to the distal end of the cholechocus

- When the dilated choledochus is intensely inflamed and extensively adhesive, its anterior wall is opened, and then the dissection of dilated choledochal wall from the portal vein is carried out carefully while viewing the dilated choledochus internally and externally. After dividing the midportion of the dilated choledochus, the upper and lower parts of the dilated choledochus are removed as described above.
- The Roux limb is passed through a window in the transverse mesocolon to the porta hepatis. The jejunum is opened longitudinally on the antimesenteric border a few millimeters from the end of the Roux loop. Hepaticojejunostomy is fashioned using two running sutures of 5/0 PDS. (Interrupted sutures are used when the diameter of the common hepatic duct is less than 1.0 cm.) Sutures are inserted from the left to the right with 3-mm instruments. Ductoplasty is performed by opening the common hepatic duct and incising the left hepatic duct longitudinally for a variable distance if the common hepatic duct is too small.
- Mesenteric defects in the transverse mesocolon and small bowel mesentery are closed with sutures.
- The gallbladder is detached from its bed and surrounding tissues. Different parts of the dilated choledochus and gallbladder are removed through the umbilicus. The operative field is washed with warm saline. A subhepatic drain is inserted.

25.6 Laparoscopic Complete Removal of Dilated Choledochus and Hepaticoduodenostomy

The excision of dilated choledochus is carried out as described above. The duodenum is mobilized, and a hepaticoduodenostomy is constructed 2.0–3.0 cm from the pylorus.

25.7 Transumbilical Laparoendoscopic Single-Site Surgery with Conventional Instruments

The periumbilical incision is made then the periumbilical skin is detached from the fascia. Two 5-mm trocars (one long and one short) and one short 3-mm trocar are placed in a triangular fashion within the range of the skin incision. The conventional 5-mm 30 laparoscope and laparoscopic straight instruments are used. A transabdominal suspending suture is made to lift the hepatic round ligament to the abdominal wall. A second suspending suture is performed to lift the gallbladder to the abdominal wall on the right. The cystic artery is cauterized, and the cystic duct is exposed, clipped, and divided. A third suspending suture is made to lift the anterior wall of the choledochus to the abdominal wall. The distal part of the choledochus is dissected. More suspending sutures can be added to facilitate dissection of the choledochus if necessary. The rest of the operation is performed similar to the operation with four incisions [20].

25.8 Intraoperative Complications

25.8.1 Injury of Hepatic Artery and the Portal Vein

In general the hepatic artery is easy to be recognized and separated from the dilated choledochus. On the contrary, separation of the choledochus from the portal vein is much more difficult that is why injury of the portal vein can happen when the dilated choledochus is intensely inflamed and extensively adhesive. This complication can be prevented by always keeping the dissection as close as on the dilated choledochal wall. When severe inflammation and adhesion around the dilated choledochus are present, the dilated choledochus should be opened at its anterior wall followed by careful separation of its left and posterior wall from the portal vein while viewing internally and externally.

25.8.2 Transection of Two Hepatic Ducts

This complication can happen when the hepatic bifurcation is situated low far from the liver hilar. This complication could be avoided by performing the first transection of the proximal part of the choledochus below the cystic duct level then identifying the orifice of the right and left hepatic ducts by internal inspection before definitive division of the choledochus from the hepatic duct.

Injury of pancreatic duct: clear anatomy of the common biliopancreatic channel obtained by MRCP, ERCP, or perioperative cholangiography is useful. Internal inspection of the distal choledochus to identify the orifice of the common biliopancreatic duct helps the surgeon to decide where the division of the distal part of the dilated choledochus can be.

Roux limb twist: this complication has been reported in hepaticojejunostomy. Inspection of the Roux limb before performing hepaticojejunostomy is mandatory to avoid this complication.

25.9 Postoperative Care and Complications

- Oral feeding is resumed after the fluid from the gastric tube becomes clear, usually on day 2 or 3 after the operation. The abdominal drain is removed on day 5 if there is no anastomotic leakage.
- Early postoperative complications include bleeding, intestinal obstruction, anastomotic leakage, and pancreatic fistula. The bilio-digestive anastomotic leakage and pancreatic fistula can be resolved with abdominal drainage, intravenous antibiotics, nasogastric decompression, and parenteral nutrition.
- Cholangitis, anastomotic stricture, and intrahepatic calculi are late complications. Cholangitis without anastomotic stricture or intrahepatic calculi is treated with antibiotics, whereas radiological intervention or surgery is considered for anastomotic stricture or intrahepatic calculi.

25.10 Outcomes

From January 2007 to October 2012, we performed laparoscopic surgery on 547 patients with dilated choledochus at the National Hospital of Pediatrics, Hanoi, Vietnam, 353 patients with removal of dilated choledochus plus hepaticoduodenostomy and 194 with removal of dilated choledochus plus hepaticojejunostomy. Mean operative time for hepaticoduodenostomy was 156 ± 47 and 210 ± 56 min for hepaticojejunostomy. Conversion to open surgery was required in two patients. Intraoperative complications included transection of two hepatic ducts in three patients, perforation of the right portal vein in one patient, and perforation of the right hepatic duct in another. Repair was successful in all patients through laparoscopy. Early postoperative complications included biliary fistula in nine patients (1.6%), with one patient requiring reoperation. Pancreatic fistula occurred in five patients (0.9%). No patients required reoperation. Mean postoperative hospital stay was 6.2 ± 0.3 days for hepaticoduodenostomy and 6.6 ± 0.5 days for hepaticojejunostomy. Follow-up from 1 to 57 months was obtained in 453 patients. Eight patients had cholangitis (1.4%), six patients in the hepaticoduodenostomy group (2%) and two patients in the hepaticojejunostomy group (1.3%). The rate of gastritis due to bilious reflux in hepaticoduodenostomy group was 6.8%. Three patients required reoperation, two due to anastomotic stricture and another due to stenosis at the bifurcation of hepatic ducts.

References

1. Farello GA, Cerofolini A, Rebonato M, et al. Congenital choledochal cyst: video-guided laparoscopic treatment. Surg Laparosc Endosc. 1995;5:354–857.
2. Tan HL, Shankar KR, Ford WD. Laparoscopic resection of type I choledochal cyst. Surg Endosc. 2003;17:1495.
3. Tanaka M, Shimizu S, Mizumoto K, et al. Laparoscopically assisted resection of choledochal cyst and Roux-en-Y reconstruction. Surg Endosc. 2001;15:545–52.
4. Li L, Feng W, Jing-Bo F, et al. Laparoscopic-assisted total cyst excision of choledochal cyst and Roux-en Y hepatoenterostomy. J Pediatr Surg. 2004;39:1663–5.
5. Lee H, Hirose S, Bratton B, et al. Initial experience with complex laparoscopic biliary surgery in children: biliary atresia and choledochal cyst. J Pediatr Surg. 2004;39:804–7.
6. Jang JY, Kim SW, Han HS, et al. Totally laparoscopic management of choledochal cyst using a four-hole method. Surg Endosc. 2006;20:1762–5.
7. Laje P, Questa H, Bailez M. Laparoscopic leak-free technique for the treatment of choledochal cyst. J Laparoendosc Adv Surg Tech A. 2007;17:519–21.
8. Aspelund G, Ling SC, Ng V, et al. A role for laparoscopic approach in the treatment of biliary atresia and choledochal cysts. J Pediatr Surg. 2007;42:869–73.
9. Hong L, Wu Y, Yan Z, et al. Laparoscopic surgery for choledochal cyst in children: a case review of 31patients. Eur J Pediatr Surg. 2008;18:67–71.
10. Liem NT, Dung LA, Son TN. Laparoscopic complete cyst excision and hepaticoduodenostomy for choledochal cyst: early results in 74 cases. J Laparoendosc Adv Surg Tech. 2009;19(s1):s87–90.
11. Liem NT, Hien PD, Dung LA, et al. Laparoscopic repair for choledochal cyst: lessons learned from 190 cases. J Pediatr Surg. 2010;45:540–4.
12. Liem NT, Pham HD, Dung le A, et al. Early and intermediate outcomes of laparoscopic surgery for choledochal cysts with 400 patients. Laparoendosc Adv Surg Tech A. 2012;22(6):599–603.
13. Chokshi NK, Guner YS, Aranda A, et al. Laparoscopic choledochal cyst excision: lessons learned in our experience. J Laparoendosc Adv Surg Tech A. 2009;19:87–91.
14. Lee KH, Tam YH, Yeung CK, et al. Laparoscopic excision of choledochal cyst in children: an intermediate-term report. Pediatr Surg Int. 2009;25:355–60.
15. Miyano G, Koga H, Shimotakahara A, et al. Intralaparoscopic endoscopy: its value during laparoscopic repair of choledochal cyst. Pediatr Surg Int. 2011;27:463–6.
16. Diao M, Li L, Cheng W. Laparoscopic versus open Roux-en-Y hepaticojejunostomy for children with choledochal cysts: intermediate-term follow-up results. Surg Endosc. 2011;25:1567–73.
17. Qiao G, Li L, Li S, et al. Laparoscopic cyst excision and Roux-Y hepaticojejunostomy for children with choledochal cysts in China: a multicenter study. Surg Endosc. 2015;29(1):140–4.
18. Koga H, Okawada M, Doi T, et al. Refining the intraoperative measurement of the distal intrapancreatic part of a choledochal cyst during laparoscopic repair allows near total excision. Pediatr Surg Int. 2015;31(10):991–4.
19. Nederlandse Studiegroep voor Choledochus Cysten/malformaties (NeSCHoC), van den Eijnden MHA, de Kleine RHJ, de Blaauw I, Peeters PGJM, Koot BPG, Oomen MWN, Sloots CEJ, van Gemert WG, van der Zee DC, van Heurn LWE, Verkade HJ, Wilde JCH, Hulscher JBF. Choledochal malformation in children: lessons learned from a Dutch National Study. World J Surg. 2017;41(10):2631–7. https://doi.org/10.1007/s00268-017-4064-x.
20. Son TN, Liem NT, Hoan VX. Transumbilical laparoendoscopic single-site surgery with conventional instruments for choledochal cyst in children: early results of 86 cases. J Laparoendosc Adv Surg Tech A. 2014;24(12):907–10.

Chapter 26
How to Deal with Intrahepatic Bile Duct Stenosis in Congenital Biliary Dilatation and Pancreaticobiliary Maljunction

Hisami Ando

Abstract Congenital stenosis of the bile duct in congenital biliary dilatation is not rare and is present in almost all cases of type IV-A, and it plays a major role in the development of postoperative cholangitis, intrahepatic calculi, and/or cancer. There are two different types of stenosis: membranous stenosis and septal stenosis. When extrahepatic bile duct resection is performed without appropriate treatment of the stenosis, non-smooth bile flow affects bacterial growth through the hepaticoenteric anastomosis and leads to recurrent ascending cholangitis and intrahepatic calculus formation. Meticulous probing and excision of intrahepatic bile duct stenosis from the cut end of the common hepatic duct is effective to prevent intrahepatic calculus formation after surgery. Wide hilar hepaticoenterostomy may be a safe and durable reconstructive technique that can be performed at any age and may help to minimize the long-term risk of complications. Hepatectomy may be the treatment of choice when the stenosis is distant from the hepatic hilum or when it is impossible to reach the hepatic hilum due to severe adhesion. In any case, it is important to ensure that the stenosis is resected or reconstructed during the initial operation.

Keywords Intrahepatic bile duct stenosis · Membranous stenosis · Septal stenosis Wide hilar hepaticoenterostomy · Intrahepatic calculus formation

26.1 Intrahepatic Bile Duct Stenosis in Congenital Biliary Dilatation

Despite the standard excision of the extrahepatic bile duct in congenital biliary dilatation (CBD), a considerable number of patients, reported to account for as many as 2.0–19.8% of cases, will develop postoperative cholangitis and/or intrahepatic

---

H. Ando
Welfare Center for Persons with Developmental Disabilities, Aichi Prefectural Colony, Kasugai, Aichi, Japan
e-mail: hando@med.nagoya-u.ac.jp

T. Kamisawa, H. Ando (eds.), *Pancreaticobiliary Maljunction and Congenital Biliary Dilatation*, https://doi.org/10.1007/978-981-10-8654-0_26

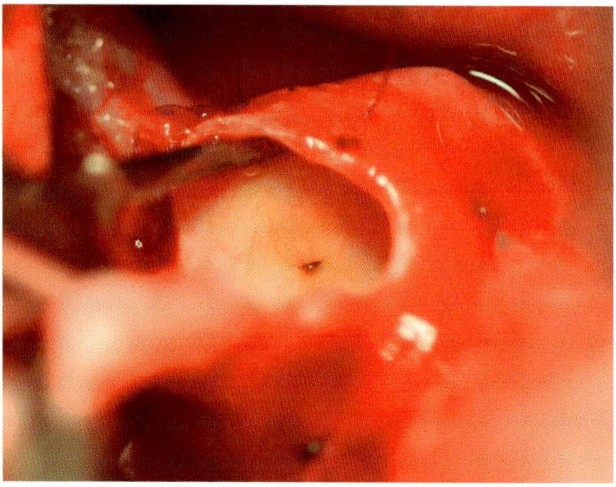

Fig. 26.1 Membranous stenosis is characterized by the presence of a thin diaphragmatic membrane

calculi or cancer after a long duration of time [1]. As a cause of postoperative cholangitis, intrahepatic calculi, and/or cancer, hepaticoenteric anastomotic stenosis may play a role [2, 3]. However, the risk of these complications further increases when stenosis and dilatation of the intrahepatic bile duct coexist [4]. Congenital stenosis of the bile duct in CBD is usually found in the bile duct near the hepatic hilum or in the intrahepatic bile duct proximal to the hepatic hilum, and it plays a major role in the development of postoperative cholangitis, intrahepatic calculi, and/or cancer [5, 6].

There have been some reports about stenosis of the intrahepatic bile duct which is usually present in the hepatic hilum or in some parts of the intrahepatic biliary tracts, and which plays an important role in postoperative cholangitis and intrahepatic calculus formation. Glenn et al. [7] reported a case of diaphragm-like obstruction at the junction of the left hepatic duct and the common hepatic duct, and Melhem et al. [8] reported on congenital diaphragm of the common hepatic duct. In these earlier reports, the stenosis was considered to result from intrahepatic calculi or repeated cholangitis, and to be very rare, but the relationship between stenosis and CBD or pancreaticobiliary malformation (PBM) was not examined. However, stenosis in CBD is not rare and is present in almost all cases of type IV-A [1, 2, 4, 6].

There are two different types of stenosis in CBD: membranous stenosis and septal stenosis [6]. Membranous stenosis consists of a narrow orifice with a smooth mucosal appearance and a diaphragm with a central orifice or semilunar valve and is characterized by a thin membrane (<2 mm) (Fig. 26.1). On the other hand, septal stenosis is characterized by a slender column which divides the bile duct, making it appear as if there are two lumens (Fig. 26.2). These stenoses are identified as the blocking of contrast medium in the intrahepatic bile ducts on preoperative or intraoperative cholangiography and confirmed by direct observation during surgery. The stenosis consists of a mucosal layer composed of a monolayer of cuboidal epithelial cells and a fibromuscular layer composed mostly of collagen fibers and elastic fibers and a few smooth muscle fibers. These histological findings show that the stenosis

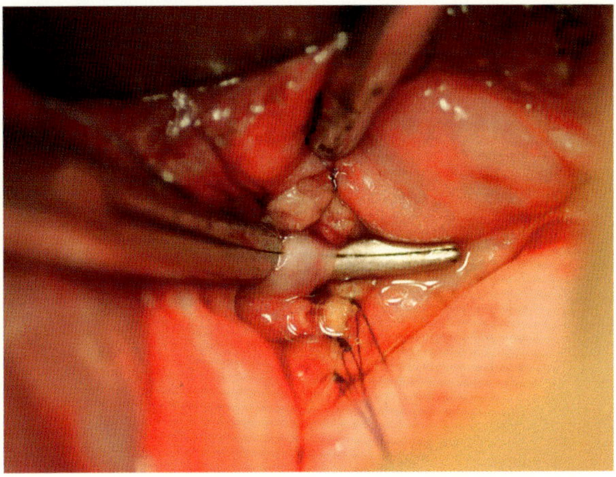

Fig. 26.2 Septal stenosis is characterized by a slender column dividing the bile duct

is not due to inflammation or acquired abnormality. The etiology of the formation of bile duct stenosis is not clear, but it is formed congenitally and has the potential for defective recanalization of the bile duct [5].

26.2 Surgical Treatment of Intrahepatic Bile Duct Stenosis in Congenital Biliary Dilatation

When extrahepatic bile duct resection is performed without appropriate treatment of the stenosis, non-smooth bile flow affects bacterial growth through the hepatico-enteric anastomosis and leads to recurrent ascending cholangitis and intrahepatic calculus formation [9]. Moreover, repeated cholangitis may be a risk factor for cancer. Standard excision of the extrahepatic bile duct alone is inadequate as a surgical procedure in particular for the treatment of type IV-A. Therefore, radical treatment of CBD should be undertaken considering bile flow disorder due to stenosis at the time of the initial operation. There are three methods in dealing with bile duct stenosis: (1) resection of the stenosis from the cut end of the common hepatic duct of the hepatic hilum, (2) incision of the lateral wall of both hepatic ducts, and (3) hepatectomy.

26.2.1 Resection of the Stenosis from the Cut End of the Common Hepatic Duct of the Hepatic Hilum

Stenosis is usually observed around the confluence of the hepatic ducts; therefore, resection of the stenosis can be performed comparatively easily. To resect the stenosis from the cut end of the common hepatic duct of the hepatic hilum, the membranous

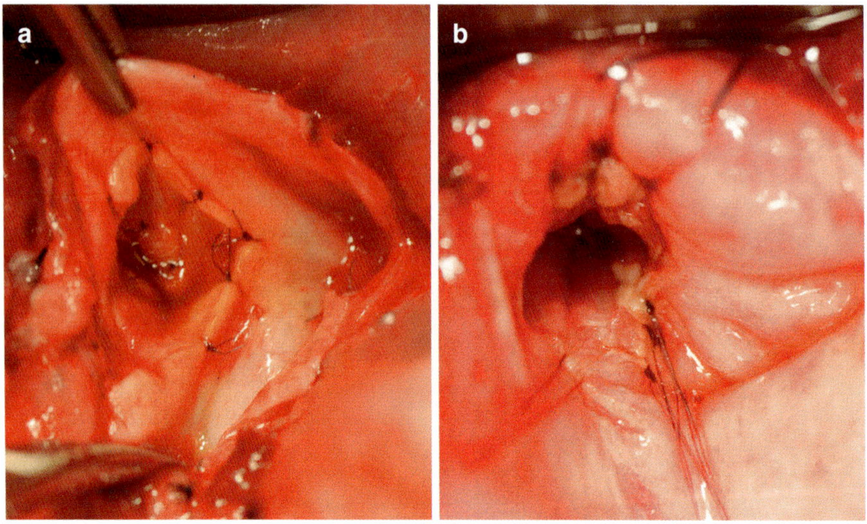

Fig. 26.3 The hepatic duct is widened by resection of the membranous stenosis or septal stenosis ((**a**) the same case as the Fig. 26.1, (**b**) the same case as the Fig. 26.2)

or septal stenosis can be hooked by right-angled forceps or surgical sonde and resected through the hepatic side cut end under direct vision [10]. The cut surface of the membrane or septum should be sutured with 5-0 absorbable material to achieve hemostasis and to prevent cicatricial stricture (Fig. 26.3). Probing and resection of the stenosis are needed to minimize the risk of ascending cholangitis, intrahepatic calculus formation, and/or cancer after long-term postoperative follow-up. All stenoses should be resected without overlooking any, because several stenoses are usually found in the hepatic ducts. Intraoperative cholangioscopy is useful for observation and evaluation of the biliary tract to eliminate possible residual stenosis in the remaining biliary tract. When the stenosis is located distant from the hepatic hilum, it is useful to grasp the membrane or septum with a grasper through the intraoperative cholangioscopy and resect it using electrocautery [11]. Resecting the stenosis from the cut end of the common hepatic duct can be performed in almost all cases by open surgery. Recently, laparoscopic surgery has been widely accepted as a technique for the excision of CBD, but the laparoscopic technique is not commonly used as a therapeutic modality for stenosis. Tanaka et al. [12] reported that bipolar micro-forceps can be used for resection of membranous or septal stenosis in small ducts, and this method is available for laparoscopic surgery.

The efficacy of resection of intrahepatic bile duct stenosis should be evaluated only after long-term follow-up. As a result of long-term follow-up, Tanaka et al. [12] reported that meticulous probing and excision of intrahepatic bile duct stenosis from the cut end of the common hepatic duct is effective to prevent intrahepatic calculus formation after surgery for CBD.

26.2.2 Incision of the Lateral Wall of Both Hepatic Ducts

Conventional hepaticoenterostomy below the hepatic hilum often requires additional procedures due to cholangitis and/or intrahepatic calculi. Therefore, Lilly [13] and Todani et al. [2] reported wide hilar hepaticoenterostomy for type IV-A. The technique of hepaticoenterostomy consists of transection of the common hepatic duct at the hilum with an incision extending approximately 5 mm along the lateral wall of both hepatic ducts to permit a wide anastomotic stoma. Stringer et al. [14] reported that wide hilar hepaticoenterostomy may be a safe, effective, and durable reconstructive technique that can be performed at any age and may help to minimize the long-term risk of complications such as ascending cholangitis and/or intrahepatic calculus formation. Furthermore, Li et al. [15] reported that ductoplasty by laparoscopic surgery was made possible by cutting the anterior wall of the right and left hepatic ducts following the method of Lilly and Todani. Long-term follow-up of wide hilar hepaticoenterostomy is necessary to evaluate a decrease in postoperative complications. Urushihara et al. [16] revealed satisfactory long-term results following wide hilar hepaticojejunostomy. On the other hand, Zheng et al. [17] reported that wide hilar anastomosis did not eliminate the propensity to develop biliary complications after the long-term observation.

26.2.3 Hepatectomy

Historically, hepatectomy including the region of the stenosis has been performed for intrahepatic calculi. In recent years, there have been an increasing number of reports of hepatectomy for children with type IV-A. Tsuchida et al. [18] reported a case of lateral segmentectomy in a 4-year-old girl, and Pal et al. [19] reported on left hepatectomy in a 5-year-old girl, a 10-year-old girl, and an 11-year-old boy and right hepatectomy in a 7-year-old boy. The procedure consists of hepatectomy including the stenotic region of the hepatic duct and resection of the extrahepatic bile duct. Because the morbidity rate of reoperation was significantly higher in cases of excision of the extrahepatic bile duct alone than in cases of liver resection, Zheng et al. [17] reported that removal of the segment including the region of the stenosis is required for type IV-A in adult patients. Meanwhile, Kawarada et al. [20] recommended total resection of the dilated bile duct with S4a+S5 hepatectomy (Taj Mahal hepatectomy) for biliary dilatation extending from the region of the right and left hepatic duct confluence.

Hepatectomy is the treatment of choice when the stenosis is distant from the hepatic hilum or when it is impossible to reach the hepatic hilum due to severe adhesion (Fig. 26.4). However, most stenoses are observed around the confluence of the hepatic ducts and can be resected from the hepatic hilum. Hepatectomy in children may have limited application but, if necessary, should be considered. In any case, it is important to ensure that the stenosis is resected or reconstructed during the initial operation.

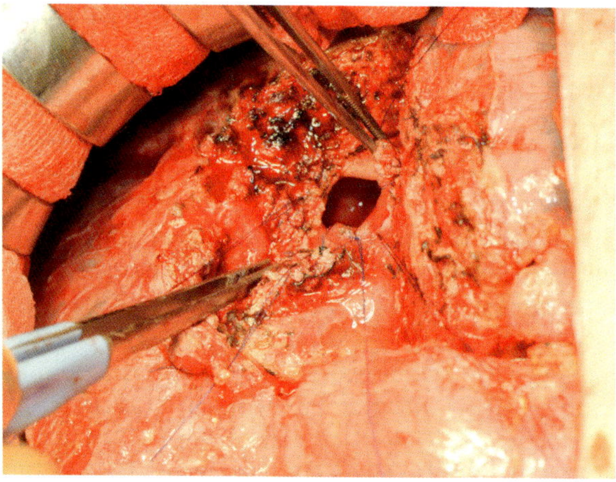

Fig. 26.4 The intrahepatic duct is opened by partial S4a hepatectomy because of severe adhesion of the hepatic hilum (the orifice of the left hepatic duct is not visible in this figure)

References

1. Chijiiwa K, Tanaka M. Late complication after excisional operation in patients with choledochal cyst. J Am Coll Surg. 1994;179:139–44.
2. Todani T, Watanabe Y, Urushihara N, et al. Biliary complications after excisional procedure for choledochal cyst. J Pediatr Surg. 1995;30:478–81.
3. Kim JH, Choi TY, Han JH, et al. Risk factors of postoperative anastomotic stricture after excision of choledochal cysts with hepaticojejunostomy. J Gastrointest Surg. 2008;12:822–8.
4. Uno K, Tsuchida Y, Kawarasaki H, et al. Development of intrahepatic cholelithiasis long after primary excision of choledochal cysts. J Am Coll Surg. 1996;183:583–8.
5. Matsumoto Y, Fujii H, Yoshioka M, et al. Biliary stricture as a case of primary intrahepatic bile duct stones. World J Surg. 1986;10:867–75.
6. Ando H, Ito T, Kaneko K, et al. Congenital stenosis of the intrahepatic bile duct associated with choledochal cysts. J Am Coll Surg. 1995;181:426–30.
7. Glenn F, Moody FG. Intrahepatic calculi. Ann Surg. 1961;153:711–24.
8. Melhem RE, Nahra K. Congenital diaphragm of the common hepatic duct. Br J Radiol. 1966;39:392–4.
9. Kaneko K, Ando H, Seo T, et al. Bile infection contributes to intrahepatic calculi formation after excision of choledochal cysts. Pediatr Surg Int. 2005;21:8–11.
10. Ando H, Kaneko K, Ito F, et al. Operative treatment of congenital stenosis of the intrahepatic bile ducts in patients with choledochal cysts. Am J Surg. 1997;173:491–4.
11. Ono Y, Kaneko K, Ogura Y, et al. Endoscopic resection of intrahepatic septal stenosis: minimally invasive approach to manage hepatolithiasis after choledochal cyst excision. Pediatr Surg Int. 2006;22:939–41.
12. Tanaka Y, Tainaka T, Sumida W, et al. The efficacy of resection of intrahepatic bile duct stenosis-causing membrane or septum for preventing hepatolithiasis after choledochal cyst excision. J Pediatr Surg. 2017;52(12):1930–3.
13. Lilly JR. Surgery of coexisting biliary malformations in choledochal cyst. J Pediatr Surg. 1979;14:643–7.
14. Stringer MD. Wide hilar hepaticojejunostomy: the optimum method of reconstruction after choledochal cyst excision. Pediatr Surg Int. 2007;23(6):529–32.
15. Li L, Liu S, Hou WY, et al. Laparoscopic correction of biliary duct stenosis in choledochal cyst. J Pediatr Surg. 2008;43:644–6.

16. Urushihara N, Fukumoto K, Fukuzawa H, et al. Long-term outcomes after excision of choledochal cysts in a single institution: operative procedures and late complications. J Pediatr Surg. 2012;47:2169–74.
17. Zheng X, Gu W, Xia H, et al. Surgical treatment of type IV-A choledochal cyst in a single institution: children vs. adults. J Pediatr Surg. 2013;48:2061–6.
18. Tsuchida Y, Taniguchi F, Nakahara S, et al. Excision of a choledochal cysts and simultaneous hepatic lateral segmentectomy. Pediatr Surg Int. 1996;11:496–7.
19. Pal K, Singh VP, Mitra DK. Partial hepatectomy and total cyst excision is curative for localized type IV-A biliary duct cysts - report of four cases and review of management. Eur J Pediatr Surg. 2009;19:148–52.
20. Kawarada Y, Das BC, Tabata M, et al. Surgical treatment of type iv choledochal cysts. J Hepato-Biliary-Pancreat Surg. 2009;16:684–7.

Chapter 27
Therapeutic Strategy for PBM Without Biliary Dilatation

Tsukasa Takayashiki, Hideyuki Yoshitomi, Katsunori Furukawa, and Masayuki Ohtsuka

Abstract Pancreaticobiliary maljunction (PBM) describes both cases in which the extrahepatic bile duct is dilated (PBM with biliary dilatation, congenital biliary dilatation) and those in which it is not dilated (PBM without biliary dilatation). A recent detailed report of extrahepatic bile duct measurements using ultrasonography has largely defined a non-dilated bile duct. According to the report, the maximum inner diameter of an extrahepatic bile duct increases according to age. Once the diagnosis of PBM is established, immediate prophylactic surgical treatment is recommended before the onset of malignant changes, even in patients without biliary dilatation. Cholecystectomy and resection of the extrahepatic bile duct, so-called flow-diversion surgery, are established standard surgical methods for PBM with biliary dilatation. As a therapeutic strategy for PBM without biliary dilatation, prophylactic cholecystectomy is also strongly recommended as standard surgical treatment for prevention of gallbladder cancer. However, whether additional prophylactic resection of the extrahepatic bile duct, as in flow-diversion surgery, should be performed for PBM without biliary dilatation remains controversial. Further investigation and surveillance are needed to clarify the appropriate surgical strategy for PBM without biliary dilatation.

Keywords Pancreaticobiliary maljunction · Biliary dilatation · Flow-diversion surgery · Prophylactic cholecystectomy · Resection of the extrahepatic bile duct · Clinical practice guidelines

Pancreaticobiliary maljunction (PBM) describes both cases in which the extrahepatic bile duct is dilated (PBM with biliary dilatation, congenital biliary dilatation) and those in which it is not dilated (PBM without biliary dilatation). Early diagnosis of PBM without biliary dilatation before onset of biliary cancer is necessary [1], and

T. Takayashiki · H. Yoshitomi · K. Furukawa · M. Ohtsuka (✉)
Department of General Surgery, Graduate School of Medicine, Chiba University, Chiba, Japan
e-mail: otsuka-m@faculty.chiba-u.jp

T. Kamisawa, H. Ando (eds.), *Pancreaticobiliary Maljunction and Congenital Biliary Dilatation*, https://doi.org/10.1007/978-981-10-8654-0_27

the committee of the Japanese study group on PBM proposed diagnostic criteria for PBM in 2013 [2]. PBM without biliary dilatation can be diagnosed with endoscopic retrograde cholangiopancreatography (ERCP) (Fig. 27.1), magnetic resonance cholangiopancreatography (MRCP) (Fig. 27.2), multi-planar reconstruction (MPR) images obtained with multi-detector row computed tomography (MDCT)

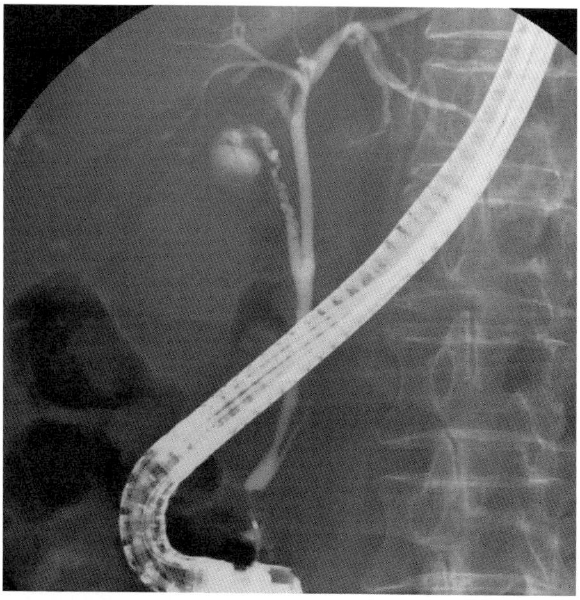

Fig. 27.1 PBM without biliary dilatation were showed in ERCP

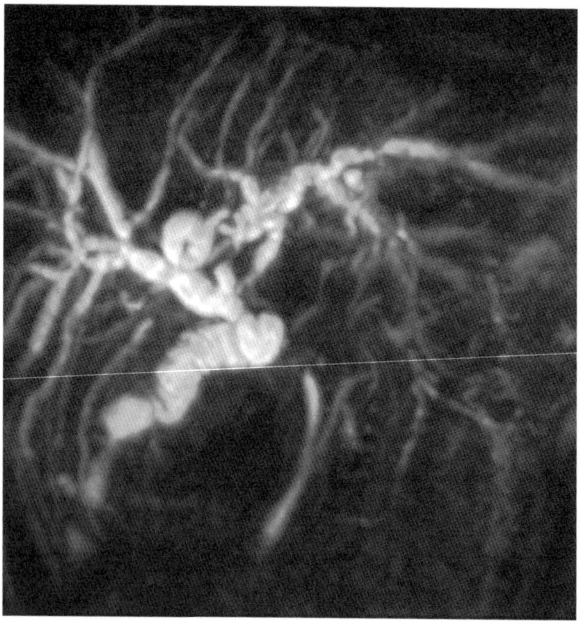

Fig. 27.2 PBM without biliary dilatation were showed in MRCP

(Fig. 27.3), and endoscopic ultrasonography (EUS) (Fig. 27.4). In adults, a common bile duct less than 10 mm in diameter has been defined as non-dilated bile duct, despite the absence of clear evidence for this determination. A recent detailed report of extrahepatic bile duct measurements using ultrasonography has largely defined a non-dilated bile duct [3]. According to the report, the maximum inner diameter of an extrahepatic bile duct increases according to age, measuring 3.9 ± 1.0 mm at age 20–29, 3.9 ± 1.2 mm at 30–39, 4.3 ± 1.2 mm at 40–49, 4.6 ± 1.3 mm at 50–59, 4.9 ± 1.4 mm at 60–69, and 5.3 ± 1.6 mm at age greater than 70 years. In future, PBM without biliary dilatation should be diagnosed according to these data. However, several authors have suggested that PBM without biliary dilatation should be defined not only by diameter of the bile duct but also by the shape of the common bile duct, changes in diameter of the bile duct, and relative stenosis; therefore, accurate diagnosis of PBM without biliary dilatation is still under discussion.

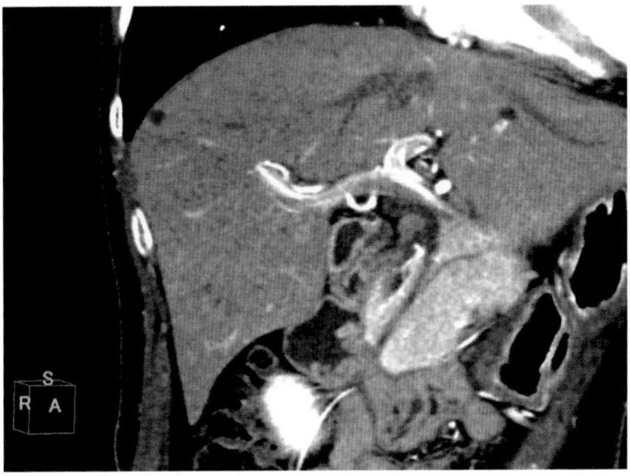

Fig. 27.3 PBM without biliary dilatation were showed in MPR from MDCT

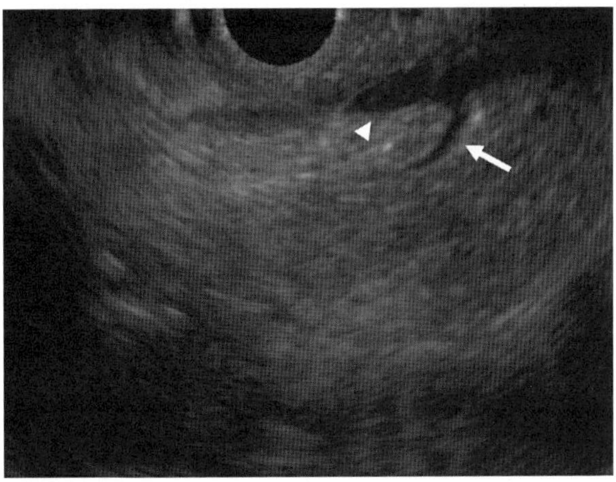

Fig. 27.4 PBM without biliary dilatation were showed in EUS. Non-dilated bile duct (*arrow head*) and pancreatic duct (*arrow*) join outside of the duodenal wall

Once the diagnosis of PBM is established, immediate prophylactic surgical treatment is recommended before the onset of malignant changes, even in patients without biliary dilatation [4]. A Japanese retrospective nationwide survey of PBM reported that the incidence of biliary tract cancer was 42.2% (218 of 514 patients) in cases of PBM without biliary dilatation, among which 37.4% were gallbladder cancers, 3.1% were extrahepatic bile duct cancers, and 1.8% were combined gallbladder and extrahepatic bile duct cancers; thus, 88.1% (192 of 218 patients) of biliary cancers in cases of PBM without biliary dilatation were gallbladder cancers [5]. Histopathological features such as a hyperplastic and atypical bile duct epithelium were only seen in dilated extrahepatic bile ducts in PBM cases [6], and point mutations of the *K-ras* oncogene, which are frequently present in biliary tract cancers, were also only seen in noncancerous mucosa of dilated extrahepatic bile ducts in PBM cases [7]. Therefore, prophylactic cholecystectomy is strongly recommended to prevent gallbladder cancer in PBM without biliary dilatation, and laparoscopic cholecystectomy might be a suitable surgical procedure, as it is less invasive [8]. In fact, many institutions have been performing prophylactic cholecystectomy alone, and they reported that no extrahepatic bile duct cancer has been developed in such PBM cases without biliary dilatation in their institutions, even after long-term postoperative follow-up [9, 10]. These data suggest that prophylactic resection of the extrahepatic bile duct and biliary diversion may be unnecessary in patients with PBM without biliary dilatation.

In contrast, some institutions have recommended that both the extrahepatic bile duct and gallbladder should be resected and that biliary diversion is necessary for PBM without biliary dilatation, because of the risk of developing both extrahepatic bile duct cancer and gallbladder cancer. An analysis of 1361 PBM cases described extrahepatic bile duct cancer as a complication, with an incidence of 4.0% in PBM without biliary dilatation, similar to the 5.2% incidence in PBM with biliary dilatation [11]. The incidence of extrahepatic bile duct cancer in PBM cases, even in those without biliary dilatation, is extremely high, when compared with the incidence of extrahepatic bile duct cancer in the general population. In addition, histopathological changes of carcinogenesis, such as hyperplasia and dysplasia, have been observed in extrahepatic bile ducts in PBM without biliary dilatation [12]. Moreover, point mutations of the *K-ras* oncogene and/or overexpression of *p53* gene products were also reportedly seen in extrahepatic bile ducts of PBM without biliary dilatation [13]. The development of extrahepatic bile duct cancer in PBM cases without biliary dilatation that have undergone cholecystectomy alone without extrahepatic bile duct resection has also been reported [14]. In addition, when resection of the extrahepatic bile duct is performed, the distal part of the common bile duct needs to be cut just above its junction with the pancreatic duct so as to leave as little of the bile duct as possible, as same as surgical methods for PBM with biliary dilatation (congenital biliary dilatation) [15], whereas there is no clear evidence for the appropriate cut line of the hepatic side of non-dilated bile duct.

The Japanese clinical practice guidelines for PBM considered the operative procedures for PBM without biliary dilatation, and stated that "There is no fixed strategy on the prophylactic resection of the extrahepatic bile duct for prevention of bile duct cancer" [16]. In addition, the clinical practice guidelines for the management of biliary tract cancers stated that "Controversy remains as to whether prophylactic bile duct excision is necessary for PBM without bile duct dilatation" [17]. Therefore, whether prophylactic resection of the extrahepatic bile duct should be performed for PBM patients without biliary dilatation remains unclear in the clinical guidelines for both PBM and biliary cancer [18].

In conclusion, prophylactic cholecystectomy and resection of the extrahepatic bile duct, so-called flow-diversion surgery, are established standard surgical methods for PBM with biliary dilatation. As a therapeutic strategy for PBM without biliary dilatation, prophylactic cholecystectomy is also strongly recommended as standard surgical treatment for prevention of gallbladder cancer. However, whether additional prophylactic resection of the extrahepatic bile duct, as in flow-diversion surgery, should be performed for PBM without biliary dilatation remains controversial. Further investigation and surveillance are needed to clarify the appropriate surgical strategy for PBM without biliary dilatation.

References

1. Takuma K, Kamisawa T, Tabata T, Hara S, Kuruma S, Inaba Y, et al. Importance of early diagnosis of pancreaticobiliary maljunction without biliary dilatation. World J Gastroenterol. 2012;18:3409–14.
2. Kamisawa T, Ando H, Hamada Y, Fujii H, Koshinaga T, Urushihara N, et al. Diagnostic criteria for pancreaticobiliary maljunction 2013. J Hepatobiliary Pancreat Sci. 2014;21:159–61.
3. Itoi T, Kamisawa T, Fujii H, Inui K, Maguchi H, Hamada Y, et al. Extrahepatic bile duct measurement by using transabdominal ultrasound in Japanese adults: multi-center prospective study. J Gastroenterol. 2013;48:1045–50.
4. Kamisawa T, Kuruma S, Chiba K, Tabata T, Koizumi S, Kikuyama M. Biliary carcinogenesis in pancreaticobiliary maljunction. J Gastroenterol. 2017;52:158–63.
5. Morine Y, Shimada M, Takamatsu H, Araida T, Endo I, Kubota M, et al. Clinical features of Pancreaticobiliary Maljunction: update analysis of 2nd Japan-nationwide survey. J Hepatobiliary Pancreat Sci. 2013;20:472–80.
6. Noda Y, Fujita N, Kobayashi G, Ito K, Horaguchi J, Takasawa O, et al. Histological study of gallbladder and bile duct epithelia in patients with anomalous arrangement of the pancreaticobiliary ductal system: comparison between those with and without a dilated common bile duct. J Gastroenterol. 2007;42:211–8.
7. Masuhara S, Kasuya K, Aoki T, Yoshimatsu A, Tsuchida A, Koyanagi Y. Relation between K-ras codon 12 mutation and p53 protein overexpression in gallbladder cancer and biliary ductal epithelia in patients with pancreaticobiliary maljunction. J Hepato-Biliary-Pancreat Surg. 2000;7:198–205.
8. Deng YL, Cheng NS, Lin YX, Zhou RX, Yang C, Jin YW, et al. Relationship between pancreaticobiliary maljunction and gallbladder carcinoma: meta-analysis. Hepatobiliary Pancreat Dis Int. 2011;10:570–80.
9. Kusano T, Takano T, Tachibana K, Tanaka Y, Kamachi M, Ikematsu Y, et al. Whether or not prophylactic excision of the extrahepatic bile duct is appropriate for patients with pancreaticobiliary maljunction without bile duct dilatation. Hepato-Gastroenterology. 2005;52:1649–53.
10. Ohuchida J, Chijiiwa K, Hiyoshi M, Kobayashi K, Konomi H, Tanaka M. Long-term results of treatment for pancreaticobiliary maljunction without bile duct dilatation. Arch Surg. 2006;141:1066–70.

11. Funabiki T, Matsubara T, Miyakawa S, Ishihara S. Pancreaticobiliary maljunction and carcinogenesis to biliary and pancreatic malignancy. Langenbeck's Arch Surg. 2009;394:159–69.
12. Seki M, Yanagisawa A, Ninomiya E, Ninomiya Y, Ohta H, Saiura A, et al. Clinicopathology of pancreaticobiliary maljunction: relationship between alterations in background biliary epithelium and neoplastic development. J Hepato-Biliary-Pancreat Surg. 2005;12:254–62.
13. Matsubara T, Sakurai Y, Zhi L, Miura H, Ochai M, Funabiki T. K- ras and p53 gene mutations in noncancerous biliary lesions of patients with pancreaticobiliary maljunction. J Hepato-Biliary-Pancreat Surg. 2002;9:312–21.
14. Yamada S, Shimada M, Utsunomiya T, Morine Y, Imura S, Ikemoto T, et al. Hilar cholangiocarcinoma accompanied by pancreaticobiliary maljunction without bile duct dilatation 20 years after cholecystectomy: report of a case. J Med Investig. 2013;60:169–73.
15. Ando H, Ito T, Nagaya M, Watanabe Y, Seo T, Kaneko K. Pancreaticobiliary maljunction without choledochal cysts in infants and children: clinical features and surgical therapy. J Pediatr Surg. 1995;30:1658–62.
16. Kamisawa T, Ando H, Suyama M, Shimada M, Morine Y, Shimada H. Japanese clinical practice guidelines for pancreaticobiliary maljunction. J Gastroenterol. 2012;47:731–59.
17. Miyazaki M, Yoshitomi H, Miyakawa S, Uesaka K, Unno M, Endo I, et al. Clinical practice guidelines for the management of biliary tract cancers 2015: the 2nd English edition. J Hepato-Biliary-Pancreat Surg. 2015;22:249–73.
18. Kamisawa T, Ando H, Shimada M, Hamada Y, Itoi T, Takayashiki T, et al. Recent advances and problems in the management of pancreaticobiliary maljunction: feedback from the guidelines committee. J Hepatobiliary Pancreat Sci. 2014;21:87–92.

Chapter 28
Role of Endoscopic Therapy in Pancreaticobiliary Maljunction and Congenital Biliary Dilatation

Takao Itoi

Abstract Recently, interventional endoscopy has been increasingly used to treat pancreaticobiliary diseases in pancreaticobiliary maljunction (PBM)/congenital biliary dilatation (CBD) patients. However, there has been no detailed description of endotherapy for PBM/CBD thus far. Herein, we describe the role of endoscopic therapy on the biliary drainage including bile duct drainage and gallbladder drainage, stones and/or protein plugs removal, peripancreatic fluid collections, and choledochocele in PBM/CBD. In conclusion, although the fundamental therapy in PBM/CBD patients is surgical intervention, endotherapy appears to be useful for the treatment of PBM/CBD-induced complications.

Keywords Pancreaticobiliary maljunction · Congenital biliary dilatation Endoscopic retrograde cholangiopancreatography · Endoscopic ultrasonography Therapeutic endoscopy · Interventional endoscopy

28.1 Introduction

Pancreaticobiliary maljunction (PBM)/congenital biliary dilatation (CBD) is a congenital anomaly in which the junction of the pancreatic and bile ducts is located outside the duodenal wall [1]. PBM/CBD occurs predominantly in women and is often found in Asian populations. In PBM/CBD patients, as the action of the sphincter of Oddi does not functionally affect the pancreatic and bile duct junction, continuous reciprocal reflux between the pancreatic juice and the bile occurs, resulting in various pathological conditions in the biliary tract and pancreas. As the hydropressure within the pancreatic duct is usually greater than that in the bile duct, pancreatic juice frequently refluxes into the biliary duct in PBM. As a result, PBM/CBD causes various pancreaticobiliary diseases such as acute cholangitis, acute

T. Itoi
Department of Gastroenterology and Hepatology, Tokyo Medical University, Tokyo, Japan

T. Kamisawa, H. Ando (eds.), *Pancreaticobiliary Maljunction and Congenital Biliary Dilatation*, https://doi.org/10.1007/978-981-10-8654-0_28

cholecystitis, acute pancreatitis owing to pancreatic and/or biliary stone, and obstructive jaundice owing to malignant pancreaticobiliary conditions. In terms of concomitant cancers, bile duct and gallbladder cancers were found in 14% and 22% of our 49 CBD patients, respectively. Only gallbladder cancer was detected in 70% of 53 PBM patients without biliary dilatation. Thus, once PBM/CBD is diagnosed, prophylactic flow-diversion surgery (bile duct resection and bilioenteric anastomosis) or simple cholecystectomy is performed.

Recently, interventional endoscopy has been increasingly used to treat pancreaticobiliary diseases in PBM/CBD patients. However, there has been no detailed description of endotherapy for PBM/CBD thus far. Herein, we describe the role of endoscopic therapy in PBM/CBD.

28.2 Interventional Endoscopy

28.2.1 Biliary Drainage

In PBM/CBD, two-way regurgitation, pancreaticobiliary reflux, and biliopancreatic reflux occur, resulting in various pathologic conditions in the biliary tract and pancreas. Biliary tract cancers and stones are often observed under these conditions. Biliary drainage is an essential technique for the treatment of cholangitis, cholecystitis, and obstructive jaundice.

28.2.1.1 Bile Duct Drainage

At present, transpapillary bile duct drainage by endoscopic retrograde cholangiopancreatography (ERCP) is the most commonly used technique for bile duct decompression. Selective biliary cannulation is thought to be relatively easy because of the single orifice of both the bile duct and the pancreatic duct. Furthermore, the bile duct drainage technique is not different between PBM/CBD and non-PBM/CBD patients. However, the risk of pancreatitis in PBM/CBD patients may be higher than that in non-PBM/CBD patients because a large caliber biliary drainage catheter or stent may block the outflow of pancreatic juice. Thus, when placement of a large-bore stent (e.g., 10 Fr plastic stent or metal stent) is scheduled, endoscopic sphincterotomy (EST) or simultaneously placing a prophylactic pancreatic duct stent may be desirable to avoid obstructive pancreatitis.

Selective biliary cannulation by ERCP is not always successful even when performed by skilled endoscopists because of several reasons, namely, gastric outlet obstruction and surgically altered anatomy. Traditionally, percutaneous transhepatic biliary drainage or surgical intervention has been performed when ERCP fails. Recently, endoscopic ultrasonography-guided biliary drainage (EUS-BD) has been reported as a useful and safe salvage technique [2]. Although the technical success rate of those who have expertise in EUS is relatively high (>80–90%), the adverse event rate ranges from 10% to 30% including fatal cases. This adverse event rate may never be observed in conventional ERCP because of an "intraluminal procedure" but not of a "transluminal procedure." From these viewpoints, EUS-BD thus far has not apparently become a useful alternative to conventional ERCP, although it may be useful for salvage therapy [2].

28.2.1.2 Gallbladder Drainage

Acute cholecystitis is a relatively common inflammatory disease in daily practice. Based on the latest guidelines for treating acute cholecystitis, that is, "Tokyo Guidelines 2018 (TG18)," early or emergency cholecystectomy is the fundamental treatment procedure for patients with acute cholecystitis who do not respond to initial conservative treatment [3]. However, cholecystectomy is not always performed owing to several reasons, namely, severe underlying diseases or absence of a surgeon in the hospital. In such a case, percutaneous transhepatic gallbladder drainage (PTGBD) is traditionally considered a safe alternative to early cholecystectomy [4, 5].

Recently, as an alternative technique, endoscopic transpapillary gallbladder decompression by ERCP including endoscopic naso-gallbladder drainage and gallbladder stenting has been performed in acute cholecystitis [6]. As we described earlier, when placement of a large-bore stent is scheduled, EST or simultaneous placement of a prophylactic pancreatic duct stent may be desirable to avoid obstructive pancreatitis. More recently, EUS-guided gallbladder drainage has been used as a salvage therapy when ERCP fails or when PTGBD is contraindicated [7]. A new dedicated and ideal lumen-apposing metal stent has been shown to have high technical and clinical success rates and a low adverse event rate [8, 9].

28.2.2 Removal of Stones and Protein Plugs

Continuous reciprocal reflux between the pancreatic juice and the bile causes the formation of stones or protein plugs in the pancreaticobiliary system (Fig. 28.1a). Bile duct stones are found in the dilated bile duct in CBD, and the distal bile duct shows a narrow segment, causing difficulty in stone extraction from the bile duct endoscopically even by performing EST (Fig. 28.1b, c). Thus, if surgical intervention is scheduled, endoscopic stone removal is not recommended. On the other hand, protein plugs are often found in the dilated common channel and cause not only biliary complications such as obstructive jaundice but also serious pancreatic complications such as acute pancreatitis. In fact, acute pancreatitis occurs more frequently in children (30%) than in adults (9%) [10], and one of the reasons for this is increased pancreatic duct pressure by plug obstruction. Thus, even if surgical intervention is scheduled in patients with pancreatitis, endoscopic removal of the protein plugs would be desirable to avoid any delay in the operation owing to the recurrent pancreatitis.

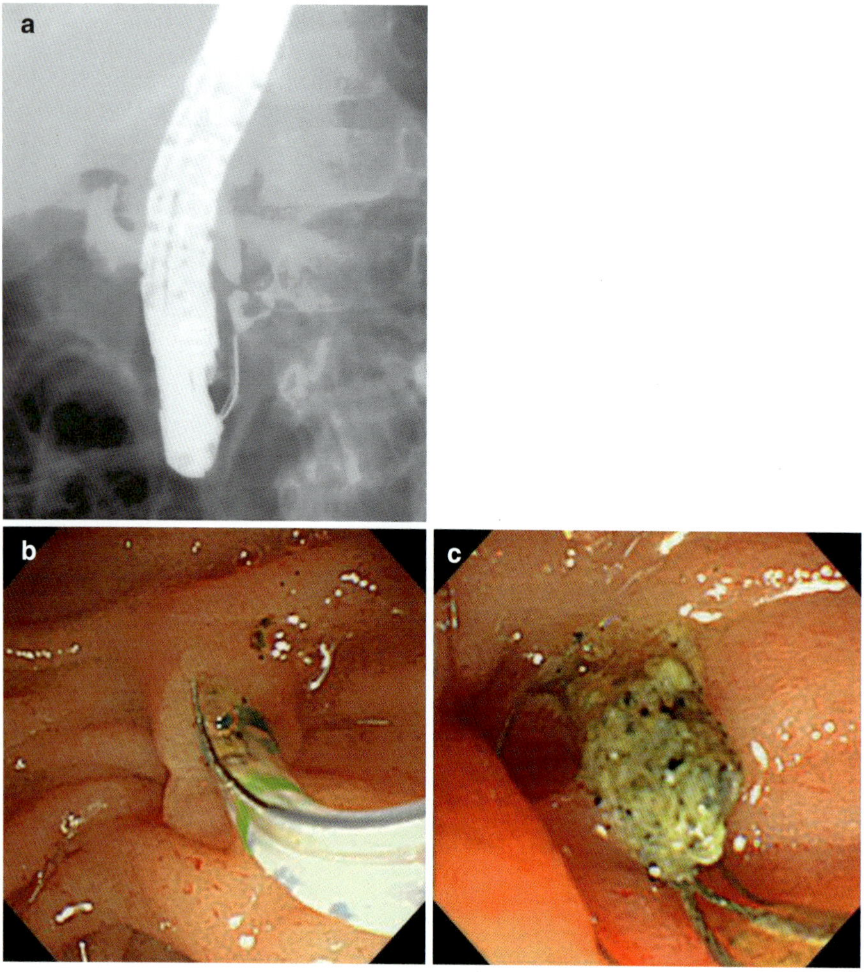

Fig. 28.1 Stone in the common channel in a 3-year-old boy with PBM. (**a**) ERCP showed stone in the common channel. (**b**) Endoscopic sphincterotomy was performed. (**c**) A stone was extracted by using a basket catheter

28.2.3 Therapy of Peripancreatic Fluid Collections

Peripancreatic fluid collections (PFCs), which include pancreatic pseudocyst and walled-off necrosis, are rare, and PFCs are more difficult to manage if they are infected. In such cases, EUS-guided drainage of PFCs is recommended [11] because it is a safer and more reliable drainage technique than surgical, percutaneous, and even endoscopic interventions using a conventional upper GI endoscope [12]. In case of walled-off necrosis, endoscopic necrosectomy following drainage is occasionally conducted. If endoscopic management is not difficult, a step-up approach using percutaneous and surgical interventions is recommended [11].

28.2.4 *Therapy for Choledochocele*

A choledochocele is a cystic dilation of the distal common bile duct (CBD). It corresponds to a type III choledochal cyst (choledochocele) according to the classification by Todani et al. [13] and is extremely rare [14]. Choledochocele causes pancreaticobiliary inflammation and occasionally obstructive jaundice. Recently, several reports have described that choledochocele may have a malignant potential because a neoplastic lesion [15] or an atypical epithelium showing K-ras mutation [16] arises in the choledochocele as a result of damage to the epithelium. Thus, endoscopic interventions would be desirable to reduce such kind of complications.

28.2.4.1 Endoscopic Sphincterotomy

EST has been performed in symptomatic choledochocele [17] (Fig. 28.2a, b). If standard EST is not possible owing to difficult cannulation, access to the bile duct can be obtained by unroofing the choledochocele with a needle-knife, the so-called infundibulotomy with or without subsequent introduction of the standard EST [18]. More recently, EUS-guided ERCP has been used as a salvage therapy in failed conventional ERCP [19].

28.2.4.2 Endoscopic Papillectomy

EST is the gold standard therapy for symptomatic choledochocele. However, the risk of intraepithelial canceration in choledochocele still remains. Thus, the ultimate therapy for choledochocele is surgical resection of the whole cele. However, this is thought to be extremely radical because of the low canceration rate. Thus, we performed endoscopic balloon-assisted choledochocele resection using a double-channel duodenoscope [16] (Fig. 28.3a–e). Interestingly, the resected specimens showed an atypical epithelium with positive K-ras mutation.

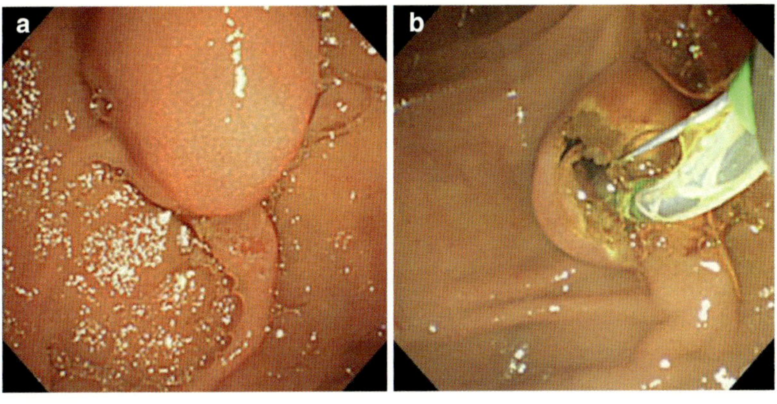

Fig. 28.2 Endoscopic sphincterotomy in a patient with a type III choledochal cyst. (**a**) Endoscopic imaging showed bulging of papillary roof, suggesting type III choledochal cyst. (**b**) Endoscopic sphincterotomy was performed

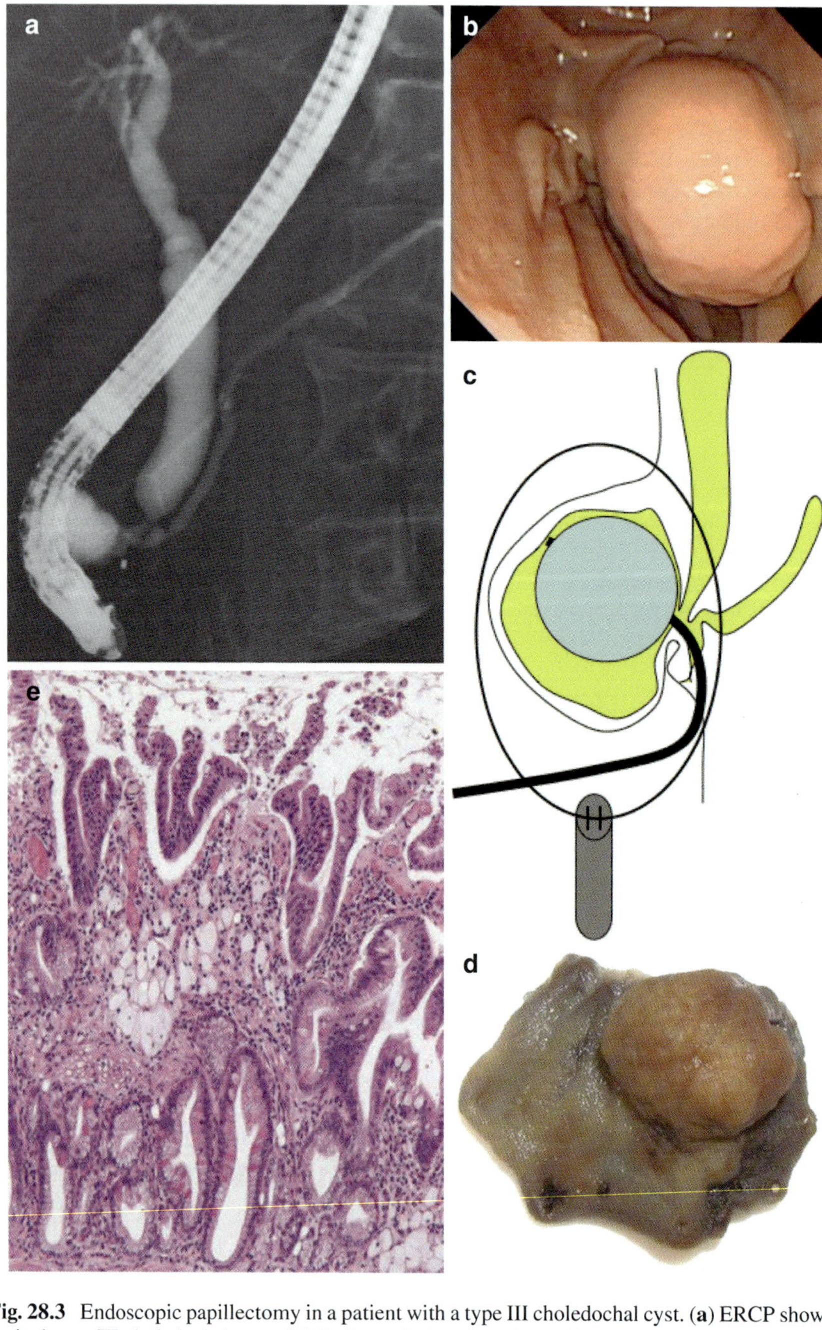

Fig. 28.3 Endoscopic papillectomy in a patient with a type III choledochal cyst. (**a**) ERCP showed typical type III choledochal cyst. (**b**) Endoscopic imaging showed bulging of papillary roof, suggesting type III choledochal cyst. (**c**) Schema of endoscopic balloon-assisted choledochocele resection using a double-channel duodenoscope. (**d**) Macroscopic imaging of resected specimen. (**e**) Histologic specimens showed atypical epithelium with positive K-ras mutation

28.3 Conclusion

Although the fundamental therapy in PBM/CBD patients is surgical intervention, endotherapy appears to be useful for the treatment of PBM/CBD-induced complications.

Acknowledgment We thank Dr. Edward Barroga (http://orcid.org/0000-0002-8920-2607) for reviewing and editing the manuscript.

References

1. Kamisawa T, Kaneko K, Itoi T, Ando H. Pancreaticobiliary maljunction and congenital biliary dilatation. Lancet Gastroenterol Hepatol. 2017;2(8):610.
2. Mukai S, Itoi T. How should we use endoscopic ultrasonography-guided biliary drainage techniques separately? Endosc Ultrasound. 2016;5:65–8.
3. Miura F, Okamoto K, Takada T, et al. Tokyo Guidelines 2018: initial management of acute biliary infection and flowchart for acute cholangitis. J Hepatobiliary Pancreat Sci. 2018;25:31–40. https://doi.org/10.1002/jhbp.509.
4. Mori Y, Itoi T, Baron TH, et al. TG18 management strategies for gallbladder drainage in patients with acute cholecystitis: updated Tokyo Guidelines 2018 (with videos). J Hepatobiliary Pancreat Sci. 2018;25:87–95.
5. Itoi T, Takada T, Hwang TL, et al. Percutaneous and endoscopic gallbladder drainage for the acute cholecystitis: international multicenter comparative study by a propensity score-matched analysis. J Hepatobiliary Pancreat Sci. 2017;24(6):362.
6. Itoi T, Kawakami H, Katanuma A, et al. Endoscopic nasogallbladder tube or stent placement in acute cholecystitis: a preliminary prospective randomized trial in Japan. Gastrointest Endosc. 2015;81:111–8.
7. Itoi T, Coelho-Prabhu N, Baron TH. Endoscopic gallbladder drainage for management of acute cholecystitis. Gastrointest Endosc. 2010;71:1038–45.
8. Itoi T, Binmoeller KF, Shah J, et al. Clinical evaluation of a novel lumen-apposing metal stent for endosonography-guided pancreatic pseudocyst and gallbladder drainage (with video). Gastrointest Endosc. 2012;75:870–6.
9. Walter D, Teoh AY, Itoi T, et al. EUS-guided gallbladder drainage with a lumen apposing metal stent; a prospective long-term evaluation. Gut. 2016;65:6–8.
10. Morine Y, Shimada M, Takamatsu H, et al. Clinical features of pancreaticobiliary maljunction: update analysis of 2nd Japan-nationwide survey. J Hepatobiliary Pancreat Sci. 2013;20:472–80.
11. Mukai S, Itoi T, Kamada K, Tanaka R, Ishii K. Successful extraction of a carelessly impacted bile duct stone using sphincterotome. Gastrointest Endosc. 2015;8:1486–7.
12. Vosoghi M, Sial S, Garrett B, et al. EUS-guided pancreatic pseudocyst drainage: review and experience at Harbor-UCLA Medical Center. MedGenMed. 2002;4:2.
13. Todani T, Watanabe Y, Narusue M, et al. Congenital bile duct cysts: classification, operative procedures, and review of thirty-seven cases including cancer arising from choledochal cyst. Am J Surg. 1977;134:263–9.
14. Yamaguchi M. Congenital choledochal cyst. Analysis of 1,433 patients in the Japanese literature. Am J Surg. 1980;140:653–7.
15. Tomoda T, Kato H, Tsutsumi K, et al. Tubular adenoma arising in a choledochocele. Gastrointest Endosc. 2016;84:1066–7.
16. Itoi T, Gotoda T, Yasuda I, et al. Balloon-catheter-assisted complete endoscopic snare resection for choledochocele by using double-channel duodenoscope (with videos). Gastrointest Endosc. 2007;66:622–5.

17. Law R, Topazian M. Diagnosis and treatment of choledochoceles. Clin Gastroenterol Hepatol. 2014;12:196–203.
18. Min Lee JM, Lee HS, Kim CD. Infundibulotomy and endoscopic retrograde cholangiopancreatography in situs inversus totalis combined with choledochocele. Dig Endosc. 2015;27:777.
19. Mangiavillano B, Parodi A, Conio M. Endoscopic ultrasound-guided ERCP in the treatment of a Todani type-III cyst causing acute necrotizing pancreatitis. Endoscopy. 2016;48:E44.

Part VII
Prognosis

Chapter 29
Postoperative Hepatolithiasis in Pancreaticobiliary Maljunction and Congenital Biliary Dilatation

Hideo Ohtsuka and Michiaki Unno

Abstract Pancreaticobiliary maljunction (PBM) is a congenital malformation in which the pancreatic duct and the bile duct join outside of the duodenal wall. Due to the reciprocating flow of the pancreatic juices and bile, various complications can develop in the biliary tree system and the pancreas. Therefore, in cases with congenital biliary dilatation, resection of the dilated extrahepatic biliary duct followed by hepaticojejunostomy (so-called flow diversion surgery) is considered to be a standard treatment. Despite being well-established as the standard treatment, complication characteristics of this disease, such as carcinogenesis and hepatolithiasis in the remnant bile duct, often develop long after the operation. In some cases, intrahepatic calculi are detected diffusely in both lobes. For the treatment of hepatolithiasis, complete removal of the calculi is recommended. However, even if the calculi are completely removed, it is not uncommon for patients to experience a recurrence. In postoperative hepatolithiasis, the percutaneous transhepatic and peroral endoscopic approaches are considered the first choices of the treatment. In cases where endoscopic therapy has been unsuccessful or liver atrophy is observed during the course of treatment, surgery is required. Combining hepatectomy with endoscopic treatment may be effective for complete removal of the intrahepatic calculi. However, there is a need for development of a consensus on the indication, timing, and the selection of the optimal surgical procedure.

Keywords Congenital biliary dilatation · Pancreaticobiliary maljunction Hepatolithiasis · Biliary tract reconstruction · Cholangitis

---

H. Ohtsuka · M. Unno (✉)
Department of Surgery, Tohoku University Graduate School of Medicine, Sendai, Miyagi, Japan
e-mail: m_unno@surg1.med.tohoku.ac.jp

T. Kamisawa, H. Ando (eds.), *Pancreaticobiliary Maljunction and Congenital Biliary Dilatation*, https://doi.org/10.1007/978-981-10-8654-0_29

29.1 Introduction

Pancreaticobiliary maljunction (PBM) is a congenital malformation in which the pancreatic duct and the bile duct join outside the duodenal wall. Due to the reciprocating flow of pancreatic juices and bile, various complications may develop in the bile duct and the pancreas [1]. In cases with congenital biliary dilatation (CBD), there is an increase incidence of extrahepatic bile duct cancer or gallbladder cancer, during the natural course. Therefore, prophylactic resection of the dilated extrahepatic biliary duct and gallbladder followed by hepaticojejunostomy (so-called flow diversion surgery) is considered as a standard treatment for CBD [2, 3]. However, despite being well-established as the standard treatment, complication characteristics for this disease, such as carcinogenesis and hepatolithiasis in the remnant bile duct, often develop long after the operation [4–6]. The process of preventing long-term complications after surgery is clinically very important in this disease, not only in children but also in adults.

For the treatment of hepatolithiasis after biliary tract reconstruction, complete removal of the stones via percutaneous transhepatic approach (percutaneous transhepatic cholangioscopic lithotomy: PTCSL) or peroral endoscopic approach (peroral cholangioscopic lithotomy: POCSL) is recommended as the first choice. However, even if the calculi are completely removed, intrahepatic calculi often recur. In cases where localized hepatic atrophy is observed during the course of treatment, surgery should be required because of high risk of carcinogenesis. In addition, in the cases where the development of carcinoma is suspected, surgical resection should be considered. However, there has not been a consensus on the timing for or the selection of the optimal surgical procedure.

In recent years, although the incidence of primary hepatolithiasis has decreased significantly in Japan, the incidence of postoperative hepatolithiasis after biliary tract reconstruction, especially in CBD, is relatively increasing. Therefore, establishment of a strategy for the diagnosis and the therapy should be important issues [7].

29.2 Incidence and Pathogenesis

In CBD, reflux of pancreatic juice to the bile duct due to PBM damages the bile duct epithelium and increases the risk of developing biliary cancer. Therefore, extrahepatic bile duct resection followed by biliary tract reconstruction is commonly regarded as standard surgical treatments. However, this surgery is often associated with complications characteristic of this disease, such as hepatolithiasis and cancer of the remnant bile duct. Postoperative hepatolithiasis is considered to be a clinically important complication due to the difficulty in its treatment. Hepatolithiasis occurs after surgical treatment for CBD in approximately 7–8% of the cases [8, 9].

Table 29.1 Postoperative long-term complications after surgery in PBM

PBM cases (2001–2015) Age: 38.6 (15–71) y.o. Male/female: 11/26		Postoperative long-term complications			
		Postoperative hepatolithiasis	Cholangitis	Pancreatitis	Cancer of the remnant bile duct
Total	37 (100%)	3 (8.1%)	7 (18.9%)	1 (2.7%)	0 (0%)
Type of CBD					
Type I	20 (54.1%)	1 (5.0%)	2 (10.0%)	1 (5.0%)	0 (0%)
Type IV-A	11 (29.8%)	2 (18.2%)	5 (45.5%)	0 (0%)	0 (0%)
Without dilatation	6 (16.2%)	0 (0%)	0 (0%)	0 (0%)	0 (0%)

Table 29.1 shows the incidence of long-term complications in 37 cases of initial surgical treatment performed at our institute from 2001 to 2015. The mean age at the time of operation was 38.6 years (15–71 years). Regarding the types of biliary dilatation (Todani classification), there were 13 cases (35.1%) of type Ic, 7 cases (18.9%) of type Ia, 11 cases (29.8%) of type IV-A, and 6 cases without dilatation. Thirty-two patients (86.5%) underwent extrahepatic bile duct resection followed by biliary reconstruction, and three patients received a pancreaticoduodenectomy. For biliary reconstruction, the Roux-en-Y method was selected in all cases. The long-term complications during postoperative follow-up (average 71.8 months) included three cases (8.1%) of intrahepatic calculus, seven cases (18.9%) of repeating cholangitis, and one case (2.7%) of pancreatitis. No occurrence of remnant cholangiocarcinoma was observed in the cases. When the incidence of long-term complications was investigated with respect to the types of dilatation, the incidence of hepatolithiasis in type IV-A (18.2%) was higher than that of type I (5.0%). In addition, the incidence of the postoperative cholangitis in type IV-A was also higher than that in type I (10.0%).

In postoperative hepatolithiasis in CBD, the calculi commonly were calcium bilirubinate gallstones. Based on this, bacterial infection in the static intrahepatic bile has been closely associated with the development of postoperative intrahepatic calculi [10]. In type IV-A, which is characterized by multiple dilatations of the intrahepatic and extrahepatic bile ducts, the incidence of postoperative hepatolithiasis is high [6]. Even in our case, the incidence was as high as 18.2%. The proposed causes of postoperative hepatolithiasis include (1) stasis in the dilated intrahepatic bile duct, (2) anastomotic stenosis after reconstruction, and (3) stasis in the section of the intestinal tract that had been used for biliary tract reconstruction [11, 12]. In type IV-A, in addition to these mechanisms, the bile duct stricture observed in the hilar region is also important. If the bile duct stricture remains after reconstruction of the biliary tract, it is likely to cause repeated episodes of cholangitis in the long-term and acutely may cause postoperative intrahepatic calculus. In order to completely remove the stricture in the hilar region, the bifurcation of the left and right hepatic ducts should be exposed from the surrounding tissues, and the removal line of the bile duct should be decided carefully. In some cases, to obtain a sufficient caliber of the duct, strictureplasty should be performed before hepaticojejunostomy [13].

Furthermore, in cases of type IV-A, congenital intrahepatic biliary strictures due to membrane-like or string-like structure characteristics for this type are commonly observed and considered important as causes of postoperative hepatic calculus [14]. Careful observation of the intrahepatic bile duct during surgery is necessary, and resection of these structures is required. In our institute, intraoperative cholangioscopy is performed in all cases to release these membrane-like or string-like structures.

As a cause of postoperative hepatolithiasis, congenitally narrowed structures such as the downstream relative stenosis of a dilated intrahepatic bile duct, or the membrane-like stenosis in the intrahepatic bile duct, are considered to be important as described above. However, even if these stenoses can be released completely, it is impossible to completely prevent their development postoperatively. In addition, because development of postoperative hepatolithiasis occurs in cases of type I without dilatation of the intrahepatic bile duct, various other factors should be identified in the development of postoperative hepatolithiasis. As the intrahepatic gallstones developed in CBD are mostly bilirubin calcium stone, its major cause is biliary infection and persistent chronic inflammation. Continuous inflammation in the epithelium of the bile duct activates protein kinase C and other inflammatory cytokines, which promote the secretion of mucin core proteins such as MUC2 and MUC5. It is speculated that these mucin core proteins increase the viscosity of bile through their gel-forming ability, which triggers the development of intrahepatic calculi [15]. At the time of surgical treatment of congenital biliary dilatation, the continuous reflux of pancreatic juices causes chronic inflammatory changes in the epithelium of bile duct. It is also speculated that these inflammatory changes could cause changes in the composition of the bile, leading to increases in the viscosity of bile such that intrahepatic calculi are likely to develop.

29.3 Diagnosis of Postoperative Hepatolithiasis

For the diagnosis of hepatolithiasis, it is important to show the presence of a calculus in the intrahepatic bile duct on an imaging examination. Imaging examinations include both noninvasive examinations such as ultrasound, computed tomography (CT), and magnetic resonance imaging (MRI) and invasive examinations such as endoscopic retrograde cholangiography (ERC) or percutaneous transhepatic biliary cholangioscopy (PTC). In order to properly diagnose and treat, it is important to understand the characteristics of the various diagnostic imaging modalities and make a plan for treatment from screening inspections using either noninvasive examination methods or invasive examination method.

29.3.1 Ultrasonic Examination

Abdominal ultrasonography is considered to be the first-line examination. It is simultaneously useful and noninvasive in detecting calculus and dilated bile ducts. For bilirubin/calcium stones, the typical ultrasound image is of an equivalent intensity to the liver parenchyma with weak acoustic shadow. In cholesterol stones, the typical image has a high echoic intensity with strong acoustic shadows. Other findings suggesting the presence of hepatolithiasis are expansion or stenosis of the intrahepatic bile duct, atrophic regions in the liver, decreased regional blood flow on Doppler ultrasonography, and intrahepatic microcalcifications. However, it is important to note that stones are not accompanied by acoustic shadowing in all cases. In addition, in cases where the bile duct is filled with numerous calculi, or in cases of calculi that show equivalent intensity to the liver parenchyma, detection of the calculi is extremely difficult.

29.3.2 Computed Tomography (CT) Examination (*Fig. 29.1a*)

Abdominal computed tomography (CT) examinations are useful in the detection of the intrahepatic calculus, as well as for detecting dilatation and stricture of the intrahepatic bile duct, or thickening of the wall of the bile duct. In general, bilirubin/calcium stones are recognized as high absorption masses in the bile duct.

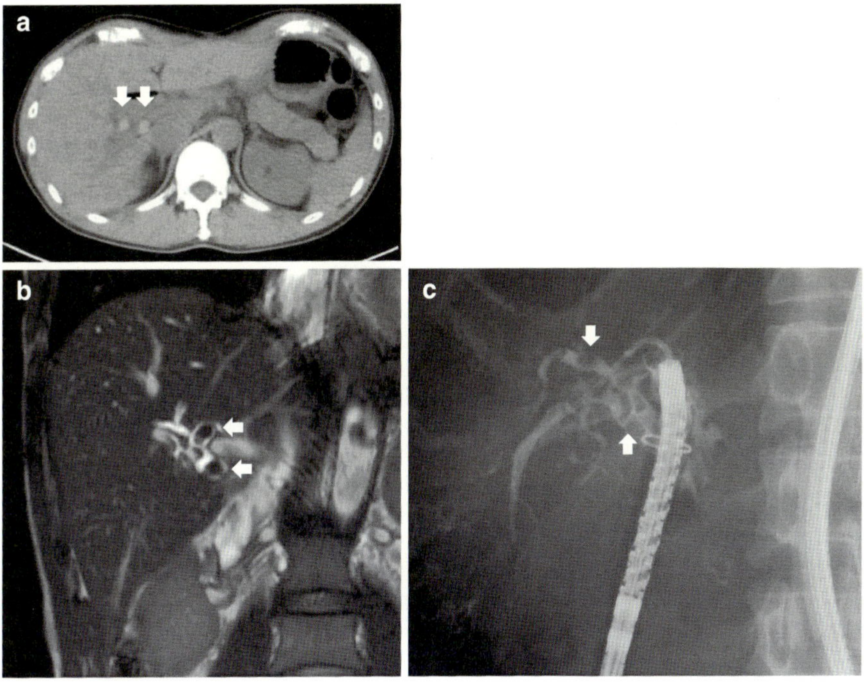

Fig. 29.1 CT, MRI, and direct cholangiography findings of postoperative hepatolithiasis in CBD (**a** abdominal simple CT examination, **b** MRI T2-weighted image, **c** peroral direct cholangiography). CT examination revealed a high absorption structure (*white arrow*) due to calculus in the posterior brunch of the intrahepatic bile duct. In the MRI T2-weighted image and the direct cholangiography, it is depicted as a shadow defect (*white arrow*) in the bile duct

However, because intrahepatic calculi have a low calcium content, CT examinations often show similar absorption values to the surrounding bile. In drip infusion cholangiography (DIC)-CT, calculi are detected as filling defects in the bile duct, so that the ability to detect the intrahepatic calculus increases. However, in the atrophic region, or the area with severe cholestasis, the bile duct may not be detected because discharge of the contrast agent into the bile duct is suppressed.

As it is known that cholangiocarcinoma may combine with hepatolithiasis, this should be taken into consideration at the time of examination. If bile duct wall thickness or stenosis is detected in the intrahepatic bile duct, it should be closely investigated as to whether cancer is developing simultaneously. Previous reports indicated that CT is useful for distinguishing those lesions from bile duct cancer. The soft tissue density shadow spread surrounding the bile duct, the contrast effect in the bile duct wall in the portal phase, and the obstruction of the portal vein are often found in cases of bile duct carcinoma. However, it is generally difficult to distinguish this combination of conditions from bile duct cancer alone, using CT examination. Further investigations such as bile duct biopsy during endoscopic retrograde cholangiography should be undertaken.

29.3.3 Magnetic Resonance Imaging (MRI) (Fig. 29.1b)

MRI is one of the most important examinations because it is both minimally invasive and has superior ability to detect calculus and bile duct stricture, compared to other imaging modalities. The calculus is detected as an area filling defect in the bile, which is displayed as a high-signal area in the T2-weighted image. However, in cases with biliary tract pneumobilia, commonly observed after biliary reconstruction, bubbles are also depicted as filling defects in the bile duct.

29.3.4 Direct Cholangiography (Fig. 29.1c)

Direct cholangiography imaging, such as endoscopic retrograde cholangiography (ERC) and percutaneous transhepatic cholangiography (PTC), has been carried out less often due to its invasiveness and due to advancements in other noninvasive diagnostic modalities. However, it is an indispensable examination for the accurate identification of the segment of bile duct in which a calculus exists. In recent years, ERC has often been enforced as the first-line test choice instead of PTC. In cases where biliary duct stenosis and wall thickening are detected on CT, and bile duct cancer is suspected, intraluminal ultrasound inspection (IDUS) and bile duct biopsy under ERC are extremely important for discrimination.

29.4 Treatment for Postoperative Hepatolithiasis

Postoperative hepatolithiasis often complicates acute cholangitis at the time of diagnosis. Biliary drainage through a peroral endoscopy or percutaneous transhepatic approach is the first step in the treatment of postoperative hepatolithiasis. At the same time, an accurate evaluation for the position of the intrahepatic calculi and accompanying bile duct stenosis is required. At the site of stenosis, the possibility of coincident and complicating bile duct cancer should be evaluated. After the evaluation, removal of any intrahepatic calculi should be attempted using the same approach. Conventionally, it has been difficult to approach this area via peroral endoscopy following a biliary tract reconstruction. Thus, the percutaneous transhepatic approach was regarded as the primary choice. However, in recent years, with advances in the equipment, the balloon endoscope has become useful for the removal of intrahepatic calculi [16, 17]. It is also advantageous to be able to observe the state of the bile duct on the lower side where the stone exists from a peroral endoscopic approach. In our institute, the cases in which peroral endoscopic approach are performed have been increasing in recent years because the procedure is minimally invasive. Table 29.2 shows the cases in which postoperative hepatolithiasis developed and were treated in our department. The cases include seven patients who had received an initial surgical consultation at other hospitals but were referred to our institute for the treatment of hepatolithiasis. In five cases, the calculi were detected diffusely in both lobes, and in the other five cases, the calculi were localized to one leaf or one section. The peroral endoscopic approach was performed in three cases. In one case, a recurrence of the calculus was observed after PTCSL, and the peroral endoscopic approach was performed. After the treatment with peroral endoscopic approach, relapse was observed in one case, and no relapse occurred in the other two cases. However, the number of cases is small, and long-term outcome should be examined in future larger studies.

When an attempt to remove the intrahepatic calculi through either the peroral or percutaneous transhepatic approach fails, surgery should be considered. Surgical operation was performed in six cases in our institute. In all cases, attempts to remove the calculi with percutaneous transhepatic approach or peroral endoscopic approach had been performed several times prior to the patients' presentation at our institute. In two cases (cases 5 and 6), resection of the residual bile duct and removal of the calculi were performed using an intraoperative cholangioscopy. However, in both cases, recurrence of calculi occurred within 2 years after surgery. A hepatectomy was performed in four of those cases. In case number 10, intrahepatic calculi were observed in both the left and right lobes, and a PTCSL was attempted from the right lobe. After the treatment, the calculi in the right lobe were removed, but the calculi remained in situ in the left lobe. In addition, atrophy was also observed in the left lobe so that left hepatectomy was performed. In three of four cases in which hepatectomy was per-

Table 29.2 Treatment for postoperative hepatolithiasis in CBD

	Age/sex	Type of CBD	Procedure for biliary reconstruction	Time to progression	Location of the calculi	Treatment for the hepatolithiasis	
						First (result)	Second (result)
1	28/M	IV-A	Hepaticojejunostomy(Roux-en-Y)	6 years 4 months	Left	(Observation)	
2	27/M	Ia	Hepaticojejunostomy(Roux-en-Y)	9 years 3 months	Left and Right	ERC (no relapse)	
3	31/M	IV-A	Hepaticojejunostomy(Roux-en-Y)	7 years 2 months	Posterior segment	ERC (relapse)	(Observation)
4	15/F	Unknown	Hepaticojejunostomy(Roux-en-Y)	34 years	Left	PTC (relapse)	ERC (no relapse)
5	34/F	Ic	Hepaticojejunostomy(Roux-en-Y)	5 years 3 months	Left and Right	PTC (relapse)	Resection of the anastomosis and reconstruction (relapse)
6	48/F	IV-A	Choledochoduodenostomy	4 years 8 months	Left and Right	Resection of the remnant bile duct and reconstruction (relapse)	PTC (relapse)
7	33/M	Ia	Hepaticojejunostomy(Roux-en-Y)	17 years 7 months	Medial segment	Left hepatectomy (no relapse)	
8	47/F	Unknown	Choledochoduodenostomy	10 years	Posterior segment	Right hepatectomy (no relapse)	
9	45/F	IV-A	Hepaticojejunostomy(Roux-en-Y)	3 years	Left and Right	Left hepatectomy (relapse)	PTC (no relapse)
10	32/M	Ia	Hepaticojejunostomy(Roux-en-Y)	3 years 6 months	Left and Right	PTC (relapse)	Left hepatectomy (no relapse)

formed, recurrence was not recognized postoperatively. In general, when the intrahepatic calculi were localized to one lobe, especially the left lobe, hepatectomy procedures, such as a lateral segmentectomy or left hepatectomy, should be considered as the most reliable way to remove the calculi. In cases where the hepatic resection can completely remove the intrahepatic calculus in addition to the stenotic region of the intrahepatic bile duct, recurrences are rare [18]. However, with hepatolithiasis after biliary reconstruction, the calculi are commonly detected diffusely in both lobes, and it is difficult to determine the optimal surgical procedure. In patients with anastomotic strictures at a previous hepaticojejunostomy site, the removal of the calculus and reanastomosis are considered as a surgical option for the treatment. However, after these procedures, the recurrence rates were reported to be high [19]. Even in our patient population, in both patients for whom these procedures were performed, recurrence of hepatolithiasis occurred within 2 years after the operation. In our cases, hepatectomy was performed for two patients in whom calculi were found in both liver lobes. In these cases, hepatectomies were followed by an endoscopic lithotomy with percutaneous transhepatic cholangioscopic lithotomy (PTCSL) approach. In both cases, after the calculi were removed, recurrence of intrahepatic calculi was not observed after surgery. Even in cases where calculi are identified in both lobes, in order to facilitate an approach to the residual liver, surgical resection of the area in which severe biliary stenosis was located should be considered.

29.5 Conclusion

Patients with CBD often develop long-term complications after treatment with surgical excision of the dilated bile duct, including postoperative cholangitis, intrahepatic calculi, pancreatitis, and carcinogenesis in the remnant bile duct. While precise and thorough surgical treatment is necessary to prevent these complications, surgery alone will not be sufficient. In these cases, surgery must be accompanied by long-term postoperative follow-up, especially in the patients with type IV-A CBD.

In the treatment of intrahepatic calculus, endoscopic stone removal through either the peroral or percutaneous transhepatic approach is the first choice. Although the cases treated using peroral endoscopy have been increasing in recent years, the long-term outcomes of these treatment methods are unclear, and it is necessary to accumulate and analyze cases in the future. Surgical treatment is considered in cases where endoscopic treatment has failed. Even in cases where stones are detected diffusely within both lobes, effective treatment can be achieved by combining surgical resection and endoscopic treatment. In cases where hepatic atrophy is identified, surgical resection should be considered, taking into account the possibility of postoperative cancer development.

References

1. Hewitt PM, Krige JE, Bornman PC, et al. Choledochal cysts in adults. Br J Surg. 1995;82:382–5.
2. Kobayashi S, Asano T, Yamasaki M, et al. Prophylactic excision of the gallbladder and bile duct for patients with pancreaticobiliary maljunction. Arch Surg. 2001;136:759–63.
3. Kimura W. Congenital dilatation of the common bile duct and pancreaticobiliary maljunction-clinical implications. Langenbeck's Arch Surg. 2009;394:209–13.
4. Takeshita N, Ota T, Yamamoto M. Forty-year experience with flow-diversion surgery for patients with congenital choledochal cysts with pancreaticobiliary maljunction at a single institution. Ann Surg. 2011;254:1050–3.
5. Congo K, Lopes MF, Oliveira PH, et al. Outcomes of choledochal cysts with or without intrahepatic involvement in children after extrahepatic cyst excision and Roux-en-Y hepaticojejunostomy. Ann Hepatol. 2012;11:536–43.
6. Ohtsuka H, Fukase K, Yoshida H, et al. Long-term outcomes after extrahepatic excision of congenital choladocal cysts: 30 years of experience at a single center. Hepato-Gastroenterology. 2015;62:1–5.
7. Suzuki Y, Mori T, Yokoyama M, et al. Hepatolithiasis: analysis of Japanese nationwide surveys over a period of 40 years. J Hepatobiliary Pancreat Sci. 2014;21:617–22.
8. Chijiiwa K, Tanaka M. Late complications after excisional operation in patients with choledochal cyst. J Am Coll Surg. 1994;179:139–44.
9. Uno K, Tsuchida Y, Kawarasaki H, et al. Development of intrahepatic cholelithiasis long after primary excision of choledochal cysts. J Am Coll Surg. 1996;183:583–8.
10. Kaneko K, Ando H, Seo T, et al. Bile infection contributes to intrahepatic calculi formation after excision of choledochal cysts. Pediatr Surg Int. 2005;21:8–11.
11. Ohi R, Yaoita S, Kamiyama T, et al. Surgical treatment of congenital dilatation of the bile duct with special reference to late complications after total excisional operation. J Pediatr Surg. 1990;25:613–7.
12. Todani T, Watanabe Y, Toki A, et al. Reoperation for congenital choledochal cyst. Ann Surg. 1988;207:142–7.
13. Todani T, Watanabe Y, Urushihara N, et al. Biliary complications after excisional procedure for choledochal cyst. J Pediatr Surg. 1995;30:478–81.
14. Ando H, Ito T, Kaneko K, et al. Congenital stenosis of the intrahepatic bile duct associated with choledochal cysts. J Am Coll Surg. 1995;181:426–30.
15. Sasaki M, Ikeda H, Nakanuma Y. Expression profiles of MUC mucins and trefoil factor family (TFF) peptides in the intrahepatic biliary system: physiological distribution and pathological significance. Prog Histochem Cytochem. 2007;42:61–110.
16. Shimatani M, Matsushita M, Takaoka M, et al. Effective "short" double-balloon enteroscope for diagnostic and therapeutic ERCP in patients with altered gastrointestinal anatomy: a large case series. Endoscopy. 2009;41:849–54.
17. Tsujino T, Yamada A, Isayama H, et al. Experiences of biliary interventions using short double-balloon enteroscopy in patients with Roux-en-Y anastomosis or hepaticojejunostomy. Dig Endosc. 2010;22:211–6.
18. Vetrone G, Ercolani G, Grazi GL, et al. Surgical therapy for hepatolithiasis: a Western experience. J Am Coll Surg. 2006;202:306–12.
19. Otani K, Shimizu S, Chijiiwa K, et al. Comparison of treatments for hepatolithiasis: hepatic resection versus cholangioscopic lithotomy. J Am Coll Surg. 1999;189:177–82.

Chapter 30
Cholangiocarcinoma Developing from the Remnant Bile Ducts Following Cyst Excision for Congenital Biliary Dilatation

Takashi Kobayashi, Taku Ohashi, Jun Sakata, Kohei Miura, and Toshifumi Wakai

Abstract Cholangiocarcinoma developing from the remnant bile ducts following cyst excision for congenital biliary dilatation (CBD) is an increasing problem. There are some reports demonstrating that cholangiocarcinoma develops in approximately 0.7–6.5% of patients who undergo cyst excision; the incidence is 121.5 times higher than that of the general population. The cumulative incidence of cholangiocarcinoma at 15, 20, and 25 years after cyst excision for CBD is reported to be 1.6%, 3.9%, and 11.3%, respectively. Repeated cholangitis, hepatolithiasis, or remnant dilated bile ducts due to inadequate cyst excision have been reported to be risk factors for cholangiocarcinoma following cyst excision. Biliary-enteric anastomosis itself is also reported to be a risk factor for cholangiocarcinoma. The outcomes of treatment for cholangiocarcinoma developing from the remnant bile ducts following cyst excision are unfavorable. The overall cumulative survival rates at 2 and 3 years after treatment were reported to be 32% and 16%, respectively. The median survival time was 15 months. Most patients were diagnosed at the late stage of cholangiocarcinoma. Longer follow-up is needed, even after complete cyst excision, because of the lifelong risk of subsequent cholangiocarcinoma. The regular check-ups that include the evaluation of tumor markers (including CEA and CA19-9) and imaging studies, such as abdominal US and CT, are useful for the diagnosis of cholangiocarcinoma developing from the remnant bile ducts.

Keywords Cholangiocarcinoma · Remnant bile duct · Cyst excision · Congenital biliary dilatation

---

T. Kobayashi · T. Ohashi · J. Sakata · K. Miura · T. Wakai (✉)
Division of Digestive and General Surgery, Niigata University Graduate School of Medical and Dental Sciences, Niigata, Japan
e-mail: wakait@med.niigata-u.ac.jp

T. Kamisawa, H. Ando (eds.), *Pancreaticobiliary Maljunction and Congenital Biliary Dilatation*, https://doi.org/10.1007/978-981-10-8654-0_30

30.1 Introduction

Congenital biliary dilatation (CBD) is defined as a congenital malformation involving both the local dilatation of the extrahepatic bile ducts (including the common bile duct) and pancreaticobiliary maljunction (PBM) [1, 2]. CBD is frequently associated with cholangiocarcinoma. Cyst excision (extrahepatic bile duct resection) has been recommended as the best surgery for preventing malignant changes and is now the standard procedure for the treatment of CBD worldwide [3, 4]. However, a number of authors have reported cholangiocarcinoma developing from the remnant bile ducts (the intrahepatic, hilar, and intrapancreatic bile ducts) following cyst excision, and it is an increasing problem.

In this chapter, we describe the incidence, risk factors, treatment outcomes, and the postoperative follow-up of cholangiocarcinoma developing from the remnant bile ducts after cyst excision.

30.2 The Incidence of Cholangiocarcinoma Developing from the Remnant Bile Ducts

Although cholangiocarcinoma developing from the remnant bile ducts following cyst excision is observed as a late complication and is an increasing problem, there have been no major studies on this issue.

Of the 997 adult cases of CBD during the 18 years between 1990 and 2007 that were studied by Japanese Study Group on Pancreaticobiliary Maljunction, 79 (7.9%) cases had coexisting cholangiocarcinoma at the time of the diagnosis [5]; this was the rate of cholangiocarcinoma coexistence at the time of the diagnosis of CBD. On the other hand, the incidence of cholangiocarcinoma developing from the remnant bile ducts following cyst excision for CBD is reported to be 0.7–6.5% [6, 7], and the interval between cyst excision and cancer detection is reported to be 9.0–11.9 years [6, 8, 9]. The incidence of the subsequent cholangiocarcinoma following cyst excision is 121.5 times higher than that in the general population [7]. The cumulative incidence of cholangiocarcinoma at 15, 20, and 25 years after cyst excision for CBD was 1.6%, 3.9%, and 11.3%, respectively [10].

Watanabe et al. [6] reviewed the clinical data of 23 patients with cholangiocarcinoma after the excision of choledochal cysts who were reported in the English- and Japanese-language literature and the data of 1353 Japanese patients with CBD. Among the 23 patients, the mean age at cyst excision was 23.0 ± 13.7 years, and cancers were detected at the mean age of 32.1 ± 12.2 years; the mean interval between cyst excision and the detection of cholangiocarcinoma was 9.0 ± 5.5 years. Cyst excision was inadequate in nearly half of the 23 reported cases. Among the 1353 Japanese patients with CBD, 1291 underwent cyst excision for CBD. The incidence of cholangiocarcinoma developing from the remnant bile ducts after cyst excision was assumed to be 0.7% (9/1291).

Kobayashi et al. [7] reported that cholangiocarcinoma developing from the remnant bile ducts after cyst excision was detected in 3 out of 46 (6.5%) patients. The interval between cyst excision and cholangiocarcinoma detection in these patients was 29, 104, and 234 months, respectively. The incidence of cholangiocarcinoma in patients with CBD before cyst excision was 163.9 times higher than that of the general population. The incidence of cholangiocarcinoma developing from the remnant bile ducts after cyst excision for CBD was 121.5 times higher than that of the general population. Thus, after cyst excision, there was a slight decrease in the incidence from 163.9 times to 121.5 times. However, they concluded that the incidence of cholangiocarcinoma might not decrease after cyst excision.

Lee et al. [11] reported the incidence of cholangiocarcinoma in 668 patients without malignant biliary tumors who underwent cyst excision for CBD. In a Korean multicenter study, cholangiocarcinoma was reported to have developed from the remnant bile ducts in four patients (4/668, 0.6%).

Ohashi et al. [10] reported a follow-up study of 94 patients who had undergone cyst excision for CBD in a single institute. Of the 114 patients who were treated from 1971 to 2006, 20 patients who had a coexisting biliary tract cancer were excluded. The remaining 94 patients who underwent cyst excision were included in the analysis. The median follow-up time following cyst excision for CBD was 181 months (range, 7–484 months). During the follow-up period, 4 of the 94 patients (4.3%) had subsequent cholangiocarcinoma at 13, 15, 23, and 32 years, respectively, after cyst excision. The anatomic sites of cholangiocarcinoma were the intrahepatic ($n = 2$), hilar ($n = 1$), and intrapancreatic ($n = 1$) bile ducts. The cumulative incidence of cholangiocarcinoma at 15, 20, and 25 years after cyst excision for CBD was 1.6%, 3.9%, and 11.3%, respectively (Fig. 30.1).

In addition to the abovementioned cases, Kamisawa et al. reviewed 106 cases of cholangiocarcinoma developing from the remnant bile ducts following cyst excision for CBD [9]. Between 1967 and 2015, 106 cases of subsequent cholangiocarcinoma following cyst excision were reported in 30 English-language and 52 Japanese-language studies. According to Todani's classification, 63 of 106 patients (59%) were classified into type IV-A, 28 (26%) were classified into type I, and 15 (14%) were unknown. The most common site of involvement in the 106 cases was the hilar bile duct (44%, 47/106) followed by the intrapancreatic bile duct (25%, 26/106) and intrahepatic bile duct (23%, 24/106). The site was unknown in 9 cases (8%, 9/106). In these patients, cancer was detected at a mean of 11.9 ± 9.1 years after cyst excision and at a mean age of 47.1 ± 16.8 years (Table 30.1). The incidence of cholangiocarcinoma developing from the remnant bile ducts after cyst excision was 2% (46/2347) [9].

Recently, Mizuguchi et al. [12] reviewed 17 reported Japanese cases in which the patients developed cholangiocarcinoma from the remnant intrapancreatic bile duct after cyst excision. Todani's classifications of the 17 choledochal cysts were as follows: type I, $n = 9$; type IV-A, $n = 5$; and unknown, $n = 3$. The mean time to the development of subsequent cholangiocarcinoma was 13.6 years.

On the other hand, Todani et al. [13] reported that at least two-thirds of the patients who underwent internal drainage, which is not performed for CBD at

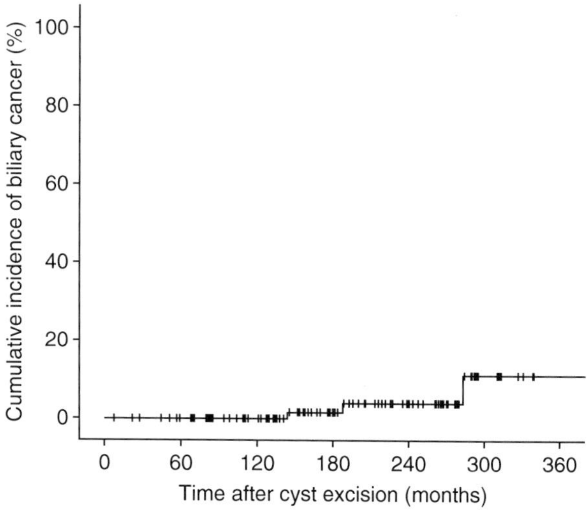

Fig. 30.1 The cumulative incidence of biliary tract cancer after cyst excision for congenital choledochal cysts among 94 patients. The cumulative incidence of biliary tract cancer at 15, 20, and 25 years after cyst excision was 1.6%, 3.9%, and 11.3%, respectively [10]

present, developed biliary tract cancer within 10 years. Moreover, at the onset of cancer, the patients who underwent an internal drainage procedure were reported to be up to 15 years younger in comparison to those who developed cancer following cyst excision. Although there was no comparison study of internal drainage versus cyst excision, it may be fair to conclude that the incidence of biliary tract cancers following internal drainage procedures is higher than that following cyst excision [3, 4].

30.3 Risk Factors for Cholangiocarcinoma Developing from the Remnant Bile Ducts

Repeated cholangitis or hepatolithiasis and Todani's type IVA were reported to be risk factors for the development of cancer of the hepatic hilum or intrahepatic bile ducts after cyst excision [6, 7, 9]. Inadequate bile duct excision is also associated with cholangiocarcinoma developing from the remnant bile ducts [9].

Todani et al. [13] reported that the risk of subsequent cholangiocarcinoma was related to dysplasia and metaplasia of the epithelium of the remnant dilated bile ducts. Thus, complete cyst excision seems to be essential for preventing subsequent cholangiocarcinoma for CBD with PBM. In type I and IV cysts (Todani's classification), cyst excision involves the complete excision of the bile duct from the confluence of the hepatic duct (proximally) up to the pancreaticobiliary junction (distally). Biliary-enteric anastomosis at the larger caliber duct is recommended for the prevention of postoperative biliary stricture and subsequent cholangiocarcinoma after cyst excision [14].

Table 30.1 The associations between the origin of cholangiocarcinoma after cyst excision and various features [9]

	Cancer origin				
	Intrapancreatic remnant bile duct	Hilar bile duct	Intrahepatic bile duct	Total	Unknown
Number of patients	26	47	24	97	9
Sex					
Female	16	27	14	57	
Male	8	10	8	26	
Unknown	2	10	2	14	
Todani's classification					
Type I	12	9	6	27	1
Type IV-A	7	31	17	55	8
Unknown	7	7	1	15	
Age at bile duct excision (years)	36.2 (20.3)	31.9 (17.2)	31.1 (16.3)	34.6 (18.4)	
Age at cancer detection (years)	48.0 (17.3)	45.1 (16.5)	44.4 (14.7)	47.1 (16.8)	
Interval between cyst excision and cancer detection (years)	11.8 (8.6)	11.5 (9.7)	13.4 (9.9)	11.9 (9.1)	
Cholangitis or hepatolithiasis after cyst excision					
Yes	3	16	11	30	
No	14	17	10	41	
Unknown	9	14	3		

The data indicate the number of patients or mean (SD). The data were obtained from 30 English-language and 52 Japanese-language publications

Kamisawa et al. [9] reported that inadequate cyst excision is probably associated with subsequent cholangiocarcinoma because in 73 of 97 cases (75%) of cholangiocarcinoma following cyst excision, the cholangiocarcinoma developed from the intrapancreatic remnant bile duct or hepatic hilum (Table 30.1). Moreover, almost half of the patients with cholangiocarcinoma developing from the remnant hilar or intrahepatic bile duct gave a medical history of cholangitis or hepatolithiasis after cyst excision (Table 30.1). Postoperative or pre-existing stenosis of the bile duct, bile stasis caused by stenosis, and chronic inflammation of the epithelium might induce carcinogenesis. Thus, wide anastomosis with free drainage of bile and the complete excision of the dilated bile duct are essential for preventing the development of cholangiocarcinoma [8].

Tocchi et al. [15] reported that the chronic inflammatory changes that occur as a consequence of biliary-enteric anastomosis for benign biliary disease should be closely monitored for the late development of cholangiocarcinoma. This suggests that the risk of subsequent cholangiocarcinoma may be associated with biliary-enteric anastomosis itself. Strong et al. [16] also reported that biliary-enteric anastomosis itself was a risk factor for subsequent cholangiocarcinoma.

30.4 The Outcomes of Treatment for Cholangiocarcinoma Developing from the Remnant Bile Ducts

The reported outcomes of treatment for cholangiocarcinoma developing from the remnant bile ducts following cyst excision for CBD were unfavorable. Ohashi et al. [10] reported that three of four patients with subsequent cholangiocarcinoma following cyst excision underwent surgical resection. The remaining one patient underwent exploratory laparotomy, which revealed carcinoma that was unresectable due to distant lymph node metastasis. The surgical resection procedures included left trisectionectomy of the liver ($n = 2$) and pancreaticoduodenectomy ($n = 1$). Adenocarcinoma was identified as the primary tumor in these three patients. They died at 9, 15, and 35 months after the surgical resection of the subsequent cholangiocarcinoma following cyst excision. One patient remained alive with intrahepatic cholangiocarcinoma after receiving chemoradiotherapy. Ohashi et al. [10] also reported an analysis of 32 reported patients with subsequent cholangiocarcinoma following choledochal cyst excision. Twelve of the 32 reported patients were treated with supportive care, and 14 patients received either surgical resection ($n = 11$), chemoradiotherapy ($n = 2$), or chemotherapy ($n = 1$). None of the 32 patients survived for 4 years. Among the 14 patients who received treatment for subsequent cholangiocarcinoma following cyst excision, the overall cumulative survival rates at 2 and 3 years after treatment were 32% and 16%, respectively, with a median survival time of 15 months (Fig. 30.2). Despite an aggressive treatment approach, subsequent cholangiocarcinoma was associated with an unfavorable outcome. These results may reflect that subsequent cholangiocarcinoma has a more aggressive biology than de novo cholangiocarcinoma. Patients undergoing resection for subsequent biliary malignancies are therefore clear candidates for adjuvant chemotherapy such as cisplatin plus gemcitabine [17].

Mizuguchi et al. [12] also reported the poor survival rate of patients who received treatment for subsequent intrapancreatic cholangiocarcinoma after cyst excision in a review of the literature. Among the 17 patients who developed subsequent cholangiocarcinoma, 16 underwent surgical treatment. Among these 16 patients, 13 underwent aggressive treatment with pancreaticoduodenectomy ($n = 6$), pylorus preserving pancreaticoduodenectomy ($n = 4$), or total pancreatectomy ($n = 3$). One patient underwent a palliative bypass procedure, and one underwent cystojejunostomy. Surgical treatment was attempted in the remaining patients but was changed to probe laparotomy because the cancer was found to be at an advanced stage. One patient underwent chemotherapy for metastatic liver cancer. Four patients received adjuvant chemotherapy after aggressive surgical treatment. The overall cumulative survival rate at 1 year after treatment was of approximately 40%, with a mean survival time of 12 months (95% confidence interval, 9.6–14.3) (Fig. 30.3).

On the other hand, Lee et al. [11] reported the importance of widespread careful long-term follow-up and the relatively early detection of subsequent cholangiocarcinoma. As a result, approximately 60% of the patients were classified as stage I or II, and the 5-year survival rate was comparable to that of cholangiocarcinoma in general.

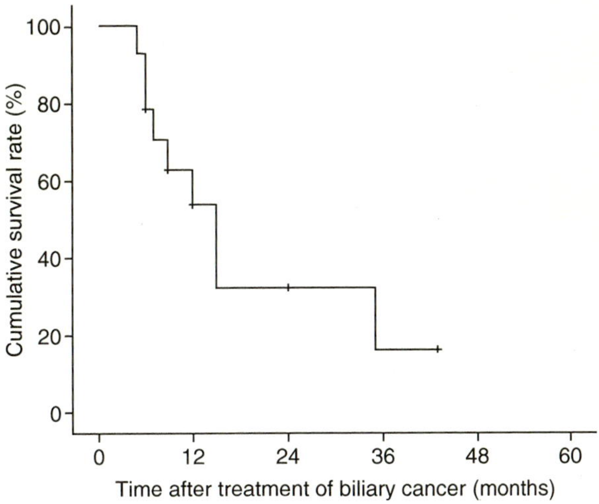

Fig. 30.2 Kaplan–Meier survival estimates in 14 cases (identified in the literature review) involving patients suffering from subsequent biliary malignancy following choledochal cyst excision in which the outcomes after treatment were documented. The overall cumulative survival rates at 2 and 3 years after treatment were 32% and 16%, respectively, with a median survival time of 15 months [10]

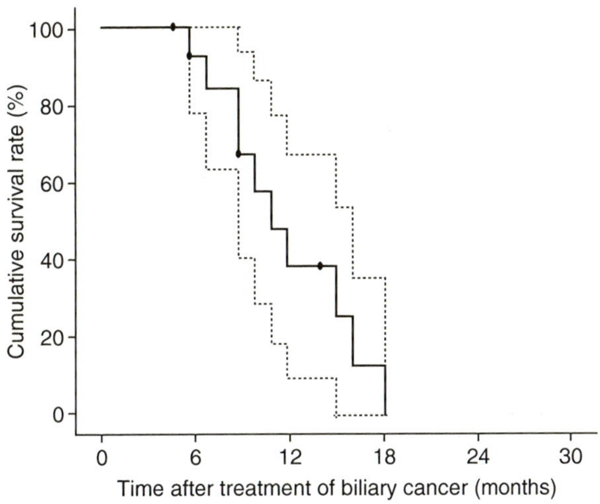

Fig. 30.3 The cumulative survival rates after the treatment of recurrence. A Kaplan–Meier analysis of the cumulative survival (*solid line*) rate with the 95% confidence interval (*dotted line*) of the 17 patients who developed subsequent cholangiocarcinoma in the remnant intrapancreatic bile duct [12]

30.5 Postoperative Follow-Up After Cyst Excision

Patients who have undergone cyst excision for CBD should be followed up for the rest of their lives [4, 8, 18, 10].

Mizuguchi et al. [12] reported on the diagnosis of subsequent cholangiocarcinoma. Thirteen of 15 patients showed abdominal symptoms (i.e., epigastralgia, fullness, and nausea). Among the two patients who had no abdominal symptoms, one patient was found to have subsequent cholangiocarcinoma after the detection of an elevated serum glucose level; in the other patient, a mass was incidentally found in the pancreatic head on US as part of a routine checkup. No patients were being followed up at the time when the subsequent cholangiocarcinoma was found. The measurement of tumor marker levels during follow-up was diagnostically useful because almost all cases (7/8) had elevated serum levels of CEA and/or CA19-9. The diagnostic imaging modalities included abdominal US, CT, MRCP, ERCP, and positron emission tomography (PET). Among these, CT detected a mass in the pancreatic head in the majority of cases (9/10).

Nishiyama et al. [19] have suggested lifelong biannual follow-up examinations with CT and the measurement of CA 19-9 in patients who are considered to be at high risk for developing cholangiocarcinoma and annual ultrasound for low-risk patients. High-risk features include the presence of dilated biliary ducts after resection and reconstruction with choledochoduodenostomy and hepatitis. The rationale behind such stringent follow-up is that resection would be more difficult or even impossible in patients with more advanced disease. The belief is that with a tighter follow-up protocol, the development of cholangiocarcinoma can be detected at an early stage, giving these patients a greater chance of a cure [20].

References

1. Hamada Y, Ando H, Kamisawa T, Itoi T, Urushihara N, Koshinaga T, Saito T, Fujii H, Morotomi Y. Diagnostic criteria for congenital biliary dilatation 2015. J Hepatobiliary Pancreat Sci. 2016;23(6):342–6.
2. Kamisawa T, Ando H, Shimada M, Hamada Y, Itoi T, Takayashiki T, Miyazaki M. Recent advances and problems in the management of pancreaticobiliary maljunction: feedback from the guidelines committee. J Hepatobiliary Pancreat Sci. 2014;21(2):87–92.
3. Ishibashi H, Shimada M, Kamisawa T, Fujii H, Hamada Y, Kubota M, Urushihara N, Endo I, Nio M, Taguchi T, et al. Japanese clinical practice guidelines for congenital biliary dilatation. J Hepatobiliary Pancreat Sci. 2017;24(1):1–16.
4. Kamisawa T, Ando H, Suyama M, Shimada M, Morine Y, Shimada H. Working Committee of Clinical Practice Guidelines for Pancreaticobiliary M, Japanese Study Group on Pancreaticobiliary M: Japanese clinical practice guidelines for pancreaticobiliary maljunction. J Gastroenterol. 2012;47(7):731–59.
5. Morine Y, Shimada M, Takamatsu H, Araida T, Endo I, Kubota M, Toki A, Noda T, Matsumura T, Miyakawa S, et al. Clinical features of pancreaticobiliary maljunction: update analysis of 2nd Japan-nationwide survey. J Hepatobiliary Pancreat Sci. 2013;20(5):472–80.
6. Watanabe Y, Toki A, Todani T. Bile duct cancer developed after cyst excision for choledochal cyst. J Hepato-Biliary-Pancreat Surg. 1999;6(3):207–12.
7. Kobayashi S, Asano T, Yamasaki M, Kenmochi T, Nakagohri T, Ochiai T. Risk of bile duct carcinogenesis after excision of extrahepatic bile ducts in pancreaticobiliary maljunction. Surgery. 1999;126(5):939–44.
8. Lee SE, Jang JY. Development of biliary malignancy after cyst excision for congenital choledochal cysts: what should we do? J Gastroenterol Hepatol. 2013;28(2):210–2.
9. Kamisawa T, Kaneko K, Itoi T, Ando H. Pancreaticobiliary maljunction and congenital biliary dilatation. Lancet Gastroenterol Hepatol. 2017;2(8):610–8.
10. Ohashi T, Wakai T, Kubota M, Matsuda Y, Arai Y, Ohyama T, Nakaya K, Okuyama N, Sakata J, Shirai Y, et al. Risk of subsequent biliary malignancy in patients undergoing cyst excision for congenital choledochal cysts. J Gastroenterol Hepatol. 2013;28(2):243–7.
11. Lee SE, Jang JY, Lee YJ, Choi DW, Lee WJ, Cho BH, Kim SW, Club KPS. Choledochal cyst and associated malignant tumors in adults a multicenter survey in South Korea. Arch Surg-Chicago. 2011;146(10):1178–84.

12. Mizuguchi Y, Nakamura Y, Uchida E. Subsequent biliary cancer originating from remnant intrapancreatic bile ducts after cyst excision: a literature review. Surg Today. 2017;47(6):660–7.
13. Todani T, Watanabe Y, Toki A, Urushihara N. Carcinoma related to choledochal cysts with internal drainage operations. Surg Gynecol Obstet. 1987;164(1):61–4.
14. Ando H, Kaneko K, Ito T, Watanabe Y, Seo T, Harada T, Ito F, Nagaya M, Sugito T. Complete excision of the intrapancreatic portion of choledochal cysts. J Am Coll Surg. 1996;183(4):317–21.
15. Tocchi A, Mazzoni G, Bettelli E, Miccini M, Giuliani A, Cassini D. Impact of axillary level I and II lymph node dissection on the therapy of stage I and II breast cancer. Panminerva Med. 2001;43(2):103–7.
16. Jonsson JR, Gill D, Hogan PG, Clouston AD, Edwards-Smith C, Griffin AD, Balderson GA, Lynch SV, Strong RW, Powell EE. Role of donor leukocyte chimerism in establishing the etiology of neutropenia after liver transplantation. Transplantation. 1999;67(10):1358–61.
17. Valle J, Wasan H, Palmer DH, Cunningham D, Anthoney A, Maraveyas A, Madhusudan S, Iveson T, Hughes S, Pereira SP, et al. Cisplatin plus gemcitabine versus gemcitabine for biliary tract cancer. N Engl J Med. 2010;362(14):1273–81.
18. Ono S, Fumino S, Shimadera S, Iwai N. Long-term outcomes after hepaticojejunostomy for choledochal cyst: a 10- to 27-year follow-up. J Pediatr Surg. 2010;45(2):376–8.
19. Nishiyama R, Shinoda M, Tanabe M, Masugi Y, Ueno A, Hibi T, Takano K, Fujisaki H, Kitago M, Itano O, et al. Intrahepatic cholangiocarcinoma arising 33 years after excision of a choledochal cyst: report of a case. Int Surg. 2011;96(4):320–5.
20. Kumamoto T, Tanaka K, Takeda K, Nojiri K, Mori R, Taniguchi K, Matsuyama R, Ueda M, Sugita M, Ichikawa Y, et al. Intrahepatic cholangiocarcinoma arising 28 years after excision of a type IV-A congenital choledochal cyst: report of a case. Surg Today. 2014;44(2):354–8.

Printed by Printforce, the Netherlands